Cardiothora
Critical Care

Cardiothoracic Critical Care

Edited by
Brigid C. Flynn, MD
Associate Professor
Division Chief, Critical Care Medicine
Department of Anesthesiology
University of Kansas Medical Center
Kansas City, KS, USA

Natalia S. Ivascu, MD
Professor of Clinical Anesthesiology
Department of Anesthesiology
Weill Cornell Medicine
New York, NY, USA

Vivek K. Moitra, MD, MHA
Allen I. Hyman Professor of Critical Care Anesthesiology
Division Chief, Critical Care Medicine
Department of Anesthesiology
Columbia University Irving Medical Center
New York, NY, USA

Alan Gaffney, MB BCh, PhD
Consultant Anesthesiologist and Intensivist
Department of Anaesthesiology & Critical Care Medicine
Beaumont Hospital
Royal College of Surgeons in Ireland Hospital Group
Dublin, Ireland

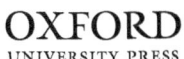

OXFORD
UNIVERSITY PRESS

Oxford University Press is a department of the University of Oxford. It furthers
the University's objective of excellence in research, scholarship, and education
by publishing worldwide. Oxford is a registered trade mark of Oxford University
Press in the UK and certain other countries.

Published in the United States of America by Oxford University Press
198 Madison Avenue, New York, NY 10016, United States of America.

© Oxford University Press 2020

All rights reserved. No part of this publication may be reproduced, stored in
a retrieval system, or transmitted, in any form or by any means, without the
prior permission in writing of Oxford University Press, or as expressly permitted
by law, by license, or under terms agreed with the appropriate reproduction
rights organization. Inquiries concerning reproduction outside the scope of the
above should be sent to the Rights Department, Oxford University Press, at the
address above.

You must not circulate this work in any other form
and you must impose this same condition on any acquirer.

Library of Congress Cataloging-in-Publication Data
Names: Flynn, Brigid C., editor. | Ivascu, Natalia S., editor. |
Moitra, Vivek K., editor. | Gaffney, Alan, editor.
Title: Cardiothoracic critical care / edited by Brigid C. Flynn, Natalia S.
Ivascu, Vivek K. Moitra, Alan Gaffney.
Other titles: Cardiothoracic critical care (Flynn) | What do I do now?
Description: New York : Oxford University Press, 2020. |
Series: What do I do now, critical care | Includes bibliographical references and index.
Identifiers: LCCN 2020009276 (print) | LCCN 2020009277 (ebook) |
ISBN 9780190082482 (paperback) | ISBN 9780190082505 (epub) |
ISBN 9780190082512
Subjects: MESH: Cardiac Surgical Procedures | Critical Care | Thoracic
Diseases | Heart Diseases | Postoperative Care | Case Reports
Classification: LCC RD598 (print) | LCC RD598 (ebook) | NLM WG 169 |
DDC 617.4/12028—dc23
LC record available at https://lccn.loc.gov/2020009276
LC ebook record available at https://lccn.loc.gov/2020009277

This material is not intended to be, and should not be considered, a substitute for medical or other
professional advice. Treatment for the conditions described in this material is highly dependent on
the individual circumstances. And, while this material is designed to offer accurate information with
respect to the subject matter covered and to be current as of the time it was written, research and
knowledge about medical and health issues is constantly evolving and dose schedules for medications
are being revised continually, with new side effects recognized and accounted for regularly. Readers
must therefore always check the product information and clinical procedures with the most up-to-date
published product information and data sheets provided by the manufacturers and the most recent
codes of conduct and safety regulation. The publisher and the authors make no representations or
warranties to readers, express or implied, as to the accuracy or completeness of this material. Without
limiting the foregoing, the publisher and the authors make no representations or warranties as to the
accuracy or efficacy of the drug dosages mentioned in the material. The authors and the publisher do
not accept, and expressly disclaim, any responsibility for any liability, loss, or risk that may be claimed
or incurred as a consequence of the use and/or application of any of the contents of this material.

9 8 7 6 5 4 3 2 1

Printed by Marquis, Canada

Contents

Preface ix

Contributors xi

1. **Risk Assessment Scores in Cardiac Surgery** 1
   Matthew Hulse and Stuart Lowson

2. **Pulmonary Artery Catheterization in Cardiac Surgery** 13
   Daniel L. Jacobs and Brigid C. Flynn

3. **Oxygen Consumption and Delivery in Critical Illness** 25
   Hans Tregear and Brigid C. Flynn

4. **Glycemic Control After Cardiac Surgery** 37
   Casey Shelley and Katherine Palmieri

5. **Post-Thoracotomy Care** 47
   Martin De Ruyter and Laura McKenzie

6. **Pulmonary Embolism and Postoperative Care** 59
   Daniel Haines and Joel Grigsby

7. **Respiratory Acidosis in the Intensive Care Unit** 73
   Jared Staab

8. **Metabolic Acidosis in the Cardiothoracic Intensive Care Unit** 85
   Paul D. Weyker and Christopher Webb

9. **Rhabdomyolysis Due to Extracorporeal Membrane Oxygenation** 97
   Candice Metzinger and Aaron LacKamp

10. **Postoperative Septic Shock** 111
    James E. Littlejohn

11. **Postoperative Right Ventricular Failure** 121
    Marguerite Hoyler and Natalia S. Ivascu

12 **Postoperative Atrial Fibrillation**   129
    Liang Shen

13 **QTc Prolongation and Torsades de Pointes**   137
    Ankur Srivastava and James E. Littlejohn

14 **Postoperative Ventricular Fibrillation**   143
    Gurbinder Singh and Natalia S. Ivascu

15 **Advanced Cardiovascular Life Support Post–Cardiac Surgery**   153
    Caryl Bailey and Michael Faulkner

16 **Critical Case of Aortic Stenosis**   161
    Rebecca Lee and Natalia S. Ivascu

17 **Robotic Mitral Valve Surgery and Unilateral Pulmonary Edema**   171
    Cindy Cheung and Christopher W. Tam

18 **Left Ventricular Assist Device Implantation and Management**   179
    Christopher W. Tam

19 **Left Ventricular Assist Device Troubleshooting: Hypotension**   191
    Jan M. Griffin, Bushra W. Taha, and Yoshifumi Naka

20 **Left Ventricular Assist Device Troubleshooting: Bleeding and Thrombosis**   197
    Jan M. Griffin, Bushra W. Taha, and Kelly M. Axsom

21 **Gastrointestinal Bleeding in the Setting of Left Ventricular Assist Device Support**   207
    Michael E. Kiyatkin, Adam S. Faye, and Tamas A. Gonda

22 **Right Ventricular Assist Device Therapies**   215
    Adrian Alexis-Ruiz and Marisa Cevasco

23 **A Failure to Oxygenate: A Case for Venovenous Extracorporeal Membrane Oxygenation** 221
Cara Agerstrand and Andrew Pellet

24 **Critical Concepts in Extracorporeal Life Support for Cardiogenic Shock** 231
Juan C. Diaz Soto, Justin A. Fried, and A. Reshad Garan

25 **Orthotopic Heart Transplant Management** 241
Artem Emple and Kelly M. Axsom

26 **Orthotopic Heart Transplant Rejection and Immunosuppression** 247
Kevin J. Clerkin and Maryjane A. Farr

27 **Pulmonary Infiltrates and Hypoxemia After Lung Transplantation** 257
Lauren D. Sutherland and Teresa A. Mulaikal

28 **Intra-aortic Balloon Pump** 267
Christopher Choi and Amirali Masoumi

29 **Cardiac Tamponade** 275
Christopher Read and Emer Curran

30 **Endocarditis** 283
Ruth Boylan and Ian Conrick-Martin

31 **Postoperative Pneumothorax** 297
Aoife Doolan and Gerard Curley

32 **Postoperative Cerebrovascular Injury** 307
Naomi Quigley and Ruth-Aoibheann O'Leary

33 **Coagulopathy in Cardiac Surgery: Etiology and Treatment Options** 313
Dana Teodorescu and Caroline Larkin

34 **Postoperative Diastolic Heart Failure** 323
Éimhín Dunne and Niall Fanning

35 **Postoperative Vasodilatory Shock** 333
Fiona Roberts and Alan Gaffney

36 **Postoperative Cardiogenic Shock** 343
Maurice Hogan

37 **Cardiac Surgery–Associated Acute Kidney Injury** 353
Coilin Smyth and Sinead Galvin

Index 367

Preface

Practicing critical care entails understanding human physiology, pharmacokinetics, and molecular pathways in concert with adherence to evidence-based literature. Some may say combining all of these entities into practice creates the "art" of critical care medicine. One strategy to gain proficiency in the practice of critical care medicine is to simulate what you would do in specific problem-based scenarios. That is the aim of this textbook, with each chapter asking aptly "What Do You Do Now?" This text focuses on cardiothoracic critical care and covers guidelines for evidence-based practice, respiratory and metabolic physiology, common hemodynamic perturbations, ventricular failure, and mechanical circulatory support devices. All clinicians who care for cardiothoracic patients who are critically ill can find pearls of practice wisdom complemented by literature citations within this text. So go ahead, place yourself at the foot of the bed and try to think through "What Do I Do Now?" when presented with each patient within these pages of your handheld cardiothoracic intensive care unit.

Contributors

Cara Agerstrand, MD
Division of Pulmonary, Allergy, and Critical Care Medicine
Department of Medicine
Columbia University College of Physicians and Surgeons
NewYork-Presbyterian Hospital
New York, NY, USA

Adrian Alexis-Ruiz, MD
Fellow, Critical Care Medicine
Department of Anesthesiology
Columbia University Medical Center
New York, NY, USA

Kelly M. Axsom, MD
Assistant Professor of Medicine
Columbia University Irving Medical Center
Center for Advanced Cardiac Care
New York, NY, USA

Caryl Bailey, MD
Fellow, Critical Care Anesthesiology
Department of Anesthesiology
NewYork-Presbyterian Hospital/Weill Cornell
New York, NY, USA

Ruth Boylan, BSc
Registrar in Anaesthesiology & Critical Care Medicine
Department of Anaesthesiology & Critical Care Medicine
Mater Misericordiae University Hospital
Dublin, Ireland

Marisa Cevasco, MD
Assistant in Clinical Surgery
Division of Cardiothoracic Surgery
Columbia University Medical Center
New York, NY, USA

Cindy Cheung, MD
Resident Physician
Department of Anesthesiology
NewYork-Presbyterian Hospital/Weill Cornell
New York, NY, USA

Christopher Choi, MD
Assistant Professor
Department of Anesthesiology and Pain Management
University of Texas Southwestern Medical Center
Dallas, TX, USA

Kevin J. Clerkin, MD, MSc
Assistant Professor of Medicine
Columbia University
Medical Center
New York, NY, USA

Ian Conrick-Martin, MB BCh
Consultant Anesthesiologist and
Intensivist
Department of Anaesthesiology &
Critical Care Medicine
Mater Misericordiae University
Hospital
Dublin, Ireland

Gerard Curley, MB BCh, BAO, MSc, PhD
Professor of Anesthesiology and
Critical Care Medicine, Consultant
Anesthesiologist and Intensivist
Department of Anaesthesiology &
Critical Care Medicine
Beaumont Hospital
Royal College of Surgeons in
Ireland Hospital Group
Dublin, Ireland

Emer Curran, MB BCh
Consultant Anesthesiologist and
Intensivist
Department of Anaesthesia
University Hospital Galway
Galway, Ireland

Martin De Ruyter, MD
Professor
Department of Anesthesiology
Kansas University Medical Center
Kansas City, KS, USA

Juan C. Diaz Soto, MD
Department of Anesthesiology
Division of Critical Care Medicine
Columbia University
Medical Center
New York, NY, USA

Aoife Doolan, MB BCh
Fellow in Critical Care Medicine
Department of Anaesthesiology &
Critical Care Medicine
Beaumont Hospital
Royal College of Surgeons in
Ireland Hospital Group
Dublin, Ireland

Éimhín Dunne, MB BCh
Fellow in Cardiac Anaesthesiology
Department of Anaesthesia,
Intensive Care and Pain Medicine
at St James Hospital
Dublin, Ireland

Artem Emple, MD
Department of Anesthesiology,
Division of Critical Care
NewYork-Presbyterian Columbia
University Irving Medical Center
New York, NY, USA

Niall Fanning, MB BCh
Consultant Anesthesiologist
Department of Anaesthesia,
Intensive Care and Pain Medicine
at St James Hospital
Dublin, Ireland

Maryjane A. Farr, MD, MSc
Associate Professor of Medicine
Medical Director, Adult Heart
Transplant Program
Columbia University
Medical Center
New York, NY, USA

Michael Faulkner, MD
Assistant Professor of
Anesthesiology
Oakland University, William
Beaumont School of Medicine
William Beaumont Hospital
Royal Oak, MI, USA

Adam S. Faye, MD
Division of Digestive and Liver
Diseases, Department of Medicine
Columbia University
Medical Center
NewYork-Presbyterian Hospital
New York, NY, USA

Brigid C. Flynn, MD
Associate Professor
Division Chief, Critical Care
Medicine
Department of Anesthesiology
Kansas University Medical Center
Kansas City, KS, USA

Justin A. Fried, MD
Division of Cardiology,
Department of Medicine
Columbia University
Medical Center
New York, NY, USA

Alan Gaffney, MB BCh, PhD
Consultant Anesthesiologist and
Intensivist
Department of Anaesthesiology &
Critical Care Medicine
Beaumont Hospital
Royal College of Surgeons in
Ireland Hospital Group
Dublin, Ireland

Sinead Galvin, MB BCh
Consultant Anesthesiologist and
Intensivist
Department of Anaesthesiology &
Critical Care Medicine
Beaumont Hospital
Royal College of Surgeons in
Ireland Hospital Group
Dublin, Ireland

A. Reshad Garan, MD
Division of Cardiology,
Department of Medicine
Columbia University
Medical Center
New York, NY, USA

Tamas A. Gonda, MD
Division of Digestive and Liver
Diseases, Department of Medicine
Columbia University
Medical Center
NewYork-Presbyterian Hospital
New York, NY, USA

Jan M. Griffin, MB BCh
Assistant Professor
Department of Medicine
NewYork-Presbyterian Columbia
University Irving Medical Center
New York, NY, USA

Joel Grigsby, MD
Assistant Professor
Department of Anesthesiology
University of Kansas
Medical Center
Kansas City, KS, USA

Daniel Haines, MD
Resident
Department of Anesthesiology
University of Kansas
Medical Center
Kansas City, KS, USA

Maurice Hogan, MB BCh, MSc, MBA
Consultant Cardiac Intensivist,
Cardiac Anesthesiologist, Section
Head, Cardiothoracic Intensive
Care Unit
Critical Care Institute, Cleveland
Clinic Abu Dhabi
Abu Dhabi, UAE

Marguerite Hoyler, MD
Resident Physician
Department of Anesthesiology
NewYork-Presbyterian Hospital/
Weill Cornell
New York, NY, USA

Matthew Hulse, MD
Assistant Professor
Department of Anesthesiology,
Division of Critical Care
University of Virginia
Health System
Charlottesville, VA, USA

Natalia S. Ivascu, MD
Professor
Department of Anesthesiology
Weill Cornell Medicine
New York, NY, USA

Daniel L. Jacobs, DO
Resident
Department of Anesthesiology
Kansas University Medical Center
Kansas City, KS, USA

Michael E. Kiyatkin, MD
Assistant Professor
Department of Anesthesiology
Columbia University
Medical Center
NewYork-Presbyterian Hospital
New York, NY, USA

Aaron LacKamp, MD
Assistant Professor
Division of Critical Care
Anesthesiology
Department of Anesthesiology
The University of Kansas School of
Medicine
Kansas City, KS, USA

Caroline Larkin, MB BCh
Consultant Anaesthesiologist and
Intensivist
Department of Anaesthesiology &
Critical Care Medicine
Beaumont Hospital
Royal College of Surgeons in
Ireland Hospital Group
Dublin, Ireland

Rebecca Lee, MD
Fellow, Critical Care
Anesthesiology
Department of Anesthesiology
NewYork-Presbyterian Hospital/
Weill Cornell
New York, NY, USA

James E. Littlejohn, MD, PhD
Assistant Professor of
Anesthesiology
Division of Critical Care Medicine,
Department of Anesthesiology
Weill Cornell Medicine
New York, NY, USA

Stuart Lowson, MBBS
Professor
Division of Critical Care
Department of Anesthesiology
University of Virginia
Health System
Charlottesville, VA, USA

Amirali Masoumi, MD
Assistant Professor of Medicine,
Interventional Cardiology |
Advanced Interventional, Heart
Failure, Transplant & Mechanical
Circulatory Support
Center for Interventional Vascular
Therapy | Interventional Heart
Failure Program, NewYork-
Presbyterian Hospital
Columbia University College of
Physicians & Surgeons
New York, NY, USA

Laura McKenzie, DO
Fellow, Regional Anesthesia
Department of Anesthesiology
Kansas University Medical Center
Kansas City, KS, USA

Candice Metzinger, BS
The University of Kansas School of
Medicine
Kansas City, KS, USA

Teresa A. Mulaikal, MD
Assistant Professor of Anesthesiology, Anesthesiology Residency Program Director
Division of Cardiothoracic and Critical Care
Department of Anesthesiology
Columbia University Medical Center
New York, NY, USA

Yoshifumi Naka, MD, PhD
Professor
Department of Cardiac Surgery
Director of Cardiac Transplantation and Mechanical Circulatory Support
Columbia University Medical Center
NewYork-Presbyterian Hospital
New York, NY, USA

Ruth-Aoibheann O'Leary, MB BCh
Consultant Anesthesiologist and Intensivist
Department of Anaesthesiology & Critical Care Medicine
Beaumont Hospital
Royal College of Surgeons in Ireland Hospital Group
Dublin, Ireland

Katherine Palmieri, MD
Associate Professor
Department of Anesthesiology
University of Kansas Medical Center
Kansas City, KS, USA

Andrew Pellet, MD
Division of Critical Care Medicine
Department of Anesthesiology
Columbia University College of Physicians and Surgeons
NewYork-Presbyterian Hospital
New York, NY, USA

Naomi Quigley, BM BS
Registrar in Anaesthesiology & Critical Care Medicine
Department of Anaesthesiology & Critical Care Medicine
Beaumont Hospital
Royal College of Surgeons in Ireland Hospital Group
Dublin, Ireland

Christopher Read, MB ChB
Registrar in Anaesthesiology & Critical Care Medicine
Department of Anaesthesia
University Hospital Galway
Galway, Ireland

Fiona Roberts, MB BCh
Registrar in Anaesthesiology &
Critical Care Medicine
Department of Anaesthesiology &
Critical Care Medicine
Beaumont Hospital
Royal College of Surgeons in
Ireland Hospital Group
Dublin, Ireland

Casey Shelley, DO
Resident
Department of Anesthesiology
University of Kansas
Medical Center
Kansas City, KS, USA

Liang Shen, MD
Assistant Professor
Department of Anesthesiology
Weill Cornell Medicine
New York, NY, USA

Gurbinder Singh, DO
Critical Care Anesthesiologist
Anesthesia Specialists of Bethlehem
Bethlehem, PA, USA

Coilin Smyth, MB BCh
Registrar in Anaesthesiology &
Critical Care Medicine
Department of Anaesthesiology &
Critical Care Medicine
Beaumont Hospital
Royal College of Surgeons in
Ireland Hospital Group
Dublin, Ireland

Ankur Srivastava, MD
Critical Care Fellow
Department of Anesthesiology
NewYork-Presbyterian Hospital/
Weill Cornell
New York, NY, USA

Jared Staab, DO
Assistant Professor
Department of Anesthesiology
University of Kansas
Medical Center
Kansas City, KS, USA

Lauren D. Sutherland, MD
Fellow, Adult Cardiothoracic
Anesthesia
Department of Anesthesiology
Columbia University
Medical Center
New York, NY, USA

Bushra W. Taha, MD
Division of Critical Care
Department of Anesthesiology
NewYork-Presbyterian Columbia
University Irving Medical Center
New York, NY, USA

Christopher W. Tam, MD
Associate Professor
Department of Anesthesiology
Weill Cornell Medicine
New York, NY, USA

Dana Teodorescu, MD
Registrar in Anaesthesiology &
Critical Care Medicine
Department of Anaesthesiology &
Critical Care Medicine
Beaumont Hospital
Royal College of Surgeons in
Ireland Hospital Group
Dublin, Ireland

Hans Tregear, MD
Resident
Department of Anesthesiology
University of Kansas School of
Medicine
Kansas City, KS, USA

Christopher Webb, MD
Participant Physician, Director of
Graduate Medical Education
The Permanente Medical Group of
Northern California
Assistant Clinical Professor
Department of Anesthesia &
Perioperative Care
University of California San
Francisco School of Medicine
San Francisco, CA, USA

Paul D. Weyker, MD
Associate Physician, Director of
Perioperative Medicine
Department of Anesthesiology,
Critical Care Medicine, Pain
Medicine
The Permanente Medical Group of
Northern California
San Francisco, CA, USA

1 Risk Assessment Scores in Cardiac Surgery

Matthew Hulse and Stuart Lowson

An 80-year-old female is brought to the emergency department after complaining of 2 weeks of worsening chest pain with exertion, shortness of breath, and weakness which has prevented her from getting around her house. Her family members state that while these symptoms are new, she has had balance issues for the past year and now ambulates with a walker. During this time she also had 10 pounds of unintentional weight loss. After reviewing her transthoracic echocardiogram, you note that the patient has a mildly reduced left ventricular ejection fraction at 40%–45% and severe calcific aortic stenosis with a valve area of 0.8 cm^2. Unfortunately, based on her anatomy, she is not a candidate for transcatheter aortic valve replacement (TAVR) and instead is scheduled for an urgent, surgical aortic valve replacement (SAVR) with cardiac surgery. Prior to surgery, her family members pull you aside, concerned about the risk of the procedure. They ask you what the chances are of her dying in the hospital.

What do you do now?

DISCUSSION

The Need for Risk Assessments

Cardiac surgical risk scoring models have been utilized to classify risk to adult patients for over 3 decades. These scores first came into construct in the 1980s when the rate of mortality following coronary artery bypass graft (CABG) surgery began to increase. From a mortality rate of 1%–2%, clinicians began seeing a 5%–6% mortality rate and needed to assess the reasons for this increase. Meaningful analysis required creation of multi-institutional databases whereby risks could properly and statistically be studied.

Since this time, numerous scoring systems have been developed to define patient risk factors. Early scoring systems attempted to identify solely the risk of mortality. Later adaptations provide the additional risk assessments of various surgical morbidities. This is important as patients rightfully wish to know not only their chances of survival after cardiac surgery but also their chances of prolonged hospitalization and physical limitations after surgery. As patients presenting for cardiac surgery are becoming older and more vulnerable, scoring systems allow for thoughtful discussions with patients and families concerning which risks are acceptable and which risks are not acceptable.

In fact, risk scores may actually prompt long-term planning discussions between patients and families. With data-driven knowledge, patients and families can together analyze associated risks of a proposed procedure during a family conversation. This discussion will allow the family and healthcare providers to hear the patient's specific desires for end-of-life healthcare. Such conversations are commonly had when discussing procedures for aortic valve replacement and deciding whether a TAVR is more beneficial versus an open SAVR, which is the decision to be made in this case.

Additionally, prediction of operative mortality and major morbidity are important to not only patients but also healthcare systems. A secondary benefit of broadly employed risk models involves improvements in outcomes. Because of the ability to compare and analyze various practices, risk models act as an important part of the algorithm when providing quality control in the care of cardiac surgical patients seen throughout the world. Thus, risk calculators not only help patients with individual decisions but are helping patients survive on a global level.

However, clinicians must realize an inherent risk associated with all risk assessment scoring systems. All systems are based on large database populations of patients and may not equate to the risk of an individual patient. Likewise, all scoring systems may not be applicable to certain hospitals or certain parts of the world. Thus, appropriate assessment and care must always be individualized for each patient, care team, and hospital practice concomitantly.

Common Risk Assessment Systems

It is likely, because of the inherent flaws of scoring systems, that there are currently approximately 20 different scoring systems in the adult cardiac surgery literature attempting to correctly assign risk for individual patients. With each validated risk score, there are numerous investigations comparing the performance of these scoring systems in regard to specified patient risk factors.

The first widely used risk model was the initial Parsonnet score, developed in 1989. The Parsonnet score predicted cardiac surgical mortality based on preoperative risk factors thought to be clinically significant. The scoring system was simple and additive and graded the severity of illness of patients into 5 groups of predicted mortality. However, this score left certain patient and surgical characteristics at the discretion of clinicians, which decreased its reliability. The Parsonnet score was later modified to a much longer version, eliminating discretionary assessment and providing clinical definitions of risk factors.

Numerous other scoring systems have been developed since the development of the Parsonnet score. Notable risk models include the Cleveland Clinic score, the Mayo Clinic model, the Bayes model, and the Northern New England score. These scores all have commonalities and differences and have been validated in various forms and in head-to-head comparisons. Some are only validated for CABG procedures, such as the Northern New England and Bayes scores. All include basic demographic data, left ventricular function, and renal disease. However, all of these scores have by and large been replaced by much more encompassing and validated risk assessments throughout the world.

The most commonly used risk assessment tools for cardiac surgical patients in the modern era are the European System for the Cardiac Operative Risk Evaluation (EuroSCORE) and the Society of Thoracic Surgeons (STS) risk score. Both of these systems were initially developed in 1999. The EuroSCORE is most commonly used in Europe and Canada, making it the most common cardiac risk calculator worldwide. The STS score is the commonest score used in the United States. Both scoring systems allow for free online access to the respective risk calculators.

Both the EuroSCORE and the STS scoring systems rely on complex prediction systems using advanced computer statistical models utilizing logistic regression analysis in hopes of correctly analyzing numerous patient variables. These scores are well validated but will still inevitably arrive at differing predictions of morbidity and mortality in a given patient. Common "inaccuracies" are typically found when there are variations between complex patients in subgroups of elective, semi-urgent, and urgent procedures performed in both low-risk and high-risk surgical patients.

The EuroSCORE was modified into its present form, EuroSCORE II, in 2011, due to the finding that the original EuroSCORE likely overestimated mortality risk. There are 18 items in the EuroSCORE II (Table 1.1), and all elements can be assessed using the additive EuroSCORE II method or the logistical regression method via the online calculator on the EuroSCORE website. The logistical regression method may be more precise in risk analysis but cannot simply be calculated at the bedside.

Conversely, the STS score not only has been validated as a mortality risk assessment but has been widely validated as a reliable morbidity risk assessment tool. This is an advantage over the EuroSCORE II, which is less validated in terms of major morbidities. The STS score is validated for certain types of cardiac surgical procedures but not for all (Table 1.2). However, many reports continue to establish that the STS scoring system may be meaningful in other surgical procedures not yet included in the STS scoring system, such as TAVR procedures. The STS score is more complicated than the EuroSCORE II, involving more than 40 data elements and various degrees for each of the data elements.

There are a few other major differences between the EuroSCORE II and the STS score. Firstly, as previously mentioned, the STS score is only validated in the cardiac surgical procedures listed in Table 1.2. Thus,

TABLE 1.1 **The Metrics Assessed by EuroSCORE for Calculation of Perioperative Mortality Risk Following Cardiac Surgery**

EuroSCORE
Age
Gender
Renal impairment
Extracardiac arteriopathy
Poor mobility
Previous cardiac surgery
Chronic lung disease
Active endocarditis
Critical preoperative state
Diabetes on insulin
New York Heart Association Heart Failure Classification
Angina at rest
Left ventricular function
Recent myocardial infarction
Pulmonary hypertension
Urgency
Type of procedure
Surgery on thoracic aorta

multiple valve surgery or any surgery replacing or repairing the tricuspid valve is not amenable to risk calculation. However, the EuroSCORE II simply asks for the number of procedures involved in the surgery and, thus, can be used in most every surgical situation. Secondly, when compared head-to-head, the EuroSCORE II typically overestimates perioperative risk,

TABLE 1.2 **Overview of the Society of Thoracic Surgery Scoring System for the Risk of Mortality and Various Morbidities Following Cardiac Surgery**

Types of Cardiac Surgical Procedures	Risks Assessed
Isolated CABG	Mortality
Isolated aortic valve replacement	Renal failure
Isolated mitral valve replacement	Permanent stroke
Aortic valve replacement + CABG	Prolonged ventilation
Mitral valve replacement + CABG	Deep sternal wound infection
Mitral valve repair	Reoperation
Mitral valve repair + CABG	Morbidity or mortality
	Short length of stay
	Long length of stay
	Long length of stay

whereas the STS score has been reported to underestimate perioperative risk, especially in frail patients.

Neither score identifies right ventricular failure as a risk factor. Clinicians know that right ventricular failure can greatly alter outcomes after cardiac surgery and increase mortality substantially. Unfortunately, grading right ventricular failure is difficult by echocardiographic assessment due to the unique composition and shape of the right ventricle. Both scores utilize pulmonary hypertension as a presumed surrogate for right ventricular function. However, this is known to be a poor surrogate for right ventricular function as pulmonary pressures do not uniformly predict right ventricular function. In fact, pulmonary pressures may be inversely related to the function of the right ventricle.

Lastly, the STS score does not assess the severity of physical limitations prior to surgery. This is important to acknowledge as recent literature reports the association of poor preoperative functional status to mortality and major morbidity after cardiac surgery, including minimally invasive cardiac surgical procedures. Some studies cite the importance of *prehabilitation* to lessen the risk of cardiac surgery associated with a sedentary lifestyle as evidenced by poor gait speed and frailty scores. The EuroSCORE II does assess for mobility, defining this as "severe impairment of mobility secondary to musculoskeletal or neurological dysfunction" as a "yes/no" question. Obviously, this definition may not necessarily impart cardiac risk since immobility may be due to other etiologies. While this definition may not fully capture how frail or vulnerable a patient may be, it does at least broach the subject. This may be a data element that will be modified in future iterations of the EuroSCORE II or added to the STS risk score.

Interestingly, there are very few cardiac surgical risk assessment tools developed outside of North America and the United States. The Sino System for Coronary Operative Risk Evaluation has been published in China but is not popular outside of China. However, it remains unknown if well-established scoring systems, such as the EuroSCORE II and the STS score, can be extrapolated to all ethnicities and cultures. For example, the age at which cardiovascular disease develops, the angiographic disease patterns, and the types of cardiac diseases may be quite different depending on cultural variables. Societal risk factors may play a role in disease development. As we learn more about the impact of genetics on cardiovascular disease states, these may need to be factored into reliable risk assessment tools.

Frailty as a Risk Factor
The patient in this clinical scenario represents a fairly typical profile of a preoperative patient with severe aortic stenosis. Frailty is a common trait that is rarely assessed for in a preoperative cardiac surgical evaluation. *Frailty* is an umbrella term that encompasses multiple patient factors including muscle wasting, malnutrition, limited mobility, and cognitive state and tries to describe a patient's reserve and ability to overcome a physiological stress such as a concurrent illness or surgery (i.e., the patient's vulnerability). Some authors describe frailty as the inability to maintain homeostasis. This is an especially concerning definition in regard to cardiac surgery where cardiopulmonary bypass and general anesthesia are known to disrupt homeostasis even in the healthiest of patients.

The average age and risk profile of patients undergoing cardiac surgery are steadily increasing, with more than half of procedures being performed in patients aged 75 years and older. While frailty is not confined to the elderly, its prevalence does increase with age. This presents new sets of challenges to surgical and postoperative care. While both the EuroSCORE II and STS score take the chronological age of the patient into consideration and the EuroSCORE II accounts for mobility, neither major scoring system assesses frailty.

While it has become increasingly popular to perform a preoperative assessment of frailty, there is no consensus as to how frailty should be assessed. Reports from both US and European societies of geriatric medicine recommend that patients greater than 70 years of age be assessed for frailty; however, multiple scoring systems exist, and none have been uniformly recommended. Simple and fast tests include the Clinical Frailty Score (Figure 1.1), the 5-meter gait speed, the "get up and go" test, and the Fried frailty phenotype. More complex indices based on multiple factors exist; however, there is no evidence to date that increased complexity increases reliability.

Frailty in general surgery patients is consistently associated with a greater risk of surgical complications, increased length of hospital stay, and discharge to a rehabilitation facility rather than home. In some studies, frailty has been found to be an independent predictor of hospital mortality. In addition, frail patients are at a higher risk for readmission, suffer from lower quality of life following general surgery, and end up paying higher overall costs for their care.

Systematic reviews have confirmed that a diagnosis of frailty increases the risk of mortality after TAVR. There is strong evidence that frailty is associated with all-cause mortality and major cardiovascular and cerebrovascular events following TAVR. Frailty prior to TAVR is also associated with worsening functional decline after the procedure. The exact etiology for these findings is unclear. Until recently, patients receiving TAVR procedures were too sick to be considered for SAVR procedures. Thus, it is possible that there was a bias in studies assessing postoperative outcomes based on frailty in this specific population. It will be interesting to assess the association of frailty and poor outcomes in TAVR patients as the approval for TAVR procedures allows for healthier patients to undergo this procedure. In fact, frailty may not be as important a risk factor as noted previously.

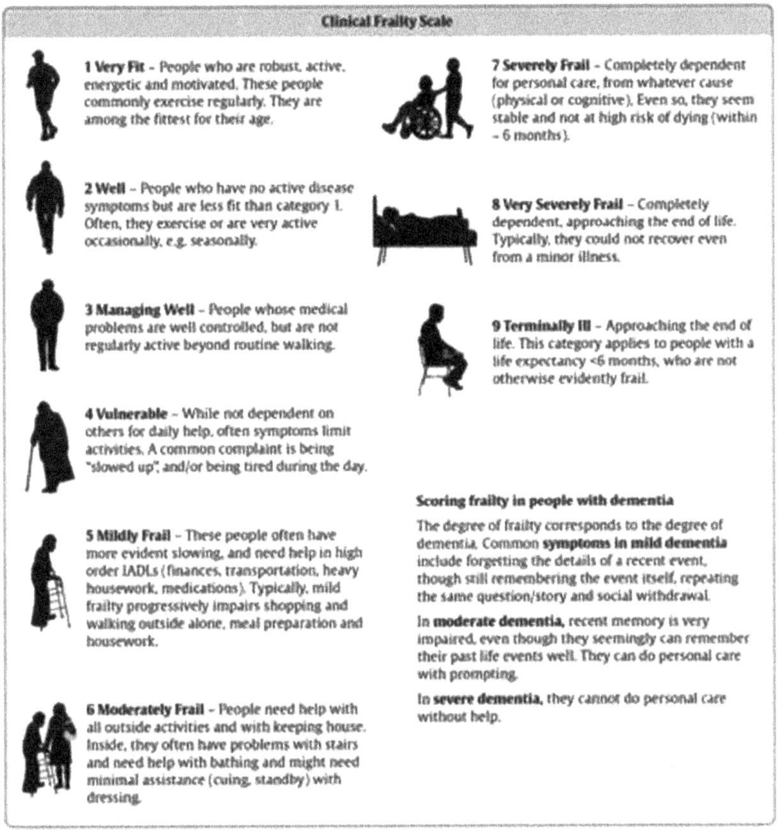

FIGURE 1.1 The Clinical Frailty Scale.
Reprinted from public domain.

Studies assessing frailty and outcomes in patients undergoing open cardiac surgical procedures have been more difficult to interpret. Some authors have demonstrated that frailty when measured via typical scoring systems is associated with in-hospital mortality, 1-year mortality, and prolonged institutional care, while others have shown that frailty measured only through gait speed was associated with mortality or major morbidity and that other measures of frailty were not associated with poor outcomes. It is important to note that the majority of these studies failed to perform a comprehensive preoperative assessment of functional ability and quality of life with which to compare postoperative metrics.

One recent study may provide clarification as to why postoperative functional outcomes are vastly different in open cardiac surgery depending on the study. Miguelena-Hycka et al. showed that, ironically, patients with a preoperative diagnosis of "frail" or "prefrail" actually had the greatest improvement in quality of life after cardiac surgery, while "robust" patients had the least improvement. This study also confirmed the well-established significant relationship between frailty and increased mortality and major morbidity after cardiac surgery but suggested that frail patients, if they survive, actually derive the greatest quality-of-life benefit from the surgery. Perhaps this should not be so surprising if the cardiac pathology was the major cause of the patient's preoperative disability.

CASE RESUMES

The family in this case was asked to participate in the conversation concerning risk assessment with the patient. They were counseled utilizing the STS risk score algorithm concerning her risk of mortality and of major morbidities. Her risk of mortality was cited at 3.2%. Her highest morbidity risk was permanent stroke at 2.1%. Her weight loss, weakness, and need for a walker were also discussed as potential risk factors for a decline in her functional status following SAVR, although the evidence is less clear concerning these factors. Ultimately, the patient decided that she felt much of her deconditioning was a result of her valvular problem and wished to proceed with SAVR. She made her wishes known to her surgeon and to her family if she should become extremely debilitated or have major morbidities following surgery.

As patients present for cardiac surgery at increasingly older ages, meaningful metrics like "did the patient return home" or survival at 1 year may become increasingly utilized during preoperative visits instead of metrics such as 28-day survival. In the setting of cardiac surgery, understanding which burdens can be attributed to and, thus, repaired with cardiac surgical interventions will be key in improving the quality of life of patients.

KEY POINTS TO REMEMBER

1. Multiple cardiac scoring systems exist which attempt to incorporate similar yet varied metrics to predict postoperative morbidity and mortality.
2. Scoring systems are derived from logistical regression of risk factors from large database cohorts and, thus, may not be accurate for individual patients.
3. Two of the most commonly used scoring systems, the STS score and the EuroSCORE II, lack right ventricular dysfunction as a risk metric.
4. The STS score and the EuroSCORE II differ in that the EuroSCORE incorporates mobility as a marker for patient frailty.
5. Frailty is consistently associated with a greater risk of morbidity and mortality in patients undergoing TAVR procedures; however, the risk associated with frailty following open cardiac surgical procedures is less clear.

Suggested Reading

1. Shroyer AL, Plomondon ME, Grover FL, Edwards FH. The 1996 coronary artery bypass risk model: the Society of Thoracic Surgeons Adult Cardiac National Database. *Ann Thorac Surg.* 1999;67:1205–1208.
2. Nashef SAM, Roques F, Michel P, Gauducheau E, Lemeshow S, Salamon R. European system for cardiac operative risk evaluation (EuroSCORE). *Eur J Cardiothorac Surg.* 1999;16:9–13.
3. Geissler HJ, Hölzl P, Marohl S, et al. Risk stratification in heart surgery: comparison of six score systems. *Eur J Cardiothorac Surg.* 2000;17:400–406.
4. Afilalo J, Sharma A, Zhnag S, et al. Gait speed and 1-year mortality following cardiac surgery: a landmark analysis from the Society of Thoracic Surgeons Adult Cardiac Surgery Database. *J Am Heart Assoc.* 2018;7(23):e010139.
5. Sepehri A, Beggs T, Hassan A, et al. The impact of frailty after cardiac surgery: a systemic review. *J Thorac Cardiovasc Surg.* 2014;148:3110–3117.
6. Miguelena-Hycka J, Lopez-Menendez J, Prada P-C, et al. Influence of preoperative frailty on health-related quality of life after cardiac surgery. *Ann Thorac Surg.* 2019;108(1):23–29.

2 Pulmonary Artery Catheterization in Cardiac Surgery

Daniel L. Jacobs and Brigid C. Flynn

A 75-year-old male presents to the cardiac surgical intensive care unit (ICU) following a 3-vessel coronary artery bypass graft (CABG) procedure. Prior to his surgery, the anesthesiologist placed a right radial arterial line, an introducer into the right internal jugular vein, and floated a pulmonary artery catheter (PAC). Upon arrival to the ICU, the patient is sedated, is intubated, and has stable vital signs. He is on a dobutamine infusion at 3 mcg/kg/min due to decreased ejection fraction estimated at 40% coming off cardiopulmonary bypass. His past medical history is significant for paroxysmal atrial fibrillation, hypertension, tobacco abuse, and obesity. Shortly after arrival, you notice that his electrocardiogram (ECG) rhythm strip shows several beats of recurrent ventricular ectopy appearing to be premature ventricular complexes (PVCs), and his pulmonary artery diastolic pressure waveform and numerical values decrease. The patient is now having decreased blood pressure.

What do you do now?

DISCUSSION

Ventricular Ectopy

Ventricular ectopy after CABG is not uncommon; however, it should be taken very seriously. PVCs occur when the impulse arises in the ventricle; thus, they are not associated with a P wave (Figure 2.1). These beats have a widened QRS and a large T wave in the opposite direction of the QRS wave. If these beats are monomorphic and less than 8 beats/min, they rarely cause instability. However, PVCs can lead to more serious dysrhythmias and accordingly should be monitored and treated if signs of hemodynamic instability occur. Sustained ventricular tachycardia is less common after cardiac surgery than PVCs but is life-threatening when it occurs.

First and foremost, with ventricular ectopy beats, ventricular ischemia should be ruled out with a formal ECG. The ECG may also aid in deciphering the origin of the ventricular ectopy and allows for calculation of intervals. Patients with preexisting atrial or ventricular ectopy due to scar or known conduction disturbances will likely have postoperative ectopy. Antidysrhythmic medication withdrawal may be one etiology, and these medications should be resumed without alteration in schedule as able intravenously or with a gastric tube.

Inotropic medications, such as dobutamine in this case, increase arrhythmogenic potential commonly by beta receptor agonism. Additionally, surgical manipulation and cardiac edema around nerve bundles exacerbate ectopy in the postoperative period. Clinicians must evaluate if there are hemodynamic changes associated with ectopic beats such as decreased blood pressure due to loss of atrial kick and atrial-ventricular dysynchrony resulting in decreased cardiac output. Lastly, PAC placement should be checked to ensure that the catheter is not misplaced into the right ventricle, which would lead to endocardial irritation and result in ventricular ectopy. Risk factors and therapies for ventricular ectopy in the ICU and potential therapies are listed in Table 2.1.

PACs

PACs provide various pressure measurements and associated waveforms including right atrial pressure or central venous pressure, right ventricular pressure, pulmonary artery pressure, and pulmonary artery occlusion

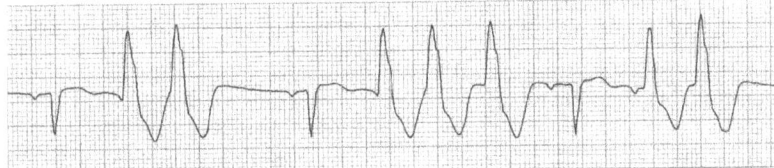

FIGURE 2.1 An ECG strip showing premature ventricular contractions.

pressure (wedge pressure), which represents left ventricular end-diastolic pressure (Figures 2.2 and 2.3). Table 2.2 provides normal values for each of these pressures within the cardiopulmonary system.

PACs also offer the opportunity to calculate an intermittent cardiac output measurement via the thermodilution technique. Thermodilution measurements of cardiac output are still considered the gold standard in the ICU setting. It is the cardiac output measuring mechanism to which newer cardiac output measurement devices are compared. Thermodilution measurement of cardiac output is accomplished by injection of cold fluid into the right atrium or central venous port of the PAC. PACs have a distal heated filament, which allows automatic heating of the blood. A thermodilution tracing is shown on the monitor based on the computer-calculated rate of fall in temperature. The lower the cardiac output, the slower the rate of temperature change. This relationship is given by the Stewart-Hamilton equation, which is the quantity of the indicator fluid divided by the area under the dilution curve. With these data along with the intracardiopulmonary pressures already mentioned, many other hemodynamic assessments can be made concerning the patient. Table 2.3 lists these.

The proper placement of the PAC is in the main pulmonary artery, which can be identified most accurately through waveform analysis. On chest X-ray, the tip of the PAC typically rests near the midline of the spine. When a PAC inadvertently floats back into the right ventricle, the waveform will be the first indicator. As expected, the waveform will appear as a right ventricular pressure waveform instead of the pulmonary artery pressure waveform (Figures 2.2 and 2.3). The right ventricular waveform differs from the pulmonary artery pressure waveform in 3 ways in that the right ventricular waveform has (1) a decreased diastolic pressure, (2) no dicrotic notch, and (3) an upsloping of the diastolic part of the tracing due to atrial

TABLE 2.1 **Risk Factors and Treatments for Ventricular Ectopy**

Risk Factor	Treatment
Nonmodifiable risk factors in the ICU • Age >65 years • Female • Body mass index <25 kg/m^2 • Preoperative decreased ventricular function • Prolonged cardiopulmonary bypass	External cardioversion should occur for shockable rhythms of unstable ventricular tachycardia and/or ventricular fibrillation with significant hypotension or cardiac arrest
Myocardial ischemia • Inadequate myocardial protection • Myocardial reperfusion • Grafting non-collateralized occluded vessel	• Ensure adequate oxygen delivery (check blood gas) • Ensure adequate coronary artery perfusion (check blood pressure and monitor left ventricular end diastolic pressure) • Obtain echocardiography looking for new regional wall motion abnormalities
PAC misplacement into right ventricle	Repeat flotation of the PAC to proper pulmonary artery position
Preexisting scar tissue	Ensure adequate oxygen and coronary blood flow to newly vascularized tissue
Hemodynamic instability	Consider adding pressor agent if hypotensive
Electrolyte abnormalities	Obtain lab values and correct, especially magnesium and potassium
Drugs • Sympathomimetics • Inotropes • Withdrawal of antidysrhythmic	• Consider decreasing sympathomimetic medications and resume antidysrhythmic as able • Consider amiodarone or lidocaine therapy
Surgical inflammation	Ensure adequate oxygen and coronary blood flow while swelling naturally subsides

TABLE 2.1 **Continued**

Risk Factor	Treatment
R-on-T	May occur when the cardiac conduction system is being paced while the patient is having native beats
Sepsis	Monitor for signs of infection and treat accordingly

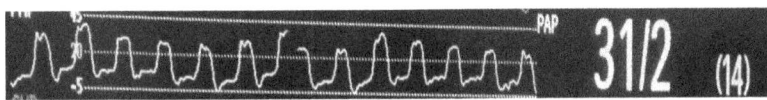

FIGURE 2.2 An ICU monitor with the pulmonary artery catheter tracing and pressure reading.

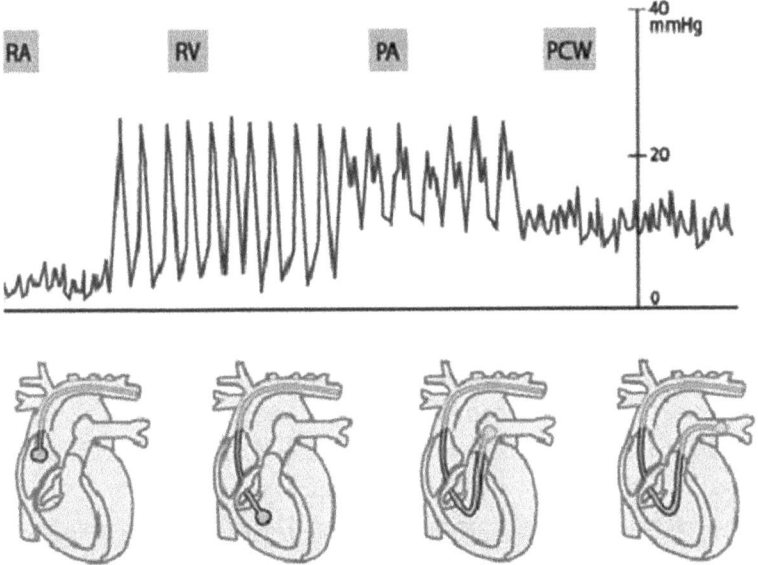

FIGURE 2.3 Typical waveforms seen in correlation with each cardiac chamber as a pulmonary artery catheter is advanced into proper position. PA, pulmonary artery; PCW, pulmonary capillary wedge; RA, right atrial; RV, right ventricular.

Reprinted with permission from Mathews L. Paradigm shift in hemodynamic monitoring. *Internet Journal of Anesthesiology.* 2006;11[2]. https://ispub.com/IJA/11/2/13289. Accessed July 28, 2020.

TABLE 2.2 **Normal Intracardiopulmonary Pressures Obtained from a PAC**

Location	Mean Pressure (mm Hg)	Range (mm Hg)
RAP	5	0–10
RVP	25/5	15–30/0–8
PAP	23/9	15–30/5–15
PAOP	10	5–15
LVEDP	8	4–12

LVEDP, left ventricular end-diastolic pressure; PAOP, pulmonary artery occlusion pressure; PAP, pulmonary artery pressure; RAP, right atrial pressure; RVP, right ventricular pressure.

contraction. The pulmonary artery waveform has a downsloping during diastasis as it does not fill like the right ventricle during this time.

Besides attention to the waveforms on the monitor, displacement of the PAC into the right ventricle may be noticed by ventricular arrhythmia. Ventricular ectopy is caused by direct contact of the tip of the PAC with ventricular nerve conduction fibers, as occurred in this case. Repeat flotation of the PAC with the balloon carefully inflated by an experienced practitioner can be attempted with watchful monitoring of the waveforms. The risk of attempting this is pulmonary artery rupture if the pulmonary artery occlusion waveform is not noticed and further advancement occurs.

Utility of PACs

The benefit of the PAC weighed against the potential for harm remains debatable. In 2005, a randomized controlled trial in the United Kingdom, dubbed the *PAC-Man trial*, examined outcomes in 1014 ICU patients treated with or without a PAC. Clinical management after insertion was at the discretion of the attending physician. Their findings showed no evidence of benefit or harm with utilization of the PAC in the treatment of critically ill patients. The authors suggested that PACs may be a redundant technology not necessary in modern ICUs.

The ESCAPE trial, also published in 2005, randomized 433 patients with heart failure to treatment either with or without a PAC and reported no difference in mortality (10% versus 9%) or the length of hospital stay

TABLE 2.3 **Values Derived from a PAC Utilizing Equations**

Value	Normal Value
CI = CO/BSA	2.8–4.2 L/min/m²
SV = CO/HR or SV = LVEDV − LVESV	60–110 mL/beat
LVEF = SV/LVEDV	55%–65%
SI = SV/BSA	30–65 mL/beat/m²
RVEF = SV/RVEDV	55%–60%
RVSW = (mean PAP − CVP) × SV × 0.0136	8–16 grams-m/beat
RVSWI = (mean PAP − CVP) × SI × 0.0136	5–10 grams-m/m²/beat
LVSW = (MAP − PAOP) × SV × 0.0136	58–104 grams-m/beat
LVSWI = (MAP − PAWP) × SI × 0.0136	50–62 grams-m/m²/beat
SVR = (MAP − CVP) × 80/CO	900–1200 dyn · s/cm⁵
SVRI = SVR/BSA	1500–2200 dyn · s/cm⁵
PVR = (mean PAP − PAOP) × 80/CO	100–200 dyn · s/cm⁵
PVRI = PVR/BSA	250–400 dyn · s/cm⁵

BSA, body surface area; CI, cardiac index; CO, cardiac output; CVP, central venous pressure; HR, heart rate; LVEDV, left ventricular end-diastolic volume; LVEF, left ventricular ejection fraction; LVESV, left ventricular end-systolic volume; LVSW, left ventricular stroke work; LVSWI, left ventricular stroke work index; MAP, mean arterial pressure; PAOP, pulmonary artery occlusion pressure; PAP, pulmonary artery pressure; PAWP, pulmonary artery wedge pressure; PVR, pulmonary vascular resistance; PVRI, pulmonary vascular resistance index; RVEDV, right ventricular end-diastolic volume; RVEF, right ventricular ejection fraction; RVSW, right ventricular stroke work; RVSWI, right ventricular stroke work index; SI, stroke index; SV, stroke volume; SVR, systemic vascular resistance; SVRI, systemic vascular resistance index.

(8.7 days versus 8.3 days) between the 2 groups. The authors encouraged noninvasive assessments for volume assessment in heart failure patients.

The most recent Cochrane systematic review on the subject of PAC utility was published in 2016 and included 13 randomized controlled trials and 5686 ICU patients. All studies had randomization of patients to either PAC placement and use or control groups. The authors found no statistically significant increase in mortality between the PAC and control groups. Furthermore, there was no difference in ICU length of stay or hospital length of stay.

Despite a recent trend of increased use of the PAC, worldwide the use of the PAC is decreasing. This may be due to clinician discomfort in placing and/or interpreting the data from a PAC. However, certain patient populations may benefit from management decisions based on PAC data. Use among cardiac surgical and heart failure patients remains high. Currently, the American College of Cardiology/American Heart Association guidelines recommend using PAC for heart failure patients with cardiogenic shock or those on mechanical circulatory support (class 1, level of evidence C).

While clinicians understand that the evidence suggests that use of the PAC may not improve mortality or decrease hospitalization, the data provided by the PAC are difficult to reliably obtain through other means on a continuous basis. Surface echocardiographic imaging can be challenging to interpret in ventilated patients, those with surgical dressings, and those on mechanical circulatory support. Transesophageal echocardiography can provide similar information to a PAC but requires specific training. Importantly, an indwelling PAC gives real-time numbers, which can be followed to track the effectiveness of interventions on a beat-by-beat basis.

Additionally, the PAC waveforms, can provide hemodynamic information, notwithstanding the numerical values, that cannot be found elsewhere. Indeed, waveform interpretation of the central venous tracing, the pulmonary artery tracing, and the pulmonary artery occlusion pressure tracing can provide invaluable insight into the isolated right ventricular function and left ventricular function and information about the pericardial sac and space. Information about the fluid status of each compartment of the heart can be gained. Notably, in critically ill patients, the fluid status of different chambers of the heart is often quite different from the fluid status of the lungs, which is in turn quite different from the fluid status of the kidneys, which may be quite different from the fluid status of the rest of the body. Understanding these differences with data provides a setting for educated clinical decision-making regarding fluid resuscitation, fluid removal, and inotropic medication titration.

Furthermore, echocardiography does not allow for obtainment of blood samples from inside the cardiopulmonary system as does the PAC.

A mixed venous blood gas can be drawn from the pulmonary artery port of the PAC. This venous blood gas will reveal the mixed venous oxygen saturation, which is an indicator of whole-body oxygen delivery and consumption. Many therapies can be titrated based on this value with reliability.

With many newer technologies, such as the pulse wave contour analysis devices, thoracic bioimpedance devices, and advancements in surface echocardiography, the future of the PAC remains uncertain. Some studies have claimed that pulse wave contour analysis devices and thoracic bioimpedance devices can provide the same numerical data that a PAC can provide, including cardiac output, systemic vascular resistance, and stroke volume variation. Pulse wave contour analysis devices typically only require an arterial line or alternatively a finger probe blood pressure cuff. Thoracic bioimpedance devices are completely non-invasive and rely upon adhesive patches placed on the patient. Because of this, authors may advise use of these non-invasive or minimally invasive devices.

However, the methods used and the results identified in these studies must be analyzed. In healthy patients, these devices likely work quite well. In critically ill patients with large volume shifts, aortic disease, vasodilatory shock, cardiogenic shock, and rapidly changing hemodynamics due to bleeding, the accuracy of the data is likely not reliable. When interpreting these studies, one must pay close attention to the patient population selected and the sponsoring or funding source responsible for the study. Newer studies are now surfacing to support the discrepancies between these monitors and the current gold standard hemodynamic monitoring tool, the PAC.

Some clinicians raise concern that with limited exposure to the PAC due to decreased placements, expertise in both the placement and the interpretation of the data provided by the PAC will be lost. This could impart poor decision-making and actually may harm patients. If PACs are warranted, which they are for many clinical situations, clinicians trained and skilled in the use of PACs need to be placing and making clinical decisions with the data. Understanding the limitations of the catheter, the risks to patients, and how to troubleshoot problems is imperative to managing patients with a PAC safely and effectively.

CASE RESUMES

Based on the waveforms seen in the pulmonary artery pressure tracing, the PAC in this case was suspected to be have been pulled back to the right ventricle. This is a common cause of ventricular ectopy as the PAC abuts the right bundle or the Purkinje fibers. This situation can lead to a right bundle branch block and if the patient were to have a preexisting left bundle branch block, could lead to complete heart block. Ventricular ectopy may begin with premature ventricular complexes that will likely lead to hypotension during those beats. If the ectopy degrades into a sustained ventricular tachycardia, life-threatening hemodynamic instability can ensue.

The treatment for catheter-induced ventricular ectopy is to remove the catheter from the ventricular wall. This usually fixes the problem. If not, electrolytes should be optimized, fluid status should be evaluated, and possibly an antidysrythmic medication, such as amiodarone, should be initiated. In this case, the PAC balloon was checked for deflation and the PAC pulled back until the right atrial pressure waveform was seen. The ectopy ceased with this maneuver. The balloon was then reinflated, and the PAC was then floated through the right ventricle without ectopy and into the pulmonary artery. The patient tolerated this well, and the ectopy did not return.

> **KEY POINTS TO REMEMBER**
> 1. PACs provide information such as central venous pressure, pulmonary artery pressure, and pulmonary capillary wedge pressure with pertinent waveform analysis plus the ability to obtain an intermittent cardiac output via thermodilution.
> 2. There are numerous causes of ventricular dysrhythmia following cardiac surgery that all require different treatments in cardiothoracic patients.
> 3. The PAC still has a place in monitoring critically ill patients, especially those with cardiac impairment or on circulatory assist devices.

4. Understanding the risks associated with PAC use and obtaining the skill set necessary to safely interpret the data provided by these devices are the crux of optimal PAC utilization.

Suggested Reading
1. El-Chami MF, Sawaya FJ, Kilgo P, et al. Ventricular arrhythmia after cardiac surgery: incidence, predictors, and outcomes. *J Am Coll Cardiol.* 2012;60(25):2664–2671.
2. De Backer D, Vincent JL. The pulmonary artery catheter: is it still alive? *Curr Opin Crit Care.* 2018;24(3):204–208.
3. Yancy CW, Jessup M, Bozkurt B, et al. 2013 ACCF/AHA guideline for the management of heart failure: executive summary: a report of the American College of Cardiology Foundation/American Heart Association Task Force on practice guidelines. *Circulation* 2013;128:1810–1852.
4. Harvey S, Harrison DA, Singer M, et al. Assessment of the clinical effectiveness of pulmonary artery catheters in management of patients in intensive care (PAC-Man): a randomized controlled trial. *Lancet* 2005;366:472–477.
5. Binanay C, Califf RM, Hasselblad V, et al.; ESCAPE Investigators and ESCAPE Study Coordinators. Evaluation study of congestive heart failure and pulmonary artery catheterization effectiveness: the ESCAPE trial. *JAMA.* 2005;294(13):1625–1633.

3 Oxygen Consumption and Delivery in Critical Illness

Hans Tregear and Brigid C. Flynn

A 73-year-old male arrives to the cardiothoracic intensive care unit (ICU) following coronary artery bypass graft surgery. His past medical history is significant for ischemic cardiomyopathy with an ejection fraction of 40%, chronic obstructive pulmonary disease, hypertension, and diabetes mellitus type 2. Physical examination on arrival to the ICU is unremarkable. Initial ICU laboratory values are significant for a mixed venous saturation of 43% and a lactate of 3.2 mg/dL. He is initiated on inotropic support in the form of dobutamine of 3 mcg/kg/min. Over the next 24 hours, he is extubated and appears well. His mixed venous oxygen saturation, or SvO_2, on the dobutamine inotropic support was 64%.

With numerous parameters demonstrating hemodynamic stability, his pulmonary artery catheter (PAC) was removed, and he remained with his central venous sheath access. However, his lactate continued to rise despite gentle fluid resuscitation. You check his central venous saturation, or $ScvO_2$, which was 52%.

What do you do now?

DISCUSSION

SvO_2 is the percentage of oxygen bound to hemoglobin returning to the pulmonary artery after nearly all tissues have extracted oxygen. Thus, this measurement gives insight as to the oxygen consumption, along with oxygen delivery, occurring in vivo. SvO_2 can be measured from a blood draw from the distal port of the PAC, which is located in the pulmonary artery via flotation through the right side of the heart. A normal SvO_2 value is approximately 75%. In order to understand the implications of this, the concept of oxygen consumption must be understood by utilizing the Fick equation.

The amount of oxygen consumed, or VO_2, is dependent upon the oxygen that is being delivered, or DO_2. This dependence is greatest in times of decreased oxygen delivery such as in critical illness or with myocardial depression. One can only consume what is delivered. An important example of this concept is the myocardium. The heart extracts 70%–80% of the oxygen delivered to it in order to maintain adequate function and to deliver oxygen to the rest of the body. While impossible to obtain in an ICU patient, if one were to check an SvO_2 of the heart alone, it would be around 30% due to this high oxygen consumption. Thus, in times of decreased delivery, the heart cannot increase oxygen extraction much more than is already being accomplished. This is the reason that many instances of whole-body oxygen debt result in angina and subsequent end-organ failure.

Oxygen delivery is accomplished by the heart pumping the arterial oxygen content, or CaO_2, to all tissues. The cardiac output (CO) multiplied by the CaO_2 determines the oxygen available to be consumed by all organ systems. CaO_2 is determined by 2 major components: (1) the hemoglobin oxygen carrying capacity, which in times of health is around 1.39 mg/dL of oxygen per hemoglobin molecule, and (2) the arterial oxygen saturation, or SaO_2. The partial pressure of oxygen in the arterial system is represented by PaO_2 and is then multiplied by the constant, 0.003, which is the solubility coefficient of oxygen in human plasma. This leaves PaO_2 in such low amounts that it is unnecessary to add to the calculation. To enhance understanding of these concepts, one can calculate CaO_2 with "normal" clinical values of SaO_2 of 100%, SvO_2 of 75%, hemoglobin of 15 gm/dL, and CO of 5 L/min or 50 dL/min.

$$DO_2 = CO \times CaO_2$$

$$CaO_2 = (SaO_2 \times \text{hemoglobin} \times 1.39) + (PaO_2 \times 0.003)$$

For example, $CaO_2 = 1 \times 15 \text{ gm/dL} \times 1.39 = 20 \text{ mL/dL}$

Thus, $DO_2 = 50 \text{ dL/min} \times 20 \text{ mL/dL}$
$= 1000 \text{ mL oxygen/min delivered to tissues}$

However, to ascertain the state of oxygen excess or debt within the body, we need to know the amount of oxygen that is consumed. If the body is in oxygen debt, energy will need to be generated via anaerobic pathways, leading to an accumulation of lactate. Oxygen consumption, or VO_2, can be calculated with minor alterations of the DO_2 calculation. Likewise, since mixed venous oxygen tension, or PvO_2, is such a small number, it can be omitted.

$$VO_2 = CO \times (CaO_2 - CvO_2), \text{ where}$$

$$CvO_2 = (SvO_2 \times \text{hemoglobin} \times 1.39) + (PvO_2 \times 0.003)$$

For example, using "normal" values, mixed venous oxygen content, or CvO_2, can be calculated:

$$CvO_2 = 0.75 \times 15 \text{ gm/dL} \times 1.39 = 15 \text{ mL/dL}$$

Thus,

$$VO_2 = 50 \text{ dL/min} \times (20 \text{ mL/dL} - 15 \text{ mL/dL})$$
$$= 250 \text{ mL/min of oxygen consumed}$$

Other quick equations can be applied in healthy individuals, such as VO_2 is 3.5 mL O_2/kg/min or 125 mL O_2/m of body surface area. However, these assumptions will likely not represent the VO_2 of ICU patients accurately due to vasoactive medications, anemia, mechanical ventilation, and numerous other processes that will alter oxygen delivery and consumption in ICU patients.

As the equations demonstrate and quite remarkably, a healthy body delivers 1000 mL/min of oxygen and only consumes 250 mL/min! In other words, under normal resting conditions, the body extracts only around 25% of the oxygen delivered to it. Therefore, the venous blood is left over with 75% oxygen saturation before entering the lungs (i.e., a normal SvO_2 = 75% of original DO_2). That's quite an excess of oxygen! However, critical illness can lead to oxygen debt despite this seemingly excess surplus of oxygen. Once this occurs, the body goes into anaerobic metabolism, with the creation of lactate as a by-product. This formation of lactate makes it a useful marker of the degree to which anaerobic metabolism, or oxygen debt, is occurring in ICU patients.

One also modify the aforementioned equations to calculate SvO_2:

$$SvO_2 = SaO_2 - [VO_2/(\text{hemoglobin} \times 1.36 \times CO)]$$

SvO_2 is a valuable marker of oxygen consumption and delivery in an ICU patient. However, it needs to be recognized that there are numerous causes of elevated or decreased SvO_2 that may not be strictly associated with oxygen debt. Tables 3.1 and 3.2 list these.

Thermodilution Measurements of Cardiac Output

If SvO_2 is known, the above equation can be modified to solve for CO. Alternatively, if SvO_2 is unknown, one must obtain a CO value in order to calculate it. CO measurements can be obtained with a PAC by injecting 10 mL of cooler-than–body temperature fluid into the right atrium, or the central venous pressure port of the PAC. PACs have a distal heated filament, which allows automatic heating of the blood. The amount of time it takes for washout of the injectate measured via temperature change identifies the CO of the right side of the heart. This is called a "thermodilution measurement" of CO. A thermodilution tracing is shown on the monitor based on the computer-calculated rate of fall in temperature. The lower the CO, the slower the rate of temperature change.

Since thermodilution measurements of CO are only completely accurate during conditions of constant flow, respiration-induced changes in flow can cause error in CO measurement. It is standard practice to measure the CO at end-expiration since this is when intrapleural pressure is closest to

TABLE 3.1. **Causes of Increased in SvO$_2$**

Causes of Increased SvO$_2$	Etiology
Arterial–venous fistula or left-to-right shunt	Mixture of oxygenated and deoxygenated blood
Cirrhosis	Increased cardiac output and oxygenated blood delivery
Cyanide poisoning, carbon monoxide toxicity, methemoglobinemia	Inability of cells to utilize the delivered oxygen
Hypothermia	Decreased oxygen consumption
Sepsis	Inability of mitochondria to utilize delivered oxygen
Overwedged PAC	Sampling of more oxygenated blood of capillaries
Inotropic medications	Increased cardiac output

TABLE 3.2. **Causes of Decreased in SvO$_2$**

Causes of Decreased SvO$_2$	Etiology
Decreased hemoglobin	Decreased oxygen carrying capacity
Decreased oxygen saturation	Less oxygen delivered
Decreased cardiac output	Decreased oxygen delivery
Hypovolemia	Decreased oxygen delivery
Sepsis	Increased oxygen consumption
Exercise	Increased oxygen consumption
Shivering	Increased oxygen consumption
Malignant hyperthermia	Increased oxygen consumption
Thyroid storm	Increased oxygen consumption
Seizure	Increased oxygen consumption

zero. Also, measuring at one point in the respiratory cycle gives consistency among different operators. Furthermore, if the injectate is not exactly 10 mL, CO determinations will be proportionately inaccurate such that a 0.5 mL error in injectate volume will result in a 10% error in the calculated CO. Also, injection times less than 2 seconds produce optimal results. Falsely low measurements occur with prolonged injection times greater than 4 seconds.

Patient position can impact the thermodilution CO measurement. The supine position has a 30% higher CO than the semi-erect position secondary to increased preload when supine. Other infusions being simultaneously administered through a central venous port can also cause altered results and should be momentarily stopped, if safe to do so, while the CO measurement is being obtained. Tricuspid regurgitation usually causes underestimation of the true CO due to recirculation of the indicator and underestimation of forward flow. Similarly, recirculation of blood flow via intracardiac shunts will also alter the CO measurement. Even with fastidious adherence to proper thermodilution technique, consecutive measurements may differ by as much as 10%–20% with the same operator.

Other Oxygen Delivery Assessments

Important to note is the usefulness of a critical care physical examination in critically ill patients with suspected oxygen debt. Cool extremities, poorly palpable pulses, and skin mottling are signs of malperfusion. Complementary to physical examination is the prominence of point of care cardiac ultrasound (POCUS). This tool is very helpful when attempting to identify the etiology of hemodynamic instability and causes of low oxygen delivery. In the hands of a trained provider, POCUS can ascertain biventricular dysfunction, presence of a pericardial effusion, pneumothorax, pleural effusions or hemothorax, and decreased volume status.

Hyperlactatemia

In the event that an elevated lactate remains despite adequate oxygen delivery and a normalizing SvO_2, hypoxic causes of hyperlactatemia, or type A lactic acidosis, are less likely. Non-hypoxic lactic acidosis, or type B lactic acidosis, should be considered (Table 3.3). Type B lactic acidosis can be caused by delayed clearance of lactic acid that is constantly being produced

TABLE 3.3. **Causes of Hyperlactatemia**

Type A Lactatemia (Hypoxic)	Type B Lactatemia (Non-hypoxic)
Systemic hypoperfusion	Underlying disease or organ dysfunction
Asthma exacerbation	Alcoholic or diabetic ketoacidosis
Carbon monoxide poisoning	Human immunodeficiency virus
Cardiac arrest	Malignancy
COPD exacerbation	Renal or hepatic dysfunction
Cyanide toxicity	Short bowel syndrome
Hypovolemia	Thiamine deficiency
Sepsis	Liver deficiency
Severe anemia	Drugs or toxins
Seizure	Epinephrine
Trauma	Linezolid
Local hypoperfusion	Metformin
Arterial embolism	Propofol infusion syndrome
Limb ischemia	Retroviral drugs
Mesenteric ischemia	Congenital defects
	Mitochondrial myopathy
	Pyruvate dehydrogenase

COPD, chronic obstructive pulmonary disease.

by the body via aerobic mechanisms or, alternatively, was produced during a hypoxic event that has now resolved. Underlying liver disease, liver congestion, or malignancy with metastases to the liver could decrease this clearance.

Other causes of type B lactic acidosis include drugs or toxins like ethanol, salicylates, or sorbitol. Congenital metabolic defects have also been known to cause hyperlactatemia, and it is most often related to a mitochondrial disorder. In patients with malignancy, the Warburg effect describes the preference of cancer cells for metabolism via aerobic glycolysis rather than the much more efficient oxidative phosphorylation pathway. Thus, tumor cells produce energy through lactic fermentation instead of through oxidative phosphorylation, resulting in a high amount of lactic acid, even in non-hypoxic conditions. In the setting of thiamine deficiency, pyruvate dehydrogenase requires thiamine to function appropriately in the conversion of pyruvate to acetyl-coenzyme A. A deficiency of thiamine leads to excessive pyruvate levels, which is converted to lactate by lactate dehydrogenase. Epinephrine increases hepatic glycogenolysis and gluconeogenesis with subsequent increases in pyruvate. Increased blood levels of pyruvate may be so high that pyruvate dehydrogenase is overwhelmed and pyruvate cannot be adequately converted to acetyl-coenzyme A through aerobic oxidation. Excess pyruvate is then converted to lactate. It is also possible that epinephrine inhibits the action of pyruvate dehydrogenase.

The oral diabetic medication metformin has been shown to decrease the ability of the liver to clear lactate. This drug has been associated with metabolic acidosis due to this mechanism. In children, and to a lesser extent in adults, propofol infusions may cause propofol infusion syndrome (PRIS). A major component of PRIS is lactic acidosis secondary to an imbalance between energy demand and utilization due to impairment of mitochondrial oxidative phosphorylation and free fatty acid utilization.

Utility of ScvO$_2$

ScvO$_2$ was established as one of the goals of early goal-directed therapy in the landmark paper concerning resuscitation in septic patients by Rivers et al. This study showed a 16% decrease in mortality if this ScvO$_2$ goal of 65% was met, along with other goals, including central venous pressure 8–12 mm Hg, mean arterial pressure >65 mm Hg, and urine output >0.5 mL/kg/h in the first 6 hours of critical illness. While no one would argue that having an ScvO$_2$ of 65% is a harmful measure in and of itself, one must understand the limitations in using this marker alone in guiding resuscitation.

Firstly, the location from which ScvO2 and SvO$_2$ are taken is important to understand, as depicted in Figure 3.1. SvO$_2$ is collected from the most distal port of the PAC, located in the pulmonary artery. A blood sample for ScvO$_2$ is collected via a catheter, not necessarily a PAC, located in the superior vena cava, right atrium, or inferior vena cava. Thus, ScvO$_2$ drawn from

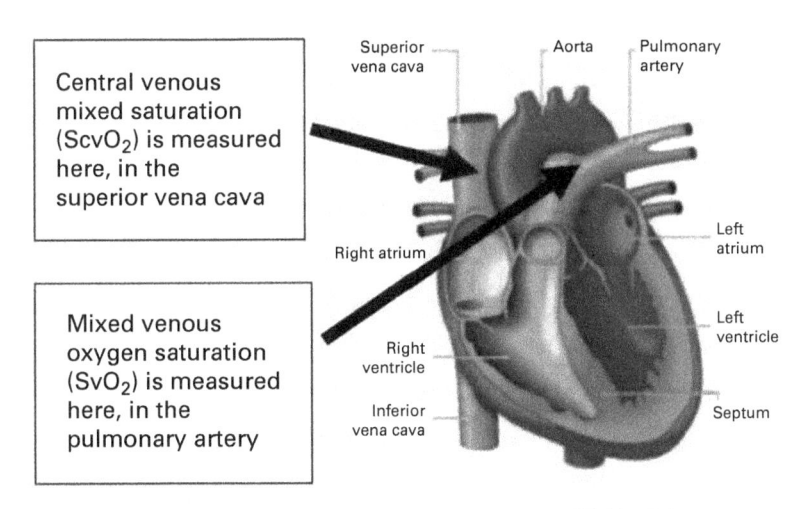

FIGURE 3.1 Sampling locations for ScvO$_2$ and SvO$_2$ measurements. BG, blood glucose.

the superior vena cava will be representative of the oxygen saturation in the upper body. Notably, the brain is a large oxygen consumer. ScvO$_2$ drawn from the inferior vena cava will be representative of the oxygen saturation in the lower body, which may be higher than actual if mesentery vasoconstriction is occurring due to shock. This is due to the body responding to shock with significant splanchnic and renal vasoconstriction in order to decrease intra-abdominal oxygen consumption. This in turn allows more blood to be delivered to the upper body, allowing perfusion of more vital organs, such as the heart and brain.

ScvO$_2$ drawn from the right atrium will reflect both the properties of the superior and the inferior vena cava, plus the blood draining directly from the myocardium via the coronary sinus. The conglomeration of saturations from all of these blood sources is what is represented in the SvO$_2$ sample in the pulmonary artery and will vary when compared to each of the individual sources. In summary, ScvO$_2$ may only reflect the oxygen delivery to consumption ratio of one part of the body, whereas SvO$_2$ is the best estimate of the oxygen delivery to consumption ratio of the body as a whole.

Notably, there are a few sources of shunt such as the Thebesian veins and the bronchial veins, which drain directly into the arterial system and are not accounted for in the SvO$_2$ measurement. Lastly, one must understand that each organ system has a differing set point of oxygen consumption even in times of health. This was previously discussed concerning the high oxygen extraction necessary for normal heart function. Another example, on the other end of the spectrum, is the oxygen consumption of the kidneys. The kidneys are extremely efficient and only utilize around 8% of the oxygen delivered. This utilization can be decreased to even lower amounts if loop diuretics are given that inhibit $Na^+/K^+/Cl^-$ cotransporter function, which is the largest source of energy utilization in the kidney!

In healthy individuals, $ScvO_2$ and SvO_2 do not differ much. However, in critically ill patients the differences increase. Depending on the body's physiological response to shock or which organ is consuming the most oxygen due to injury, $ScvO_2$ can be 20% different from SvO_2. Therefore, a clear understanding of the sampling location is as important as understanding the significance of the abnormal values and the appropriate treatments. Most clinicians believe that $ScvO_2$ can be used as a trend monitor during resuscitation but not as an actual reflection of SvO_2.

CASE RESUMES

The patient in this case had an $ScvO_2$ result of 52%, which was lower than his SvO_2 measurement. It is possible, that the patient decompensated somewhat with decreased oxygen delivery or increased oxygen consumption following his SvO_2 measurement of 64%. However, it is also possible that a sampling difference occurred. In any event, further investigation may be warranted.

In this case, the lactate level also remained elevated, prompting a liver ultrasound and an echocardiogram. Liver congestion was present, likely due to increased right ventricular dysfunction seen on echocardiogram. The team employed right ventricular support in the form of diuresis and continued inotropic support with dobutamine. Central venous pressures were monitored along with liver function tests. Over the next 24 hours, right ventricular function normalized, lactate decreased to normal values, and the patient was discharged from the ICU on postoperative day 3.

KEY POINTS TO REMEMBER

1. Identifying the oxygen delivery and oxygen consumption balance in critically ill patients allows for thoughtful management.
2. Organ perfusion can be improved by optimizing all components of the oxygen delivery calculation and decreasing oxygen consumption, if indicated.
3. Several tools that aid in this assessment include PAC-derived mixed venous oxygen saturation, central venous line–derived central venous saturation, cardiac ultrasonography, laboratory values such the arterial blood gas, and lactate levels.
4. Hyperlactatemia can be due to anaerobic metabolism, or type A lactic acidosis, or aerobic metabolism, or type B lactic acidosis.

Suggested Reading

1. Suehiro K, Tanaka K, Matsuura T, et al. Discrepancy between superior vena cava oxygen saturation and mixed venous oxygen saturation can predict postoperative complications in cardiac surgery patients. *J Cardiothorac Vasc Anesth*. 2014;28(3):528–533.
2. Vincent JL, Abraham E, Kochanek P, Moore F, Fink M, eds. *Textbook of Critical Care*. 6th ed. Philadelphia, PA: Elsevier Saunders; 2011.
3. Marino, P. *Marino's The ICU Book*. 4th ed. Philadelphia, PA: Wolters Kluwer/Lippincott Williams & Wilkins; 2014.
4. Holm J, Håkanson E, Vánky F, Svedjeholm R. Mixed venous oxygen saturation predicts short- and long-term outcome after coronary artery bypass grafting surgery: a retrospective cohort analysis. *Br J Anaesth*. 2011;107(3):344–350.
5. Rivers E, Nguyen B, Havstad S, et al. Early goal-directed therapy in the treatment of severe sepsis and septic shock. *N Engl J Med*. 2001;345(19):1368–1377.
6. Schuh AM, Leger KJ, Summers C, Uspal NG. Lactic acidosis in a critically ill patient: not always sepsis. *Pediatr Emerg Care*. 2018;34(9):e165–e167.

4 Glycemic Control After Cardiac Surgery

Casey Shelley and Katherine Palmieri

A 63-year-old man with hypertension, hyperlipidemia, and type 2 diabetes mellitus presented with unstable angina refractory to medical management and was subsequently scheduled for 4-vessel coronary artery bypass graft (CABG) surgery. The patient's diabetes was poorly controlled with a preoperative glycosylated hemoglobin (HbA1c) of 10.9%. He had been managed by his primary care physician prior to admission with a single oral hypoglycemic agent. While in the operating room, the patient's initial blood glucose was 231 mg/dL, and a continuous insulin infusion was started prior to initiation of cardiopulmonary bypass. The insulin infusion was continued for the remainder of the surgical procedure. He required a low-dose epinephrine infusion at 0.3 mcg/kg/min for inotropic assistance upon separation from cardiopulmonary bypass. Upon arrival to the intensive care unit (ICU), the insulin infusion was infusing at a rate of 10 units/h. The patient's blood glucose was measured upon arrival to the ICU and found to be elevated at 257 mg/dL.

What do you do now?

DISCUSSION

Acute hyperglycemia is common in the cardiac surgical perioperative period and is reported in as many as 60%–80% of patients. Although many hyperglycemic patients undergoing cardiac surgery carry a preexisting diagnosis of diabetes mellitus, a significant portion will have either undiagnosed diabetes or insulin resistance. According to 2015 estimates from the American Diabetes Association, 7.2 million diabetic patients in the United States are undiagnosed (approximately 24% of the 30.3 million total number of US patients with diabetes) and an additional 84.1 million patients suffer from impaired glucose tolerance. Among cardiac surgery patients, these proportions may be higher, given the known association between hyperglycemia, diabetes, and cardiovascular disease.

Stress Hyperglycemia

The remaining cardiac surgical patients may be non-diabetic but hyperglycemic due to the stress response related to surgery. This "stress hyperglycemia" is generally defined as a transient increase in blood glucose levels that develops during illness in a non-diabetic patient. Stress hyperglycemia has been shown to affect approximately 40%–60% of the surgical population.

Stress hyperglycemia results secondarily to impairments of both glucose production by the liver and glucose utilization by peripheral tissues during and after acute stress of surgery or critical illness. These impairments are mediated by activation of the central nervous system and the hypothalamic–pituitary–adrenal axis, which leads to increased levels of glucose counterregulatory hormones, including cortisol, catecholamines, growth hormone, and glucagon. Pro-inflammatory cytokines including tumor necrosis factor α, interleukin-1, and interleukin-6 are also released and activated. The complex interactions of these hormones and mediators serve to increase glucose production, alter carbohydrate metabolism, inhibit insulin release, diminish glucose uptake by the peripheral tissues, and increase insulin resistance.

The degree to which a patient sustains a significant hyperglycemic stress response is directly related to the type and length of the cardiac surgical procedure. Off-pump cardiac surgery has been shown to decrease the hyperglycemic stress response when compared to procedures requiring cardiopulmonary bypass. Similarly, longer cardiopulmonary bypass times are associated with larger increases in perioperative glucose. Cardiac procedures involving CABG plus valve repair or replacement are associated with perioperative hyperglycemia when compared to isolated procedures. It is unclear if this is due to the longer bypass times commonly associated with CABG plus valvular procedures or may be an unrelated phenomenon.

While stress hyperglycemia is most pronounced on postoperative day 1 and commonly resolves in a matter of days, 30%–60% of affected surgical patients may continue to have impaired glucose tolerance after hospital discharge. A preadmission HbA1c level is helpful in distinguishing patients with stress hyperglycemia from those with undiagnosed diabetes mellitus and thus in guiding postoperative management.

Unfortunately, non-diabetic patients who develop stress hyperglycemia during hospitalization for surgery and/or critical illness actually have been shown to have worse outcomes than their diabetic counterparts. When compared to diabetic patients with adequate glucose control, non-diabetic patients with stress hyperglycemia have a 4-fold increased risk of complications and a 2-fold increased risk of death.

Perioperative Hyperglycemia and Morbidity and Mortality

Postoperative hyperglycemia following cardiac surgery is an independent predictor of morbidity and mortality, regardless of a history of diabetes. The adverse outcomes associated with hyperglycemia in the cardiac surgery patient are directly related to the degree of hyperglycemia as well as the length of time the hyperglycemia persists. However, there is also more recent evidence that patients who have a large variability in blood glucose levels may actually be at the highest risk for perioperative complications. Thus, swings in glucose levels, especially from hyperglycemia to hypoglycemia, may be the most important factor.

The mechanisms by which perioperative hyperglycemia results in worse outcomes are not completely understood. It is known that hyperglycemia has several detrimental downstream molecular effects that greatly alter the homeostatic milieu of the patient (Table 4.1). These disruptions in normal regulatory mechanisms across multiple biological processes are believed to contribute to the reported associations between hyperglycemia and post-cardiac surgical complications.

TABLE 4.1 **Mechanisms and Associations of Perioperative Hyperglycemia Following Cardiac Surgery**

Biomolecular Effects of Hyperglycemia	Reported Complications Associated with Hyperglycemia
Increases inflammatory stress	Deep sternal wound infection
Suppresses the immune system	Poor wound healing
Impairs collagen synthesis important for wound healing	Acute kidney injury and renal failure
Exacerbates ischemia/reperfusion injury	Dysrhythmia
	Heart failure
Increases reactive oxygen	Pericarditis
Endothelial dysfunction (vasoconstriction and vascular inflammation)	Myocardial infarction
	Cerebral vascular accident
Platelet activation	Delirium
Alters free fatty acid metabolism	Prolonged mechanical ventilation

The complications associated with hyperglycemia following cardiac surgery are numerous and severe and include infection, poor wound healing, thrombogenesis as manifested by stroke and myocardial infarction, acute kidney injury and renal failure, cardiac dysrhythmia, pericarditis, heart failure, prolonged mechanical ventilation, and postoperative cognitive dysfunction (Table 4.1). Further, these complications act to increase short- and long-term mortality, length of hospital stay, readmission rates, and hospital costs.

The damaging effects of hyperglycemia in the cardiac surgical patient begin in the operating room. Elevated blood glucose levels during cardiopulmonary bypass are an independent risk factor for morbidity and mortality in all patients regardless of a preoperative history of diabetes. In a retrospective analysis of 409 cardiac surgery patients, Gandhi et al. found that for each 20 mg/dL increase in mean intraoperative glucose levels beyond 100 mg/dL, the risk of adverse events, including death, increased by more than 30%. The risk increased further as mean blood glucose levels rose, with the highest adverse event rate (76%) noted in those patients with a mean blood glucose of 200 mg/dL or more intraoperatively.

Diabetes versus HbA1c and Outcomes

The presence or absence of a diagnosis of diabetes is likely not the most important factor concerning outcomes. Indeed, many studies demonstrate that patients who have been previously diagnosed with diabetes have an increased risk of mortality and major morbidities, such as longer hospital stays, higher readmission rates, and higher rates of stroke, renal failure, and sternal wound infection following cardiac surgery. However, it is theorized that when assessing the risk of perioperative adverse outcomes, the adequacy of preoperative glucose control trumps the diagnosis of diabetes. Poorly controlled diabetes, defined by elevated HbA1c ≥6.5%, in most studies, is associated with an increased risk of early adverse outcome, early mortality, superficial wound infection, and decreased 3- and 5-year survival. Conversely, well-controlled diabetes, defined as HbA1c <6.5%, has been shown to be associated with outcomes on par with those seen in patients without diabetes.

Treatment Guidelines

The Society of Thoracic Surgeons (STS) clinical practice guidelines recommend that diabetic patients undergoing cardiac surgery have a preoperative HbA1c level measured. Patients with elevated HbA1c levels may need further interventions in order to optimize perioperative glycemic management pre-, intra-, and postoperatively. This guideline also recommends that insulin infusions be initiated in the operating room for all diabetic patients to maintain blood glucose levels ≤180 mg/dL for at least 24 hours postoperatively.

Regarding non-diabetic patients, the STS guideline recommends that blood glucose levels also be maintained ≤180 mg/dL, but an insulin infusion is not required if this goal can be achieved with intermittent intravenous insulin rather than a continuous infusion. Finally, the guideline goes on to recommend that all diabetic patients receive disease education prior to discharge and are scheduled for outpatient follow-up and that appropriate communication is made with their primary care physician. A summary of the complete STS recommendations concerning perioperative glucose control is presented in Box 4.1.

STS guidelines notwithstanding, there is currently no solid consensus regarding the optimal perioperative glucose management strategy in the

> **BOX 4.1 Summary of the STS Guidelines Concerning Glycemic Control in the Perioperative Cardiac Surgical Period**
>
> Summary of the STS Clinical Practice Guidelines for Blood Glucose Management During Adult Cardiac Surgery and in the ICU
> Management of perioperative hyperglycemia
>
> - Glycemic control is best achieved with continuous insulin infusions
> - An insulin infusion should be started in the operating room for all diabetic patients and continued for at least 24 h to maintain serum glucose levels ≤180 mg/dL
>
> Preoperative management of diabetic patients
>
> - An HbA1c level should be checked in all diabetic patients and those at risk of hyperglycemia
> - Scheduled insulin should be used to achieve glycemic control for patients awaiting surgery
> - It is reasonable to maintain a blood glucose target of ≤180 mg/dL
> - All doses of oral hypoglycemic agents and insulin should be reviewed on an individual basis prior to surgery
>
> Intraoperative recommendations
>
> - Continue any preoperative intravenous insulin infusion during the intraoperative and postoperative periods to maintain glucose levels ≤180 mg/dL
> - Non-diabetic patients on cardiopulmonary bypass may have glucose levels >180 mg/dL treated with bolus insulin, although a continuous insulin infusion should be started if glucose remains persistently elevated
>
> Postoperative recommendations in the ICU
>
> - Insulin infusions should be initiated for persistently elevated blood glucose levels to maintain glucose levels ≤180 mg/dL for the duration of the ICU stay
> - Patients requiring ≥3 d in the ICU due to mechanical ventilation, intra-aortic balloon pump or left ventricular assist device placement, inotropic support, anti-arrhythmics, or renal replacement therapy should have an insulin infusion to maintain glucose levels ≤150 mg/dL
> - Patients should be transitioned to a subcutaneous insulin schedule before discontinuing insulin infusions

cardiac surgical population, despite numerous studies conducted in an effort to address this issue. Most of these studies conclude that there is little to no difference in complication rates using "intensive" blood glucose management when compared to more "conventional" targets. Intensive glycemic control has been defined as targeting blood glucose levels in the range of 80–120 mg/dL, while conventional glucose targets are in the range of 140–180 mg/dL.

A large, international, randomized trial involving 6104 critically ill patients found that intensive glucose control (81–108 mg/dL target) increased mortality among adults in the ICU. The study was titled "Normoglycemia in Intensive Care Evaluation and Surviving Using Glucose Algorithm Regulation (NICE-SUGAR)" and spanned 42 ICUs throughout the world. This increase in mortality did not differ among surgical versus medical ICU patients. The authors of this trial recommend targeting glucoses levels of <180 mg/dL in the ICU, which is in line with STS guideline recommendations. It remains unclear if the increased mortality in this study was a result of the reduced targeted blood glucose level, the increased administration of insulin, or the occurrence of iatrogenic hypoglycemia.

One of the commonly believed etiologies imparting increased risk of mortality observed in NICE-SUGAR and other large trials is that when utilizing intensive glucose control, patients typically have a higher incidence of hypoglycemic episodes. In the ICU literature, this association remains causal, but it is known that glucose is required for major organ system function. Hypoglycemia leads to decreased "brain fuel" as glucose is the main energy source for the brain. Hypoglycemia is also associated with adverse cardiovascular outcomes, including vascular tone abnormalities and dysrhythmias.

The specific method by which surgeons and intensive care physicians manage perioperative glucose targets following cardiac surgery is generally driven by institution-specific, continuous insulin infusion protocols. There is no clear evidence that any one protocol has benefits over another or that any one protocol is superior. The most effective protocols are thought to be those that include frequent glucose monitoring. Glucose levels should be checked hourly until they stabilize and then every 2–3 hours thereafter. Effective protocols should consider the current infusion rate, the current glucose value, the previously measured glucose value, as well as the rate of

BG 75-99 mg/dL	BG 100-139 mg/dL	BG 140-199 mg/dL	BG ≥ 200 mg/dL	INSTRUCTIONS*
		BG ↑ by > 50 mg/dL/hr	BG ↑	↑ INFUSION by "2Δ"
	BG ↑ by > 25 mg/dL/hr	BG ↑ by 1-50 mg/dL/hr OR BG UNCHANGED	BG UNCHANGED OR BG ↓ by 1-25 mg/dL/hr	↑ INFUSION by "Δ"
BG ↑	BG ↑ by 1-25 mg/dL/hr, BG UNCHANGED, OR BG ↓ by 1-25 mg/dL/hr	BG ↓ by 1-50 mg/dL/hr	BG ↓ by 26-75 mg/dL/hr	NO INFUSION CHANGE
BG UNCHANGED OR BG ↓ by 1-25 mg/dL/hr	BG ↓ by 26-50 mg/dL/hr	BG ↓ by 51-75 mg/dL/hr	BG ↓ by 76-100 mg/dL/hr	↓ INFUSION by "Δ"
BG ↓ by > 25 mg/dL/hr see below†	BG ↓ by > 50 mg/dL/hr	BG ↓ by > 75 mg/dL/hr	BG ↓ by > 100 mg/dL/hr	HOLD x 30 min, then ↓ INFUSION by "2Δ"

†D/C INSULIN INFUSION; √BG q 30 min; when BG ≥ 100 mg/dL, restart infusion @75% of most recent rate.

*CHANGES IN INFUSION RATE ("Δ") are determined by the current rate:

Current Rate (U/hr)	Δ = Rate Change (U/hr)	2Δ = 2X Rate Change (U/hr)
< 3.0	0.5	1
3.0 - 6.0	1	2
6.5 - 9.5	1.5	3
10 - 14.5	2	4
15 - 19.5	3	6
20 - 24.5	4	8
≥ 25	≥ 5	10 (consult MD)

FIGURE 4.1 The Yale Insulin Infusion Protocol is an example of bedside titration for continuous insulin infusion management of perioperative hyperglycemia.

change of glucose level when making rate adjustment recommendations. A commonly utilized protocol for perioperative glucose control in cardiac surgical patients is the Yale Insulin Infusion Protocol, shown in Figure 4.1.

Continuous insulin infusions are preferred over subcutaneous insulin in patients undergoing cardiac surgery. This is due to the fact that the pharmacokinetics of subcutaneous insulin are unreliable in the context of significant fluid shifts, hemodynamic changes, changes in patient temperature, the use of inotropes, and lengthy operative times. Conversely, insulin infusions are reliable and rapidly titratable, resulting in shorter times to achieve glucose goals and lower mean glucose levels than can be obtained with either intermittent intravenous insulin or subcutaneous insulin administration.

Even with institutional protocols and the use of moderate glucose targets, achieving glucose goals may be problematic. In a recently published analysis of data from the STS Adult Cardiac Surgery Database, it was shown that "good" glycemic control (defined as glucose levels of 70–180 mg/dL) was achieved perioperatively in just 15% of patients undergoing CABG. This study also found significant variability in performance by hospital, and while some hospitals were more successful than others, the best were able to maintain just 45.4% of patients in the targeted glucose range within the first 24 hours postoperatively.

CASE RESUMES

The patient was initiated on a protocolized insulin infusion to treat his glucose level of 257 mg/dL. The protocol directed administration of an intravenous insulin bolus of 3 units along with an insulin infusion to start at 3 units/h. You surmise that his increased blood glucose level is a result of his cardiopulmonary bypass time, a significant element of stress hyperglycemia, and his infusion of epinephrine. Epinephrine causes the liver to convert stored glycogen to glucose and release it, raising blood glucose levels.

His blood glucose was subsequently checked hourly, and his epinephrine was weaned slowly. His glucose level remained >200 mg/dL for the next 2 checks, and his insulin infusion was increased appropriately to 6 units/h of insulin. Upon his next check, his blood glucose level was 146 mg/dL, which was within the goal range of 140–180 mg/dL.

The insulin infusion was decreased per the protocol but remained infusing until the patient was hemodynamically stable, off epinephrine, and tolerating oral intake on postoperative day 2. At this time, the patient was transitioned to an insulin regimen consisting of a long-acting insulin analogue, insulin glargine, as basal therapy along with mealtime boluses of the rapid-acting insulin lispro. Due to the short half-life of intravenous insulin, the insulin infusion was not discontinued until 2 hours after the first dose of basal insulin glargine was administered. The patient was also restarted on his preadmission oral antihyperglycemic agent at that time. He received inpatient education on glucose monitoring, medication administration, and nutrition and lifestyle modification. Upon discharge, the patient was scheduled for a follow-up appointment with a consulting endocrinologist, and a letter was sent to his primary care physician regarding the modifications in his diabetes therapy.

> **KEY POINTS TO REMEMBER**
>
> 1. Hyperglycemia after cardiac surgery is mediated via a number of hormones and inflammatory cytokines and leads to an increase in morbidity and mortality, regardless of diabetes status.

2. Current evidence and expert opinion suggest that the most appropriate perioperative blood glucose target is between 140 and 180 mg/dL in the cardiac surgery population.
3. Intensive blood glucose goals are thought to increase the risk of hypoglycemia, which is associated with increased mortality.
4. Protocolized continuous insulin infusions should be initiated early, although there is no evidence that any one protocol is better than another.

Suggested Reading
1. Duggan EW, Carlson K, Umpierrez GE. Perioperative hyperglycemia management: an update. *Anesthesiology*. 2017;126(3):547–560.
2. Galindo RJ, Fayfman M, Umpierrez GE. Perioperative management of hyperglycemia and diabetes in cardiac surgery patients. *Endocrinol Metab Clin North Am*. 2018;47(1):203–222.
3. Gandhi GY, Nuttall GA, Abel MD, et al. Intraoperative hyperglycemia and perioperative outcomes in cardiac surgery patients. *Mayo Clin Proc*. 2005;80:862–866.
4. Lazar HL, McDonnell M, Chipkin SR, et al. The Society of Thoracic Surgeons practice guideline series: blood glucose management during adult cardiac surgery. *Ann Thorac Surg*. 2009;87:663–669.
5. Williams JB, Peterson ED, Albrecht AS, et al. Glycemic control in patients undergoing coronary artery bypass graft surgery: clinical features, predictors and outcomes. *J Crit Care*. 2017;42:328–333.
6. NICE-SUGAR Study Investigators; Finfer S, Chittock DR, Su SY, et al. Hypoglycemia and risk of death in critically ill patients. *N Engl J Med*. 2009;360:1283–1297.

5 Post-Thoracotomy Care

Martin De Ruyter and Laura McKenzie

A 68-year-old male is scheduled for an open thoracotomy due to a recent computerized tomography describing a suspicious left-upper lobe pulmonary lesion. His past medical history is significant for tobacco abuse of 2 packs/d for 40+ years, hypertension, and a prolonged history of opioid use for chronic arthralgias. He is 110 kg and 175 cm on examination with a blood pressure of 145/80, pulse of 84 beats/min, a respiratory rate of 24 breaths/min, and distant breath sounds on auscultation. Preoperatively, he is advised to quit smoking and to continue his antihypertensive medications. He is fearful of postoperative pain and asks you how his pain will be treated.

What do you do now?

DISCUSSION

Providing optimal care for patients undergoing a thoracotomy involves setting short-term and long-term goals. Key short-term goals include separation from mechanical ventilation, effective clearance of pulmonary secretions, early mobilization, and expedient hospital discharge. Post-thoracotomy patients are at higher risk of developing postoperative respiratory complications such as pneumonia because of splinting and weak cough, often associated with inadequate analgesia. These complications can be avoided by effective participation in chest physiotherapy, which includes cough, deep breathing exercises, upper limb and trunk mobility exercises, early mobilization, and chest oscillatory percussion therapy. However, these activities will be hindered in patients with poor pain control. A well-thought-out postoperative surgical plan with milestones, supportive nursing, effective analgesia, and ancillary services is key to achieving these short-term goals (Figure 5.1).

Long-term goals of postoperative care focus on measures to reduce the likelihood of patients developing the protracted pain condition commonly known as "post-thoracotomy pain" syndrome, which may develop in over 50% of these patients. Patients characterize this pain as an "aching" or "burning" along the thoracotomy scar, which is thought to result from intercostal nerve injury from rib resection or retraction. Compared to those with mild pain, patients with moderate to severe postoperative pain are more likely to develop post-thoracotomy syndrome. This observation illustrates the importance of adequate analgesia in the acute perioperative setting.

Currently, options for post-thoracotomy analgesia vary and often include neuraxial/regional techniques, intravenous (IV) or oral (per os [po]) medications including opioids, and/or infiltration with local anesthetic. More recently a collaboration of European and western hemisphere surgeons and anesthesiologists have formed the Procedure Specific Postoperative Pain Management (PROSPECT) project. This group systematically reviews studies that target postoperative analgesia techniques for various surgical procedures, including thoracotomy. The project's goal is to establish evidence-based recommendations for optimal pain management in these procedures.

Day 1
Admission to ICU/Monitored Care Unit
    CXR, Baseline ABG, Examination of chest tubes for proper function
    Assessment of respiratory status
    Pain control
Lung Protective strategies
    Mechanically ventilated patients - follow lung-protective strategies, such as reduced tidal volumes, monitor peak airway pressures, etc. and wean as appropriate Extubated patients - if require additional respiratory support, employ continuous positive airway pressure (CPAP) or other noninvasive positive pressure ventilation techniques
Chest Physiotherapy
    Goal is to start physiotherapy as soon as patient is able to participate: spirometry, deep breathing exercises, maneuvers to clear airway secretions
Early Mobilization
    Goal is to start mobilization as soon as patient is able to participate
    Mobilization can begin as early as 1 hour postoperatively, e.g. sitting, walking, stair climbing, cycling, shoulder and trunk range of motion
Glycemic control
Goal-directed fluid management
DVT prophylaxis
Analgesics
    Continue epidural/paravertebral/ IV PCA if present
    Transition to oral analgesics as able

Day 2
Chest Physiotherapy
    Start or continue physiotherapy as the patient is able to participate: spirometry, deep breathing exercises, maneuvers to clear airway secretions
Mobilization
    Start or continue mobilization as the patient is able to participate: spirometry, deep breathing exercises, maneuvers to clear airway secretions
Nutrition
    Enteral (or parenteral if indicated)
Analgesics
    Continue epidural/paravertebral catheter infusion if present
    Transition to oral analgesics as able

Day 3
    Continue chest physiotherapy and mobilization.
    Care of and removal of chest tubes as indicated
    Removal of epidural/paravertebral after discontinuation of chest tube

FIGURE 5.1 Suggested postoperative treatment pathway in the post-thoracotomy patient. ABG, arterial blood gas; CXR, chest X-ray; DVT, deep vein thrombosis; ICU, intensive care unit; IV, intravenous; PCA, patient-controlled analgesia.

Neuraxial Techniques

Thoracic epidural is an effective modality as the primary method of analgesia in post-thoracotomy patients. A combination of local anesthetics, opioids, and adjuncts including clonidine has been described. Epidural administration of opioids is associated with superior analgesia, less respiratory depression, and decreased respiratory complications in comparison to IV opioids. Preferably, the epidural should be placed preoperatively, used intraoperatively, and continued postoperatively. Epidurals may be associated with sympathectomy, motor weakness, and urinary retention. Placement and management may be complicated by the concurrent administration of perioperative anticoagulation for deep vein thrombosis prophylaxis or other preoperative comorbidities requiring anticoagulation. Unfortunately, epidurals are ineffective at providing analgesia for shoulder pain commonly associated with thoracotomy surgeries.

Other Regional Techniques

Paravertebral blocks provide reliable blockade of multiple intercostal nerves and may be used in a unilateral fashion (Figure 5.2). This block is also amenable to placement of a catheter for continuous analgesia and can serve as an equally efficacious alternative to a thoracic epidural in patients contraindicated for epidural placement. The PROSPECT group favors the paravertebral block with continuous infusion over a thoracic epidural, citing less risk of block failure and overall fewer complications such as epidural hematoma and excessive sympathectomy with resulting hypotension. The same guidelines regarding anticoagulant use in combination with epidural placement and catheter removal exist with paravertebral block.

Intercostal nerve blocks are a well-recognized historical approach and provide excellent thoracic wall analgesia. The intercostal nerves are derived from the ventral rami of T1 to T11. These blocks can be performed intraoperatively by the surgeon while the chest is exposed, or they can be performed percutaneously. Catheters can be placed to provide continuous analgesia, but effectiveness and dislodgement can become issues. Intercostal nerve blockade is effective for port incision and chest tubes/drain sites. Of important note, these blocks are associated with the highest level of

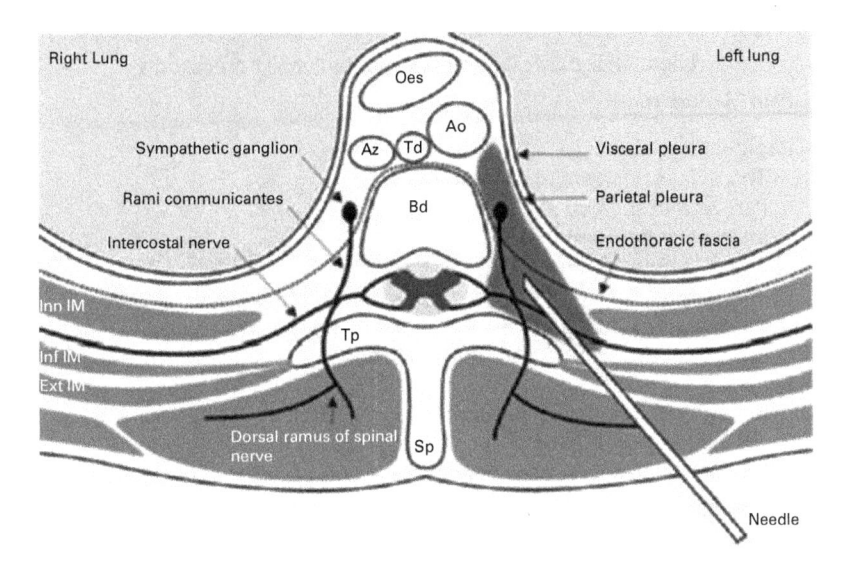

FIGURE 5.2 Schematic representation of the paravertebral space with approaching needle and surrounding vertebral body (Bd), transverse process (Tp), and spinous process (Sp). The aorta (Ao), thoracic duct (Td), azygous vein (Az), and esophagus (Oes) sit anteriorly and the innermost (Inn M), internal (Int M), and external (Ext M) intercostal muscles laterally. The shaded area represents the paravertebral space and likely the extent of spread of anesthesia. The superior costotransverse ligament is out of view but blends laterally with the external and internal intercostal muscle/membrane complex as they attach to the transverse process. Here the paravertebral space merges with the intercostal space.

Used with permission from Cowie B, et al., Ultrasound-guided thoracic paravertebral blockade: a cadaveric study. *Anesth Analg.* 2010;110[6]:1735–1739.

systemic local anesthetic absorption; thus, patients receiving these blocks are more susceptible to local anesthetic toxicity.

The widespread use of ultrasound has created new approaches for analgesic techniques that were either not described or avoided because of technical difficulty and/or risk of adverse events. Serratus anterior blocks were deemed high risk prior to the description of performing these blocks with ultrasound guidance. Recent reviews have repeatedly demonstrated the efficacy of serratus anterior blocks for treating post-thoracotomy pain. Box 5.1 summarizes common interventional analgesic options for acute postoperative thoracotomy pain.

> **BOX 5.1 Local Anesthetic Options for Acute Post-Thoracotomy Pain Management**
>
> Regional techniques
>   Thoracic (preferred) or lumbar epidural
>   Paravertebral block
>   Intercostal nerve block
>   Serratus anterior block
> Other
>   Intrapleural analgesia
>   Intraoperative local anesthetic infiltration
> For shoulder pain
>   Phrenic nerve blocks (intraoperative infiltration or interscalene or stellate ganglion blocks)
>   Intrapleural local anesthetic administration
>   Suprascapular nerve block

Opioids

Opioids provide effective pain control but are associated with several adverse side effects. Particularly in a patient undergoing thoracic surgery, the risk of respiratory depression can be extremely detrimental. IV opioid patient-controlled analgesia (PCA) is designed to decrease the inherent risk of respiratory depression associated with this drug class. Opioids generally are less effective than thoracic epidurals and, thus, are considered supplemental to primary analgesia obtained from regional techniques. Other complications include nausea, constipation, development of tolerance, and potential for abuse/addiction. However, in institutions where regional techniques are of limited availability, opioids remain an easily administered and effective modality of pain control due to shear necessity.

Multimodal Analgesia

Non-opioid adjuncts should be employed when possible. These adjuvants include non-steroidal anti-inflammatory drugs (NSAIDS), acetaminophen, gabapentinoids, ketamine, and several other agents (Table 5.1). These medications are not likely potent enough to be used as sole primary agents but can be used as part of a multimodal approach. The primary benefit of multimodal pain management is the reduction of opioid usage and an

TABLE 5.1 **Common Multimodal Agents for Postoperative Analgesia**

Medication Class	Medication	Common Dosage
NSAIDs	Celecoxib	200 mg BID
	Ketorolac	15 mg q 8 h
	Ibuprofen	800 mg
Acetyl-para-aminophenol	Acetaminophen	1000 mg q 8 h
Gapapentinoids	Gabapentin	300–1200 mg
	Pregabalin	75–150 mg
SNRI	Tramadol	100 mg BID
NMDA antagonists	Ketamine	Bolus: 0.5–1 mg/kg infusion: 0.1–0.25 mg/kg/h
	Dextromethorphan	30–60 mg po BID or TID
	Magnesium	Bolus 30–50 mg/kg
Local anesthetic	Lidocaine*	IV bolus: 1.5 mg/kg Infusion: 2 mg/kg/h
Glucocorticoids	Dexamethasone	4–10 mg
Vitamin C		2–3 g po, 50 mg/kg IV
Alpha-2 agonists	Clonidine	0.5-1 mcg/kg
	Dexmedetomidine	1 mcg/kg bolus ± infusion 0.5 mcg/kg/h

*Be cognizant of dosing if patient is receiving other routes of local anesthetic, such as nerve blocks, infiltration, and epidural infusions.
BID, 2 times per day; NMDA, N-methyl-D-aspartate; SNRI, serotonin–norepinephrine reuptake inhibitor; TID, 3 times per day.

improved safety profile, limiting unwanted opioid side effects. Additionally, these agents can be effective in treating the shoulder pain commonly associated with post-thoracotomy patients.

NSAIDS are effective pain management medications that work by blocking production of prostaglandins and, thus, producing an anti-inflammatory action. This is beneficial in the acute phase of pain as tissue damage from the procedure releases prostaglandins, histamine, and bradykinins. These mediators are the agents of peripheral sensitization to pain. Complications associated with NSAIDS include detrimental effects on the gastrointestinal system, the renal system, and platelet function.

Acetaminophen is available in both oral and IV administrations, and both are effective in reducing postoperative pain scores and opioid consumption in a variety of surgical procedures. The mechanism of action is via inhibition of synthesis of cyclooxygenase and prostaglandins, modulating serotonin pathways and inhibiting inflammatory markers such as histamine, substance P, and neurokinins. While there is yet to be a definitive comparative study of oral acetaminophen versus intravenous acetaminophen in the thoracotomy population, Uvarov and colleagues compared intravenous paracetamol versus rectal paracetamol in post-thoracotomy patients. The authors observed that both routes lead to the reduction of additional analgesics. Of note, non-thoracic procedures, such as orthopedic surgery, have not demonstrated a difference in analgesia when comparing oral versus intravenous acetaminophen.

Gabapentin and pregabalin are presynaptic calcium channel blockers, which are used to treat neuropathic pain. Studies have demonstrated the efficacy of gabapentin when implemented in a multimodal approach. Recently, Matsutani et al. studied the analgesic effects of pregabalin compared to epidurals in a prospective, randomized study of 90 thoracotomy patients. Patients receiving pregabalin reported significantly lower pain scores on postoperative days 1, 3, and 5. Pregabalin-treated patients also required significantly less rescue analgesia on days 1–5. The investigators concluded that pregabalin was superior to thoracic epidural in treating acute post-thoracotomy pain.

While ketamine infusions are becoming increasingly utilized in chronic and refractory pain, ketamine has also been used in post-thoracotomy patients experiencing pain not adequately controlled with thoracic epidurals, regional techniques, opioids, and/or NSAIDS/acetaminophen. Unlike opioids, ketamine does not cause respiratory depression but does have other side effects such as tachycardia, hyper- or hypotension, increased secretions, and delirium. Further studies are needed to stratify which patients will benefit from ketamine therapy.

Ipsilateral shoulder pain is extremely common after thoracotomy. It can impair effective breathing and delay physical therapy and is not relieved by thoracic epidural analgesia. Several mechanisms have been proposed, but a leading hypothesis suggests diaphragmatic irritation as the etiology; and with afferent pain signals traveling via the phrenic nerve (C3–5), this is interpreted by the patient as shoulder pain. Intraoperative infiltration of the phrenic nerve at the level of the diaphragm with local anesthetic is effective and supports this hypothesis, but these effects are short-lived. Interscalene blocks and stellate ganglion blocks (likely via concomitant phrenic nerve block) have shown efficacy, but some patients may not tolerate phrenic nerve paralysis; thus, these approaches may be limited. Suprascapular nerve blocks have been reported as well but are less efficacious than phrenic nerve blocks. In the context that chest tubes may contribute to the ipsilateral shoulder pain, investigators have injected intrapleural bupivacaine with mixed results. Pharmacologic treatment with NSAIDS, such as ketorolac and indomethacin, and acetaminophen have shown efficacy in relieving shoulder pain. Gabapentin has not been shown to be effective in treating this pain.

Additional Techniques

Intrapleural injection of local anesthetic at the seventh intercostal space may block multiple intercostal nerves. However, this approach requires a higher volume of injectate that may be lost via the chest tube. Additionally, distribution of the local anesthetic may be affected by patient position, empyema, fibrosis, or bronchopleural fistula. Local anesthetic infiltration at incisional sites intraoperatively by surgeons has been shown to help decrease somatic pain associated with surgical incision.

Summary

The most efficacious approach to analgesia for post-thoracotomy pain involves the employment of a multimodal approach, which utilizes the strengths of regional techniques in combination with intravenous and oral adjuncts. This multimodal pain management is designed to target the many different afferent pain pathways involved in thoracotomy pain. Techniques such as an epidural, intercostal, paravertebral, or serratus anterior blockade combined with NSAIDS, acetaminophen, opioids, gabapentinoids, and other agents are examples of this multimodal approach. Epidural and paravertebral blocks cover visceral pain and somatic chest wall pain. Intercostal nerve blockade provides analgesia for incisional and chest tube pain. NSAIDS and acetaminophen decrease shoulder pain and peripheral sensitization. Gabapentinoids help reduce the incidence of neuropathically mediated post-thoracotomy syndrome. Opioids serve as supplementary overall analgesia but with untoward side effects.

CASE RESUMES

In response to the patient's question concerning postoperative treatment for pain, he should be advised of several interventions encompassing a multimodal pain management approach with an aim at opioid reduction. These techniques will likely employ an epidural catheter or a paravertebral block and catheter with local analgesic medication infusion prior to surgery. Administration of preoperative oral agents, such as NSAIDS, acetaminophen, and/or gabapentin, should also be discussed. Continuation of the epidural or paravertebral infusion into the postoperative setting will lengthen the analgesic time. Given this patient's chronic exposure to narcotics, perioperative ketamine may be useful. Following surgery, the predefined pain relief goals should be addressed and pain psychology techniques employed as needed.

> **KEY POINTS TO REMEMBER**
>
> 1. Important goals for postoperative pain relief in patients undergoing thoracotomy include prevention of respiratory complications and post-thoracotomy pain syndrome. Both of these goals depend upon effective analgesia.
> 2. The most effective approach to analgesia is a multimodal approach, in which regional techniques are combined with systemic medications of different classes targeting various receptors.
> 3. Epidural analgesia, paravertebral nerve blocks, or serratus anterior blocks are most effective as the primary method of

analgesia. These are supported with the addition of other multimodal agents.
4. Efforts to minimize opioid consumption should be a goal, and IV PCA is the preferred method of administration for opioids.
5. Use of NSAIDS, acetaminophen, gabapentinoids, and ketamine can decrease reliance on opioids; and the use of these agents should be encouraged.

Suggested Reading
1. Uvarov D, Orlov M, Levin A, Sokolov A, Nedashkovskii E. Role of paracetamol in a balanced postoperative analgesia scheme after thoracotomy. *Anesteziol Reanimatol*. 2008;(4):46–49.
2. Matsutani N, Dejima H, Takahashi Y, Kawamura M. Pregabalin reduces post-surgical pain after thoracotomy: a prospective, randomized, controlled trial. *Surg Today*. 2015;45(11):1411–1416.
3. Slinger PD, Campos JH. Anesthesia for thoracic surgery. In: Miller, RD, ed. *Miller's Anesthesia*. 7th ed. Philadelphia, PA: Elsevier; 2015:2000–2004.
4. Pyati S, Lindsay DR, Buchheit T. Acute and chronic post-thoracotomy pain. In: Barbeito A, Shaw AD, Grichnik K, eds. *Thoracic Anesthesia*. New York, NY: McGraw-Hill Education; 2012:467–489.
5. Ökmen K, Ökmen BM. The efficacy of serratus anterior plane block in analgesia for thoracotomy: a retrospective study. *J Anesth*. 2017;31:579–585.

6 Pulmonary Embolism and Postoperative Care

Daniel Haines and Joel Grigsby

A 68-year-old male is brought to the emergency department due to rapidly progressive shortness of air over the past 24 hours. He had an uneventful elective total knee arthroplasty 5 days ago and was discharged home on postoperative day 2. His past medical history includes atrial fibrillation, hypertension, and tobacco use. Home medications include warfarin, atorvastatin, and aspirin daily.

Upon evaluation, he is tachycardic, hypotensive, and desaturating. You prescribe supplemental oxygen and give an intravenous fluid bolus with minimal improvement in his hemodynamics. Norepinephrine is initiated. Computed tomography (CT) angiography reveals a large saddle pulmonary embolus (PE) as well as lobar and segmental arterial occlusions. After a multidisciplinary discussion, the decision was made for emergent surgical pulmonary embolectomy due to unstable hemodynamics and recent surgery with concern for excess bleeding if thrombolytic therapy was attempted.

He now arrives to your intensive care unit (ICU) in cardiogenic shock with metabolic acidosis and ensuing multiorgan dysfunction.

What do you do now?

DISCUSSION

PE is an obstruction of the pulmonary circulation by an occlusive material. Figure 6.1 demonstrates the large saddle embolism described in this case. The material may be thrombus, air, tumor, or fat (Figure 6.2). PE are classified as acute, subacute, or chronic. Acute PE refers to the onset of symptoms immediately after the occlusion occurs. This can often be described very specifically by patients who typically recognize an abrupt change. Subacute refers to progressive dyspnea over days to weeks, which in some, but not all, patients can be accompanied by pleuritic chest pain and hemoptysis. Chronic PE refers to very slow development of symptoms, often over months. Patients who suffer from chronic PE often describe symptoms not specifically from the embolism itself but from the development of pulmonary hypertension and right-sided heart failure.

PE can be further classified into massive and submassive types. Submassive PE is defined as an acute PE without systemic hypotension (systolic blood pressure >90 mm Hg) but with either right ventricular (RV) dysfunction or

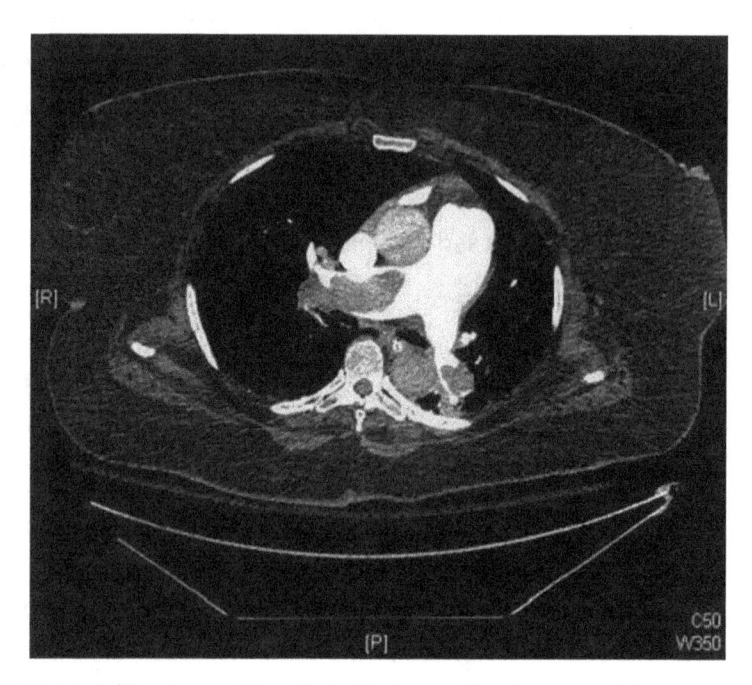

FIGURE 6.1 A CT-angiogram of the patient with a large saddle pulmonary embolus.

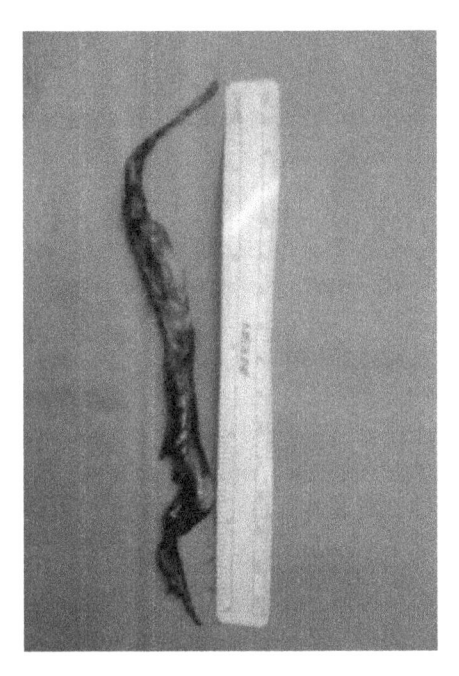

FIGURE 6.2 Large pulmonary embolus retrieved from a main pulmonary artery during surgical embolectomy.

myocardial necrosis. Massive PE is defined as an acute PE with sustained hypotension defined as systolic blood pressure <90 mm Hg for at least 15 minutes or requiring inotropic support, not due to a cause other than PE, such as arrhythmia, hypovolemia, sepsis, left ventricular (LV) dysfunction, pulselessness, or persistent profound bradycardia (heart rate <40 bpm). The patient in this case met criteria for massive PE.

Assessing RV Function in PE

One of the first assessments that should be performed in a patient with a suspected PE is assessment of cardiac function, especially that of the right ventricle. RV dysfunction has been reproducibly found to be indicative of mortality risk in both massive and submassive PE. Perhaps ironically clot burden as seen on CT imaging does not predict adverse prognosis.

Defining RV dysfunction is a clinical exercise involving both qualitative as well as quantitative assessments. Additionally, several biomarkers may aid in defining the degree of RV dysfunction present. Jaff et al. analyzed results from several studies and published a consensus statement for the American Heart Association in 2011. This statement defined RV dysfunction in the setting of acute PE as the presence of at least one of the following:

- RV dilation (apical 4-chamber RV diameter divided by LV diameter >0.9) or RV systolic dysfunction on echocardiography
- RV dilation (4-chamber RV diameter divided by LV diameter >0.9) on CT
- Elevation of brain natriuretic peptide (BNP; >90 pg/mL)
- Elevation of N-terminal pro-BNP (>500 pg/mL)
- Electrocardiographic changes (new complete or incomplete right bundle-branch block, anteroseptal ST elevation or depression, or anteroseptal T-wave inversion)

The definition of myocardial necrosis was based on elevation of troponin I (>0.4 ng/mL) or elevation of troponin T (>0.1 ng/mL).

Since this publication, other parameters of RV functional assessment have been proposed. The assessment of RV function by echocardiography relies on the assessment of size, function, and geometry. Normal RV size is accepted as an RV/LV ratio ≤0.6 in the 4-chamber view. RV dilation is considered with an RV/LV size ratio of ≥0.9–1.0. Exact measurements are often difficult by bedside echocardiography but can be assessed by CT imaging as well. In order to assess function, a fractional area change of the RV during diastole and systole can be calculated from the same view.

Functional assessments of the RV estimated by the "eyeball" technique or with descriptives such as "normal," "mildly depressed," or "severely suppressed" should be avoided as these assessments have been shown to lack reproducibility. Quantitatively, several measurements can be made. Measurement of the tricuspid annular plane systolic excursion (TAPSE) is a quick and reproducible quantitative assessment made in the 4-chamber view (Figure 6.3). A TAPSE of <17 mm is considered to be indicative of RV dysfunction.

Tissue Doppler systolic velocity of the tricuspid annulus is another measure of longitudinal RV systolic performance, similar to TAPSE. This is a reproducible and easily obtainable measure of RV systolic function. A value <9.5 cm/s is associated with RV dysfunction.

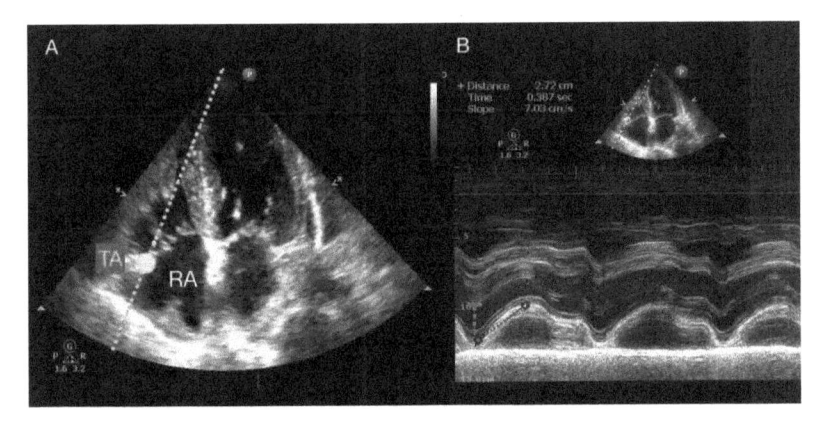

FIGURE 6.3 Apical 4-chamber view obtained via transthoracic echocardiography examination. (A) The tricuspid annulus (TA) and the correct Doppler alignment when obtaining a tricuspid annular plane systolic excursion (TAPSE) measurement. RA = right atrium. (B) M-mode representation of (A). TAPSE is measured from trough to peak within the same heartbeat (yellow dotted line).

Limitations of both TAPSE and S´ include improper Doppler angles and load dependency of the RV when performing these measurements. Additionally, these measurements may not be fully representative of global RV function as they are both measured at the tricuspid annulus.

A more advanced but recommended evaluation of RV function includes RV index of myocardial performance, or the RIMP index. RIMP is measured by tissue Doppler imaging in the same frame as the S´ measurement. A normal value is >0.54. This value represents the relationship between the ejection and non-ejection time of the heart. The "non-ejection" times are the periods when all heart valves are closed. Although RIMP avoids geometric assumptions about the RV, its use is limited by the inability to obtain clear enough Doppler images in order to assess exact contraction and relaxation times.

Finally, geometric assessment of the interventricular septum in the short-axis view will give clues as to the pressure and volume loads of the RV. In a healthy heart, the septum bows toward the RV due to higher pressure in the LV cavity. However, if the septum is flat or bows toward the left ventricle, this is abnormal. Flattening during diastole alone is consistent with volume overload of the RV. Flattening during systole is consistent with pressure overload of the RV. Flattening throughout the cardiac cycle is indicative of pressure and volume overload of the RV. While these changes are often seen in patients with PE, they are not specific for PE as many morbidities may cause the same septal findings.

Another finding oft mentioned in the setting of PE when viewing the heart with ultrasound is McConnell's sign. This refers to the finding of preserved or hyperkinetic apical function with hypokinetic RV basal segments. This is seen in any case of RV failure with preserved LV function as the left coronary artery perfuses the apex of both the left and right ventricles. McConnell's sign carries a sensitivity of 77%, a specificity of 94%, a positive predictive value of 71%, and a negative predictive value of 96%.

Severity Assessment in PE

Several scoring systems have been developed in order to assess severity and risk of mortality in patients with PE. These severity indices are important not only to guide discussions with patients and families but also to determine the best choice of intervention. The Pulmonary Embolism Severity Index (PESI) was developed by Aujesky et al. and is the most validated scoring system commonly used when predicting the prognosis of patients with PE. Since this publication, a simplified PESI score has been published and validated (Table 6.1).

Treatment of PE

Treatment of PE can be diverse and is based on the severity of the case. For a submassive PE, indicating hemodynamic stability, accepted treatment has traditionally been anticoagulation with intravenous unfractionated heparin, low–molecular weight heparin, or direct oral anticoagulants such as factor Xa inhibitors. However, there is evidence that catheter-directed thrombolytic therapy for submassive PE may be advantageous in some cases depending on the position of the PE in the pulmonary vasculature.

Massive PE requires aggressive intervention beyond anticoagulation in order to decrease the risk of mortality. However, first and foremost, stabilization of the patient with a massive PE utilizing vasopressors, inotropes, and/or pulmonary vasodilators in hopes of preventing end-organ damage is needed while further interventions are being planned. The patient in this

TABLE 6.1A Comparison of the Original Pulmonary Embolism Severity Index (PESI) and the Simplified (sPESI) Score

Variable	Score Original PESI	Score sPESI
Age >80 years	+1 per year	1
Male	+10	
History of cancer	+30	1
History of heart failure	+10	1
History of chronic lung disease	+10	
Pulse ≥110 bpm	+20	1
Systolic blood pressure <100 mm Hg	+30	1
Respiratory rate ≥30 bpm	+20	
Temperature <36°C	+20	
Altered mental status	+60	
Arterial oxygen saturation <90%	+20	1

TABLE 6.1B Mortality Risk Associated with the Original PESI Score

Original PESI Score	30-Day Mortality Rate
≤65	0–1.6%
66–85	1.7–3.5%
86–105	3.2–7.1%
106–125	4–11.4%
>125	10–24.5%

TABLE 6.1C Mortality Risk Associated with sPESI Score

sPESI Score	30-Day Mortality Risk
0	1%
≥1	10.9%

case had a massive, acute PE and thus would require treatment beyond systemic anticoagulation.

The 2 types of interventions for massive PE are thrombolysis and surgical embolectomy. Thrombolysis can be further divided into systemic thrombolysis with an intravenous agent or catheter-directed therapies. Systemic thrombolysis may be used for patients who are too critically ill to undergo transition to another location in order to receive an intervention. The most commonly utilized agent for systemic thrombolysis is recombinant tissue plasminogen activator. Obviously, patients will have significant bleeding risk with this therapy if administered systemically. Additionally, the benefits of direct clot thrombolysis are not achieved as fibrinolysis is most effective when delivered directly into the clot. Contraindications to thrombolytic therapy of either variety are recent surgery, history of bleeding dyscrasias, recent history of head trauma, or active bleeding.

Catheter-directed therapy can also attempt removal or fragmentation of the PE, called "mechanical thrombectomy." This technique can be utilized for patients who have a contraindication to thrombolytic therapy. Alternatively, mechanical thrombectomy can also be combined with catheter-directed thrombolytic therapy. Most newer catheters have the capability to remove a clot and to inject thrombolytic therapy directly onto an existing clot that cannot be removed. The most novel catheters utilize powerful jets that can both fragment the clot and then aspirate the clot fragments. These jets can likewise be used to distribute thrombolytic agents into the clot. The goal of mechanical thrombectomy or fragmentation is to decrease afterload on the right ventricle and to allow for systemic perfusion. An additional benefit of clot removal via any mechanism is the potential reduction in the long-term sequelae of chronic thromboembolic pulmonary hypertension.

The most invasive management technique concerning PE is pulmonary embolectomy via open chest surgery. Historically, this was the preferred method in hemodynamically unstable patients. Surgical embolectomy is also warranted for patients who failed thrombolytic therapy and catheter-based approaches. In experienced centers, surgical embolectomy is considered to be a safe procedure with low mortality risk. Some authors believe open chest pulmonary embolectomy provides improved postoperative RV function, decreased pulmonary pressures, and improved long-term outcomes.

Some authors advocate that surgical elimination of a large portion of the clot burden may be the only technique that saves the lives of many patients with PE. These authors advocate that this method should be considered as an initial treatment strategy in patients with massive or submassive PE with a large burden of proximal clot.

Surgical embolectomy requires the use of cardiopulmonary bypass followed by opening of the main pulmonary artery trunk and/or lobar segments to remove thrombus burden. This is done under direct visualization and often results in removing most or all of the thrombus. In some centers, this is followed by gentle attempts at more distal clot retrieval with balloon-tipped catheters passed down multiple segments of each side of the pulmonary tree. Great caution must be used with these attempts as the pulmonary vascular bed is likely very inflamed and friable at this point and excessive attempts can lead to vascular damage and potentially rupture of a pulmonary artery. This is noted by acute, large amounts of blood in the endotracheal tube of the patient. This can be managed by occluding the segmental bronchus from which the bleeding is coming, followed by rapid weaning from cardiopulmonary bypass and reversal of anticoagulation. If this is unsuccessful in terminating bleeding, resection of that portion of the lung may be required.

Postoperative Care

Postoperative management can often be quite challenging and focuses on RV function. RV dysfunction in this clinical scenario is due to the acute rise in pulmonary vascular resistance (PVR) secondary to the vascular occlusion from the large thrombus burden. The right ventricle is a thin-walled, relatively deconditioned chamber that does not respond well to rapid changes in afterload and cannot accommodate appropriately. The decreased function and increased pressure of the right ventricle also lead to increases in central venous pressure, resulting in venous congestion of the liver with resultant coagulopathy. Acute kidney injury can be caused from a low-flow, prerenal state due to decreased cardiac output and venous congestion. There may be a decrease in LV filling due to poor RV ejection, leading to decreased organ perfusion from low cardiac output, resulting in further organ damage, creating a vicious cycle.

In order to reverse this downward spiral or organ dysfunction begetting organ dysfunction, RV function must be restored or temporary mechanical circulatory support utilized. Restoring RV function involves 3 basic areas of focus: decreasing volume overload to regain native RV geometry, improving RV inotropy, and decreasing PVR to decrease RV afterload. Diuretics are generally necessary to achieve these goals. It is not uncommon for patients to diurese several liters after surgical embolectomy and to achieve marked improvement in their hemodynamics while doing so. If renal failure precludes aggressive diuresis, continuous venovenous ultrafiltration may need to be employed for a period of time.

RV function often improves with volume unloading; however, inotropic support is commonly required. Choosing a medication that assists RV contractility while decreasing RV afterload via pulmonary vasodilation is optimal. The 2 agents that provide both of these benefits are milrinone and dobutamine. Milrinone acts as a phosphodiesterase inhibitor with resultant increases in intracellular cyclic adenosine monophosphate (cAMP) levels. cAMP activates receptors for increased contractility and receptors in the pulmonary vasculature that lead to vasodilation. cAMP also acts to cause peripheral vasodilation; thus, unwanted systemic hypotension may be seen. Dobutamine improves RV function through beta-1 receptor stimulation increases in cardiac output and beta-2 receptor stimulation which will lead to pulmonary vasodilation. Beta-2 agonism may also result in systemic hypotension depending on the receptor milieu of the patient.

Milrinone and dobutamine both increase cardiac output from the right and left sides of the heart. Increased LV cardiac output aids in whole-body perfusion and, it is hoped, resolution of organ failure. However, an oft forgotten mechanism of these drugs is the reduction in PVR seen by increased RV cardiac output. Not only do these drugs have direct pulmonary vasodilatory properties but they also lead to a passive decrease in PVR in a similar manner to electrical conduction noted in Ohm's law. The law states that increases in flow in a system result in decreases in resistance.

If systemic hypotension ensues, vasopressin is the vasopressor of choice as its mechanism of action will improve systemic vascular resistance without affecting PVR. Norepinephrine and phenylephrine should be avoided if possible as the alpha-agonism provoked by both of these agents can increase PVR and further worsen RV failure. However, norepinephrine may be necessary and life-saving for hypotension due to its profound potency. Through beta-1 receptors, norepinephrine does increase heart rate, which is beneficial in most patients with RV failure, assuming dysrhythmias are not occurring.

Additionally, epinephrine can be used as a potent inotropic agent that also increases systemic blood pressure. Epinephrine is a direct beta- and alpha-receptor agonist. The alpha-agonism of epinephrine may lead to increases in PVR, but generally the overriding effect of epinephrine is an increase in cardiac output from both the left and the right ventricles. However, there are untoward side effects of epinephrine, such as hypoglycemia, hyperkalemia, and lactatemia, which need to be monitored when administering this agent.

Some centers may routinely initiate inhaled nitric oxide (iNO) on all post-embolectomy patients. iNO is a potent pulmonary vasodilator acting via the cyclic guanosine monophosphate pathway, providing substantial decreases in PVR. iNO does not cause systemic vasodilation due to the fact that it readily binds to and is inactivated by hemoglobin. This inhalational agent may also quell the compulsory ischemia–reperfusion injury in pulmonary vasculature following clot removal. Other inhaled agents include synthetic prostenoids, such as iloprost and epoprostenol, which are also effective in reducing PVR and aiding in the restoration of RV function. These agents exert their beneficial effects via cAMP stimulation. Unlike iNO, these agents do have systemic effects, including hypotension and platelet dysfunction.

Mechanical circulatory support is reserved for patients who cannot liberate from the cardiopulmonary bypass or for those who continue to worsen despite optimizing medical care. This support is often via extracorporeal membrane oxygenation or a temporary RV assist device.

CASE RESUMES

The patient in this case was managed on milrinone and vasopressin following admittance to the ICU. He was continued on a heparin infusion and iNO, which was initiated in the operating room. A furosemide intravenous infusion was initiated with brisk response. On postoperative day 2, his ischemia–reperfusion injury seemed to subside and he had diuresed approximately 6 L since surgery. His iNO followed by his ventilator support were gradually weaned. He was extubated on postoperative day 3. He was transitioned to warfarin for ongoing anticoagulation therapy and discharged home on postoperative day 7.

> **KEY POINTS TO REMEMBER**
>
> 1. Submassive PE is defined as an acute PE without systemic hypotension but with either RV dysfunction or myocardial necrosis. Massive PE is defined as an acute PE with sustained shock.
> 2. There are several strategies for treating PE depending on the stability of the patient and the location of the clot.
> 3. Systemic thrombolysis, catheter-directed thrombolysis, and catheter-directed clot removal are all treatment options, if there are no contraindications. Bleeding risk is the largest contraindication for thrombolytic therapy.
> 4. Surgical embolectomy is warranted for patients with contraindications to or failed catheter-based attempts in patients with ongoing hemodynamic instability.
> 5. RV failure is a serious complication following pulmonary embolectomy and is managed by a compilation of volume removal, inotropic support, pulmonary vasodilation, and mechanical support, if needed.

Suggested Reading
1. Jaff MR, McMurtry MS, Archer SL, et al. Management of massive and submassive pulmonary embolism, iliofemoral deep vein thrombosis, and chronic thromboembolic pulmonary hypertension: a scientific statement from the American Heart Association. *Circulation*. 2011;123:1788–1830.
2. Mitchell C, Rahko P, Blauwet L, et al. Guidelines for performing a comprehensive transthoracic echocardiographic examination in adults: recommendations from the American Society of Echocardiography. *J Am Soc Echocardiogr*. 2019;32(1):1–64.
3. Haddad F, Hunt SA, Rosenthal DN, Murphy DJ. Right ventricular function in cardiovascular disease, part I, II. *Circulation*. 2008;117:1436–1448, 1717–1731.

4. Aujesky D, Obrosky DS, Stone RA, et al. Derivation and validation of a prognostic model for pulmonary embolism. *Am J Respir Crit Care Med*. 2005;172:1041–1046.
5. Jiménez D, Aujesky D, Moores L, et al. Simplification of the pulmonary embolism severity index for prognostication in patients with acute symptomatic pulmonary embolism. *Arch Intern Med*. 2010;170(15):1383–1389.
6. Jolly M, Phillips J. Pulmonary embolism: current role of catheter treatment options and operative thrombectomy. *Surg Clin North Am*. 2018;98:279–292.

7 Respiratory Acidosis in the Intensive Care Unit

Jared Staab

You are called to a rapid response for a 64-year-old male due to altered mental status. He has a history of morbid obesity, systolic heart failure, chronic obstructive pulmonary disease (COPD), obstructive sleep apnea (OSA), anxiety, and chronic pain and was admitted for treatment of endocarditis involving his aortic valve. He is receiving the broad-spectrum antibiotics vancomycin and piperacillin/tazobactam and had just returned from a peripherally inserted central catheter (PICC) placement.

He was administered midazolam and fentanyl during the PICC line placement. He was also placed on supplemental oxygen, which was titrated to a blood oxygen saturation (SpO$_2$) of 100%. You administer flumazenil and naloxone; however, there is no improvement in the patient's mental status. An arterial blood gas (ABG) is notable for the following: pH 7.16, partial pressure of carbon dioxide (PaCO$_2$) 130 mmHg, partial pressure of oxygen (PaO$_2$) 50 mm Hg, bicarbonate 44 mmol/L, and glucose 265 mg/dL.

What do you do now?

DISCUSSION

ABG Interpretation

Interpretation of acid–base abnormalities is an essential skill required when caring for critically ill patients. Normal blood pH is 7.4. By definition, a pH below 7.35 defines acidemia, while pH above 7.45 defines alkalemia. Thus, with a pH of 7.16, the patient in this case has an acidosis. The next step is to determine what is driving the acidosis: a metabolic, respiratory, or mixed process? Table 7.1 demonstrates the 4 types of respiratory and metabolic processes involved in acid–base derangements and the common themes associated with these.

Initial ABG interpretation involves identifying the relationship between pH and $PaCO_2$. In general, patients with respiratory acidosis without compensation tend to have pH and $PaCO_2$ values altered in opposite directions. In a metabolic acidosis without compensation, the pH and $PaCO_2$ typically change in the same direction, assuming the patient is not mechanically ventilated.

Numerically, in an acute primary respiratory acidosis, the pH drops by 0.08 units and the HCO_3^- increases by 1 mEq/L per 10 mm Hg increase in $PaCO_2$ above 40 mm Hg. However, in chronic respiratory acidosis, the pH only drops by 0.03 units and HCO_3^- increases by 3–4 mEq/L per 10 mm Hg increase in $PaCO_2$. These changes are valid if metabolic compensation

TABLE 7.1 **The 4 Types of Respiratory and Metabolic Derangements and Associated Findings**

Acid–Base Disturbance	pH (Normal = 7.4)	$PaCO_2$ (normal 40 mm Hg)	Compensation
Metabolic acidosis	↓	↓	Respiratory
Respiratory acidosis	↓	↑	Renal
Metabolic alkalosis	↑	↑	Respiratory
Respiratory alkalosis	↑	↓	Renal

has not occurred. Thus, by performing these simple calculations, it can be determined if the respiratory acidosis is solely responsible for the derangement in pH or if another process is concomitantly occurring.

Renal compensation of respiratory acidosis, via HCO_3^- retention in the proximal tubules, generally peaks by 4 days. However, this attempt at normalizing pH to 7.4 is never complete; that is, the pH is never normalized with compensation. Furthermore, if the HCO_3^- is greater than 30 mmol/L, there is likely a second process such as chronic respiratory acidosis or a concomitant metabolic alkalosis occurring.

Using these equations for acute respiratory acidosis, we could expect the pH to be 6.68 if the $PaCO_2$ is 130 mm Hg (130 mm Hg is 9-fold greater than 40 mm Hg and then 0.08 × 9 = 0.72 and 7.4 – 0.72 = 6.68). In a chronic respiratory acidosis, the pH would be expected to be 7.13 (0.03 × 9 = 0.27 and 7.4 – 0.27 = 7.13).

However, the bicarbonate of 44 mmol/L in this case is higher than expected if plugged into the above equation for chronic respiratory acidosis (9 × 4 = 36 mmol/L expected HCO_3^-). Given that the measured bicarbonate of 44 mmol/L is higher than expected, we can assume that there is a secondary metabolic alkalosis. The secondary process is the body's attempt at compensation for a chronic respiratory acidosis. Past medical histories of COPD and OSA typically contribute to a chronic respiratory acidosis. Figure 7.1 displays a nomogram of expected changes in $PaCO_2$, pH, and HCO_3^- as acidosis and/or alkalosis progresses.

Assessment of Respiratory Acidosis

The differential causes of respiratory acidosis include central nervous system (CNS) depression, upper and lower airway obstruction, and hypermetabolic states with increased production of CO_2 such as malignant hyperthermia and thyroid storm. This patient has CNS depression due to administration of pain and anxiety medications to facilitate the PICC placement in conjunction with preexisting OSA and COPD. These morbidities left him with decreased tolerance to sedatives that may not cause respiratory insufficiency in most patients. Narcotics and benzodiazepines at high doses are potent respiratory depressants and have an additive effect when administered concomitantly. When combined, their individual respiratory depressant effects act synergistically to augment the respiratory depression.

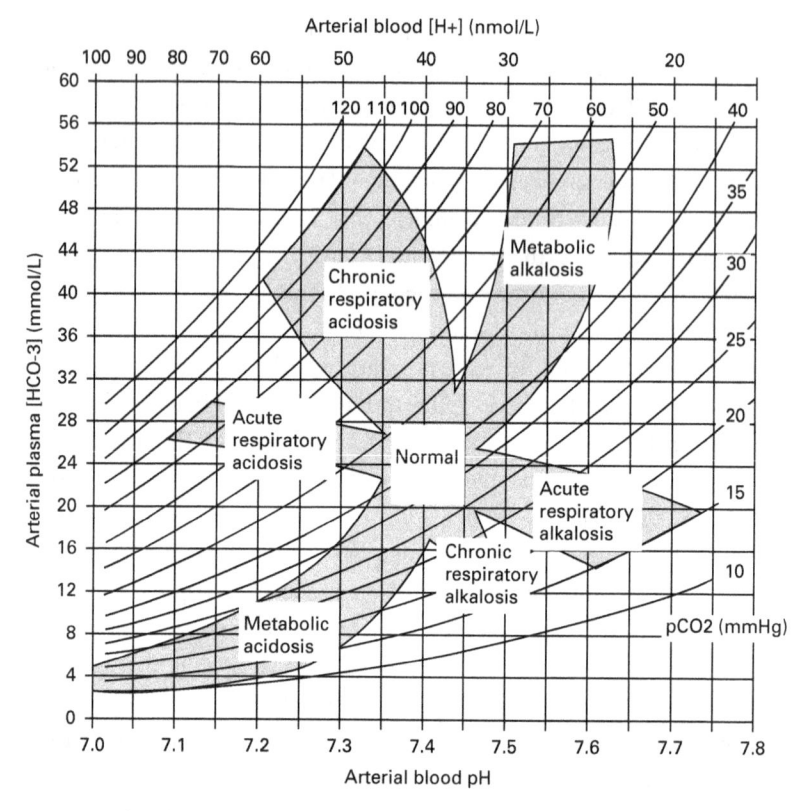

FIGURE 7.1 An acid–base nomogram for human plasma, showing the effects on the plasma pH when PaCO$_2$ (pCO$_2$, curved lines) HCO$_3^-$ occur in excess or are deficient in the plasma.
Reprinted from public domain.

A history of chronic pain syndromes, especially those treated with opiate medications, should be ascertained. It is reasonable and potentially life-saving to administer naloxone in these scenarios. If benzodiazepines have recently been administered, flumazenil intravenously should be considered.

Care should be taken with administration of these medications as unwanted side effects may occur. Naloxone is an opioid antagonist acting at the mu receptor and is administered via the intravenous, mucosal, or intramuscular route. Naloxone results in a relatively rapid reversal of opiate-induced sedation. Naloxone has a relatively short half-life compared with longer-acting opiates. Close observation and repeat administration may be required to avoid re-sedation. Large doses of naloxone can lead to tachycardia, hypertension, flash pulmonary edema, and myocardial infarction.

Flumazenil is a benzodiazepine antagonist at the gamma-aminobutyric acid (GABA) receptor. It has a short onset, allowing for rapid reversal of benzodiazepine-induced decreases in level of consciousness. Much like naloxone, the half-life may be shorter than that of the offending benzodiazepine, necessitating close observation. Flumazenil can cause serious and life-threatening seizures, especially at higher dosages.

The mechanism of respiratory depression from narcotics and benzodiazepines includes activation of the mu and GABA receptors, respectively. These medications lead to a shift of the $PaCO_2$ response curve to the right, requiring much higher $PaCO_2$ levels at the respiratory center to trigger an increase in minute ventilation (Figure 7.2). Ventilation is normally under involuntary control and relies on complex interactions of central and peripheral chemoreceptors, ventral and dorsal respiratory groups in the medulla, and apneustic and pneumotaxic centers in the pons.

CO_2 is primarily carried in the blood in the form of bicarbonate. Other forms of CO_2 include carboxyhemoglobin and dissolved CO_2. A decrease in pH caused by elevated hydrogen ion is sensed centrally in the cerebrospinal fluid and typically results in increased minute ventilation. Similarly,

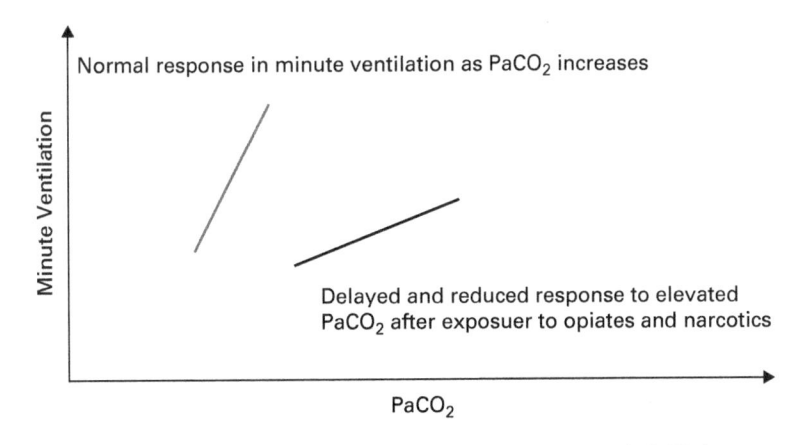

FIGURE 7.2 Graph comparing the normal response (blue line) to elevations in $PaCO_2$ in comparison to the response after exposure to opiates and narcotics (red line). The increase in minute ventilation is blunted and delayed in patients after opiate and benzodiazepine administration.

peripheral chemoreceptors, such as in the aorta, are sensitive to changes in PaO_2 and can stimulate ventilation when hypoxia is sensed. This mechanism is a potent stimulant of ventilation when the PaO_2 is less than 60 mm Hg. Figure 7.2 depicts the blunting effects on these innate mechanisms when CNS depressants are administered.

Notably, there are many causes of acutely altered mental status. With careful attention to the patient's history and physical examination, the differential diagnoses can usually be narrowed. The differential of acute mental status change includes infection, metabolic abnormalities, structural abnormalities, medications, toxins, seizure, stroke, and arrhythmia. An ABG analysis is extremely helpful in identifying the cause of altered mental status, especially if sodium, potassium, glucose, hematocrit, and lactate levels can be included. The workup must take place simultaneously with efforts to protect the patient from further harm. The patient's oxygen perfusion and hemodynamics must be ensured to be adequate. Airway protection needs to be assessed and maintained. Advanced cardiac life support should ensue if these goals cannot be met. Further testing includes a chest X-ray, complete blood count with differential, and complete blood chemistry.

Hypoxia in Respiratory Acidosis

Some authors would advocate not titrating SpO_2 to 100% in patients with COPD. Theoretically explained and clinically observed is the development of hypercarbia in these patients when "excessive" oxygen is administered. Though commonly blamed on a "blunted hypoxic respiratory drive," the more likely mechanism is related to V:Q (ventilation:perfusion) mismatching.

In disease states such as COPD, the lung architecture is disrupted, resulting in inefficient alveolar capillary interface. Hypoxic vasoconstriction is a normal response to low levels of oxygen in the lungs. This response causes blood to be shunted away from areas of poor oxygenation to areas with adequate oxygenation. Therefore, the delivery of excessive oxygen inhibits hypoxic vasoconstriction, resulting in the flow of pulmonary blood to areas of the lung which are less efficient at removing $PaCO_2$ in patients with COPD, leading to hypercarbia.

The differential for hypoxia includes V:Q mismatch as described, shunt, apnea, low inspired fraction of inspired oxygen (FiO_2), and diffusion abnormalities. The treatment for hypoxic and hypercarbic respiratory failure involves reversing the offending agents if applicable, treatment of the underlying cause, and mechanical ventilation.

Mechanical Ventilation in Respiratory Acidosis

The 2 commonly used strategies for mechanical ventilation are non-invasive ventilation with a mask and endotracheal intubation. Contraindications to non-invasive ventilation include inability to tolerate tight mask fit due to claustrophobia or anxiety, poor mask fit due to face shape or facial hair, nausea, vomiting, and full stomach with inadequate airway protection. Much of the intended airway pressure will be received by the stomach, leading to the risk of aspiration with non-invasive ventilation. If endotracheal intubation is deemed necessary to adequately treat severe respiratory acidosis, certain pitfalls should be recognized and avoided.

Caution must be taken when sedating for endotracheal intubation in patients with known to have or to be at risk of right ventricular dysfunction. In patients with respiratory acidosis requiring intubation, there are several risk factors that will precipitate right ventricular failure. Hypercarbia, acidosis, and hypoxia will increase pulmonary vascular resistance, creating increased afterload for the right ventricle. Patients with COPD and OSA are at increased risk of type III pulmonary hypertension, which implies that there is preexisting right ventricular strain. Right ventricular depression can also be caused by many of the anesthetic induction agents required for intubation. The addition of positive pressure ventilation will likewise increase right ventricular afterload. All of these factors can lead to right ventricular failure in and of themselves but, when occurring all at once, create an additive scenario for acute right ventricular failure and hemodynamic collapse.

Fortunately, patients with hypercarbia and CO_2 narcosis are somewhat anesthetized and may require less sedation. However, unless comatose, all patients will require some sedation to place the endotracheal tube, and most will need sedation to tolerate mechanical ventilation. Selection of a sedation strategy is important to increase chances of liberation from mechanical ventilation and to mitigate the risk of intensive care unit (ICU) delirium. Many strategies can be used, including but not limited to sedative hypnotics such as benzodiazepines, narcotics, propofol, ketamine, and dexmedetomidine.

Benzodiazepines are currently utilized less frequently out of concern for increased risk of ICU delirium. Although narcotics can increase the risk for delirium, inadequate pain control is also a risk factor for delirium. Dexmedetomidine is an intravenous alpha-2 agonist that offers the ability to provide sedation, anxiolysis, and pain control while minimizing respiratory depression. Sedation should be titrated with daily awakening and spontaneous breathing trials as these have been shown to allow for faster liberation from mechanical ventilation.

Mechanical Ventilation Management

The selection of ventilation strategy is dependent on numerous patient factors. Clinicians must set respiratory rate, tidal volume, positive end-expiratory pressure (PEEP), inspiratory flow, FiO_2, mode (volume versus pressure control), and the amount of assistance per breath. All need to be tailored toward each patient's specific goals. Initial ventilator settings for a patient with hypoxic and hypercarbic respiratory acidosis should focus on adequate delivery of oxygen and need for a minute ventilation high enough to reverse the hypercarbia.

Minute ventilation is determined by respiratory rate and tidal volume. Typically, initial respiratory rates are 12–20 breaths per minute, with tidal volumes of 6–8 mL/kg of ideal body weight and PEEP of 5 cmH_2O. FiO_2 is titrated to achieve PaO_2 >65 mm Hg or SpO_2 >92%, but these targets can be decreased for patients with chronic respiratory insufficiency. As for mode, volume-driven breaths provide a set tidal volume at constant flow, which may be uncomfortable and result in higher pressures and/or barotrauma. Pressure control delivers a pressure-limited breath with decelerating flow. This may help to avoid lung injury. However, in pressure control, tidal volume is dependent on compliance, and reliable tidal volumes may not be achieved on a consistent basis.

Auto-flow volume-controlled ventilation incorporates the benefits of both pressure-controlled ventilation with volume-controlled ventilation. This is a volume mode guaranteeing tidal volume but delivers each breath with a decelerating flow pattern. Auto-flow automatically regulates inspiratory flow and pressure on a breath-by-breath basis. In patients with poor lung compliance, this mode may provide benefit.

Airway Pressures

In patients with severe acidosis, there may be the temptation to hyperventilate in order to treat the hypercarbia and hypoxia as quickly as possible. This can be deleterious as high tidal volumes may lead to ventilator-induced lung injury (VILI) due to volutrauma, cytotrauma, and barotrauma.

Overzealous mechanical ventilation can also lead to increased intrathoracic pressures. This increased pressure will lead to decreased venous return to the heart. Increased intrathoracic pressures also exert pressure on the pulmonary vasculature and the right ventricle, potentially leading to hypotension. Of note, increases in pulmonary arterial pressures will also reduce pulmonary vascular blood flow. This in turn will increase dead space ventilation. Hypotension in the setting of increased airway pressures is exacerbated by hypovolemia, which may be a goal in patients in respiratory failure and right ventricular failure. The ultimate intention is to safely ventilate the patient with minimal hemodynamic perturbations.

Plateau pressure is the static pressure applied to the small airways and the alveoli during positive pressure ventilation. Plateau pressure can be measured by performing an end-expiratory pause maneuver on the ventilator. Assuming the absence of elevated intra-abdominal pressures and a non-compliant thoracic cavity, the presence of elevated plateau pressures represents a risk for VILI. In the presence of elevated peak inspiratory pressures with normal plateau pressures, the patient, the ventilator, and the endotracheal tube should be examined to rule out kinking of tubing or constriction of large airways.

Elevated airway pressures should always be investigated. Peak pressures are a measure of dynamic airway flow. Peak airway pressures in a patient with an endotracheal tube are partially determined by airway resistance of the ventilator tubing, the endotracheal tube, and the trachea. The goal is for laminar flow in these airway conduits; however, this is largely determined by the luminal radius of each. As the radius decreases, flows tend to be more turbulent, leading to higher peak airway pressures.

Elevated peak inspiratory pressures should be avoided or treated expeditiously. Breath stacking or auto-PEEP would present with elevated peak airway pressures. The risk of auto-PEEP is especially high in patients with COPD who may have intrinsically elevated PEEP or auto-PEEP occurring. Intrinsic PEEP can be measured by an end-expiratory pause maneuver on the ventilator. Increasing extrinsic PEEP applied by the ventilator to greater than 50% of the intrinsic PEEP can act as a stent, allowing the small airways to remain open, thus increasing exhalation. High minute ventilation combined with intrinsic PEEP can lead to a situation whereby the patient does not have adequate time to exhale before the next breath is delivered by the ventilator. Examination of the ventilator flow waveform would identify this, as seen in Figure 7.3.

In order to correct auto-PEEP, one could adjust the minute ventilation or adjust the inhalation:exhalation ratio, or the I:E ratio. When adjusting the I:E ratio, it is important to recognize that the largest determinants of expiration time are respiratory rate and flow rate. Increasing the respiratory rate lowers the overall expiratory time. To counteract this, one could increase the flow rate, which will decrease the inspiratory time, thus effectively increasing the time spent in expiration per breath.

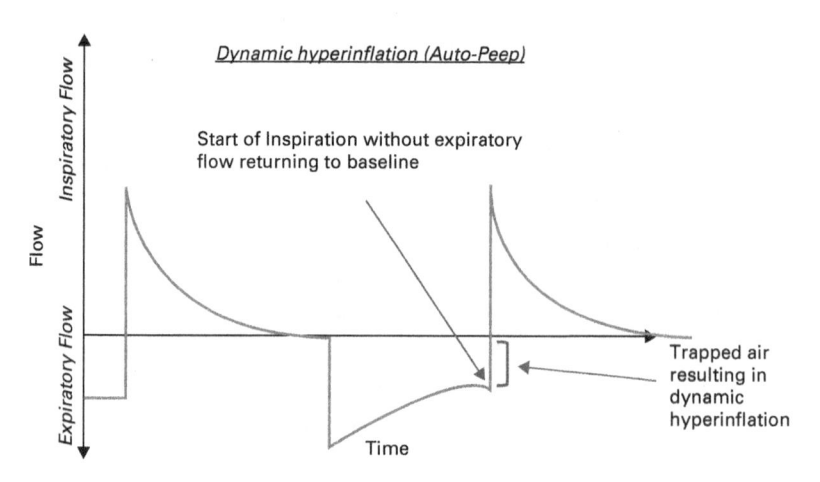

FIGURE 7.3 The ventilator waveforms depicting the phenomenon of auto-PEEP.

In clinical scenarios, auto-PEEP typically presents with increased peak airway pressures on the ventilator and, possibly, acute and complete failure of ventilation followed by sudden hypotension. The treatment in this case is to disconnect the ventilator tubing from the patient's endotracheal tube to allow for exhalation. Following this maneuver, the ventilator settings should be adjusted to avoid ongoing problems with auto-PEEP.

Other sources of increased airway pressures in patients on a ventilator include pneumothorax, bronchospasm, mainstem intubation, and kinked tubing. Rapid assessment involves physical examination of the patient with chest auscultation first and foremost. This should be performed while checking for endotracheal tube, ventilator tubing, or ventilator problems. These assessments can be followed by chest X-ray and chest ultrasonography examination, if the diagnosis remains elusive. Ultrasound examination can rule out pneumothorax with the presence of A-lines (horizontal reverberation artifacts) and lung sliding along the juxtaposed pleura. Notably, these findings only rule out pneumothorax at the level assessed.

Finally, ventilatory dysynchrony can lead to elevated peak pressures, patient discomfort, and auto-PEEP. Ensuring adequate sedation is necessary to decrease the deleterious "fighting" of the ventilator.

CASE RESUMES

Overnight the patient's level of consciousness continues to improve with associated decreases in $PaCO_2$. After several ventilator adjustments for elevated peak airway pressures, the ventilator parameters could be weaned. The next morning's ABG resulted as 7.34/64/90/46. After decreasing sedation and placing the patient on a spontaneous breathing trial, the patient is still requiring some positive pressure assistance. Since patients with COPD have been shown to benefit from early liberation from mechanical ventilation and extubation directly to non-invasive ventilation, you attempt this strategy. As such, the patient is extubated to non-invasive ventilation. The following day, he can tolerate nasal cannula oxygen delivery. He continues on aggressive pulmonary hygiene and intermittent nebulizer therapies. He is transferred to the wards and is initiated on a narcotic-sparing pain regimen, stressing the utilization of multimodal analgesia to avoid oversedation and somnolence.

KEY POINTS TO REMEMBER

1. Knowledge regarding interpretation and management of acid–base disorders is crucial for the appropriate care of the critically ill.
2. The differential etiology for respiratory acidosis includes CNS depression, upper and lower airway obstruction, and hypermetabolic states with increased production of CO_2, such as malignant hyperthermia and thyroid storm.
3. Plateau and peak pressures need to be assessed in all patients requiring mechanical ventilation with appropriate treatments initiated for elevations.
4. Auto-PEEP can be avoided by increasing expiratory time, which can be accomplished by decreasing the respiratory rate, increasing the flow rate, increasing sedation to reduce ventilator dysynchrony, and titrating extrinsic PEEP to 50% of intrinsic PEEP.
5. Patients with respiratory failure resulting from COPD benefit from non-invasive ventilation or early extubation to non-invasive ventilation when feasible.

Suggested Reading
1. Rzasa Lynn R, Galinkin JL. Naloxone dosage for opioid reversal: current evidence and clinical implications. *Ther Adv Drug Saf*. 2017;9(1):63–88.
2. An H, Godwin J. Flumazenil in benzodiazepine overdose. *CMAJ*. 2016;188(17–18):E537.
3. Mirza S, Clay RD, Koslow MA, Scanlon PD. COPD guidelines: a review of the 2018 GOLD report. *Mayo Clinic Proc*. 2018;93(10):1488–1502.
4. Nava S, Hill N. Non-invasive ventilation in acute respiratory failure. *Lancet*. 2009;374(9685):250–259.
5. Kaufman DA. Interpretation of ABGs. American Thoracic Society. Accessed March 2, 2019. www.thoracic.org/professionals/clinical-education/abgs.php.

8 Metabolic Acidosis in the Cardiothoracic Intensive Care Unit

Paul D. Weyker and Christopher Webb

A 50-year-old woman is admitted from home for combined heart–kidney transplantation secondary to non-ischemic cardiomyopathy end-stage renal disease. She is taken to the operating room with plans of performing the heart transplant followed by the renal transplant. Continuous venovenous hemodialysis (CVVHD) was initiated intraoperatively. After the cardiac graft is in place, infusions of milrinone 0.25 mcg/kg/min and epinephrine 0.03 mcg/kg/min are initiated. Due to poor graft function, the epinephrine infusion is increased to 0.1 mcg/kg/min.

Because of her hemodynamic instability, the patient is transferred to the intensive care unit (ICU) prior to performing the renal transplant. Shortly after arrival in the ICU, her arterial blood gas results were pH 7.22, partial pressure of carbon dioxide ($PaCO_2$) 44 mm Hg, partial pressure of oxygen 308 mm Hg, HCO_3^- 16.7 mmol/L, lactate 9.1 mmol/L. The surgical team wants the patient optimized with decreased pressor requirements and a normalized lactate level prior to returning to the operating room for the kidney transplant.

What do you do now?

DISCUSSION

Metabolic acidosis is a pathologic process that results in increased hydrogen ion concentration and/or decreased bicarbonate ion concentration. Acidemia is defined by a pH <7.35 and occurs when the body's natural acid/base homeostatic mechanisms are unable to compensate appropriately to the underlying cause of acidification. There are generally thought to be 3 different mechanisms that lead to the development of metabolic acidosis: increased hydrogen ion production, loss of bicarbonate, and decreased hydrogen ion excretion. Table 8.1 identifies the causes of metabolic acidosis grouped by these 3 mechanisms.

The general approach in evaluating a patient with a suspected metabolic acidosis involves obtaining a detailed history and physical exam, paying particular attention to the patient's spontaneous respiratory rate, vital signs, peripheral pulses, perfusion, and mental status. Key laboratory values include serum electrolytes, serum albumin, corrected anion gap, arterial pH, $PaCO_2$, and arterial lactate. Table 8.2 identifies several laboratory and

TABLE 8.1 **Three Mechanisms That Lead to Metabolic Acidosis and the Association with Anion Gap Presence**

Etiology of Acidosis	High Anion Gap	Normal Anion Gap
Increased H+	Lactic acidosis (types A and B), ketoacidosis ingestion/poisoning (methanol, glycols, aspirin, etc)	
Decreased HCO_3^-		Intestinal loss carbonic anhydrase inhibitors anatomical (ureteral diversion) type 2 RTA (proximal tubule)
Decreased H+ clearance	Uremic acidosis	CKD with preserved GFR type 1 RTA (distal tubule), type 4 RTA (hypoaldosteronism)

CKD, chronic kidney disease; GFR, glomerular filtration rate; RTA, renal tubular acidosis.

TABLE 8.2 **Suggested Laboratory Studies and Diagnostic Workup of Metabolic Acidosis Depending on the Anion Gap**

High Anion Gap	Normal Anion Gap	Diagnostic workup
Arterial blood gas	Arterial blood gas	Echocardiography
Serum lactate	Serum chemistry: potassium, creatinine, bicarbonate	Mixed venous oxygen saturation
Serum ketones	Urinalysis: electrolytes, osmolality, pH, BUN, glucose, fractional excretion of HCO_3^-	
Serum chemistry: creatinine chloride, bicarbonate		
Serum osmolality		
Urinalysis: ketones, organic acids, microscopy		

BUN, blood urea nitrogen.

diagnostic markers that need to be checked in order to elucidate the type of acid–base disturbance present.

Collectively, these values will assist in determining whether or not the metabolic acidosis is an isolated event or if it is part of a mixed acid–base disturbance. A mixed acid–base disturbance in metabolic acidosis would be a case in which respiratory acidosis or respiratory alkalosis is combined with a metabolic problem.

Acid–Base Equations

Henderson-Hasselbach Equation

The body has numerous compensatory mechanisms for managing metabolic derangements to maintain a homeostatic pH of 7.4. The Henderson-Hasselbalch equation calculates the pH of a system if the concentrations of acids and bases are known. This equation can be written in terms of bicarbonate as the base, $PaCO_2$ is the acid and pK_a is the dissociation constant of the acid or, in this case, $PaCO_2$, which is 6.1:

$$pH = pKa + \log_{10}([base]/[acid])$$

$$pH = 6.1 + \log_{10}([HCO_3^-]/[CO_2])$$

Winter's Formula

Winter's formula is used to predict the $PaCO_2$ which should result if there is appropriate respiratory compensation for a metabolic acidosis. The pH will be determined by the ratio of CO_2 to HCO_3^-. The initial mechanism for mitigating a metabolic acidosis is a compensatory hyperventilatory response. This increase in respirations begins within the first 30 minutes of a metabolic acidosis and persists for up to 24 hours or until the patient becomes fatigued. The hyperventilatory response leads to an initial decrease in the $PaCO_2$, which will decrease pH. Thus, it is an attempt to mitigate the acidemia associated with a metabolic acidosis. In general, a linear relationship exists between $PaCO_2$ and the serum HCO_3^- concentration and can be expressed using Winter's formula:

$$\text{Expected } PaCO_2 = 1.5(\text{measured } HCO_3^-) + 8 + 2$$

With this formula, the anticipated change in $PaCO_2$ can be calculated in order to determine if the respiratory response is an appropriate compensation for the metabolic acidosis. A $PaCO_2$ greater than expected would suggest a secondary respiratory acidosis, which can be seen in non-ventilated patients with significant underlying respiratory disease. Conversely, a $PaCO_2$ lower than expected would indicate a secondary respiratory alkalosis.

Further complicating matters, studies have demonstrated that a paradoxical renal excretion of HCO_3^- may occur. While the exact mechanism is unknown, it is thought that this paradoxical response is due to the increased minute ventilation leading to hypocapnea. While this is more commonly seen in chronic metabolic acidosis, it can occur in the acute setting and result in worsening acidemia that is independent from the primary cause of the initial metabolic acidosis.

Anion Gap

The serum anion gap analysis is one of the first steps in the diagnostic process for patients presenting with a metabolic acidosis. With a primary respiratory acidosis disturbance, the body's compensation is to renally excrete acids versus reabsorbing or producing bicarbonate. The anion gap equation calculates the unmeasured charged particles, which are a surrogate for the acids that the kidney did not excrete. By calculating the anion gap, one can narrow down the potential etiology of the metabolic acidosis. The anion gap can be calculated by:

$$\text{Anion gap} = (Na^+ + K^+) - (Cl^- + HCO_3^-)$$

Stated in words, the anion gap is the difference between the unmeasured cations and the unmeasured anions, such as albumin, phosphates, sulfates, urates, lactate, calcium, and magnesium. In general, the most common causes of an elevated anion gap metabolic acidosis in the ICU are lactic acidosis, ketoacidosis, and uremic acidosis, while the most common cause of a normal anion gap metabolic acidosis is a hyperchloremic metabolic acidosis (Table 8.1).

Normally, anion gap values range from 3 to 10 mEq/L, but they may vary based on the laboratory. For critically ill patients or patients with chronic diseases that affect the anion gap, baseline and serial measurements will provide a more accurate clinical picture. The anion gap should be corrected based on the patient's albumin and phosphate.

Hypoalbuminemia may underestimate the anion gap since albumin is a negatively charged protein and its loss from the serum results in the retention of other negatively charged ions, such as chloride and bicarbonate. Hyperphosphatemia may overestimate the anion gap by generating acidic compounds that neutralize bicarbonate. Additionally, a marked presence of cations in the blood as would occur with hypermagnesemia and hypercalcemia can lower the anion gap.

Another useful tool to help diagnose the underlying metabolic derangement is calculation of the ratio of the delta anion gap to delta HCO_3^-. In critically ill patients, multiple compensatory and pathologic processes are occurring at the same time, such that the delta anion gap to delta HCO_3^- ratio may not be 1:1, as is seen with an isolated high–anion gap metabolic acidosis. A delta anion gap to delta HCO_3^- ratio <1 can be seen in patients with a secondary normal anion gap metabolic acidosis, a high–anion gap acidosis with preserved renal function (e.g., D-lactic acidosis occurring in patients with short bowel syndrome), or a renal tubular acidosis with preserved renal function. A delta anion gap to delta HCO_3^- ratio of 1–2 can be seen in patients with a secondary metabolic alkalosis, a secondary chronic respiratory acidosis, or a high–anion gap metabolic acidosis with impaired renal function. Lastly, a delta anion gap to delta HCO_3^- ratio >2 suggests a primary high–anion gap metabolic acidosis and a secondary metabolic alkalosis or chronic respiratory acidosis.

Lactic Acidosis

Lactic acidosis represents one of the commonest types of metabolic acidosis present in cardiothoracic ICU patients. It is commonly classified as either type A or type B lactic acidosis. Type A lactic acidosis is associated with decreased perfusion and oxygen delivery to tissues. This can occur with global hypotension, profound anemia, or severe hypoxemia. Type B lactic acidosis is generally not associated with impaired oxygen delivery but is associated with either increased production or impaired metabolism of lactate. This can occur in severe liver dysfunction, in mitochondrial disorders, and with beta-adrenergic use.

Beta-adrenergic agonist medications such as intravenous epinephrine and inhaled agents such as albuterol and salmeterol can cause elevated lactate levels through an increase in metabolism. This hypermetabolic state produced by beta-agonist medications overwhelms pyruvate dehydrogenase and thus shunts the extra pyruvate to lactic acid production through the Cori cycle. Patients who have malignancy with high cellular turnover are similarly in a hypermetabolic state, and type B lactic acidosis may occur. In a similar yet unrelated mechanism, thiamine deficiency leads to type B lactic acidosis since pyruvate dehydrogenase is dependent upon thiamine for proper functioning. Table 8.3 lists common differential diagnoses for elevated lactate in the post-cardiac surgical patient.

TABLE 8.3 **Potential Causes and Pathophysiology of Hyperlactatemia Following Cardiac Surgery**

Etiology	Pathophysiology
Impaired oxygen delivery during CPB	Tissue hypoxia
Decreased cardiac output	Tissue hypoxia
Anemia	Tissue hypoxia
SIRS	Tissue hypoxia, accelerated glycolysis

Medications/Fluid:
  epinephrine, isoproterenol
  sodium nitroprusside
  propofol syndrome
  lactate buffered renal replacement
  lactated Ringer's
	Accelerated glycolysis
	Tissue hypoxia
	Type B lactic acidosis
	Type B lactic acidosis
	Type B lactic acidosis

Organ/limb ischemia (hepatic, mesenteric, limb)	Tissue hypoxia, reduced hepatic clearance
Septic shock	Tissue hypoxia, accelerated glycolysis
Seizures	Accelerated glycolysis
Renal failure	Decreased clearance

CPB, cardiopulmonary bypass; SIRS, inflammatory response syndrome.

Assessment of Metabolic Acidosis

Metabolic acidosis following cardiac surgery can have several detrimental effects in critically ill patients. Acidosis results in myocardial depression, which will limit cardiac output and oxygen delivery. Acidosis also leads to arterial vasodilation and resultant hypotension. Importantly, decreased pH and increases in $PaCO_2$ are independent potent pulmonary vasoconstrictors. Pulmonary vasoconstriction leads to increased right ventricular afterload, to which the right ventricle may not be accustomed. Ensuing right ventricular dysfunction can lead to more profound debt of oxygen delivery and further acidosis. Lastly, severe acidosis is associated with decreased vascular responsiveness to catecholamine medications such as norepinephrine.

Alternatively, the pressor effect of vasopressin is generally thought to be independent of pH and may be quite useful in these situations.

Determining the underlying cause of metabolic acidosis in the ICU is imperative in order to guide appropriate therapies. Following heart transplantation, lactic acidosis is well documented and typically clears in the next several hours. ICU patients with normal liver function and without a hypermetabolic state will have lactate clearance in the next several hours after adequate oxygen delivery is restored. It is expected that lactate clearance will be followed by normalization of the acid–base status, unless other processes are occurring.

However, if acidosis does not resolve and lactate levels continue to increase, intensivists must never lose sight of more catastrophic causes of lactic acidosis in ICU patients. Lactic acidosis resulting from myocardial dysfunction, hypovolemia, mesenteric ischemia, and cardiac tamponade should remain in the differential diagnosis. There should be a low threshold of performing echocardiography to assess for cardiac function and to rule out tamponade. Chest tube output should be monitored closely for signs of ongoing blood loss and hemorrhagic shock as the cause of metabolic acidosis. Serial physical examinations should always be followed and may be the first indication of embolic phenomena either to a limb or to the mesentery. The extremities are important to examine for temperature and coloration in order to assess the adequacy of oxygen delivery.

The balance of the oxygen delivery and oxygen consumption of the patient can be ascertained via information collected from a pulmonary artery catheter. Data obtained from a pulmonary artery catheter are valuable in assessing not only cardiac function but also filling pressures of both sides of the heart. Numeric data along with waveform analysis should be examined dutifully by providers skilled in these assessments. Trending cardiac indices obtained from thermodilution measurements as well as mixed venous oxygen saturation drawn directly from the pulmonary artery are both extremely helpful in guiding therapies in the setting of acidosis. These data can be used in conjunction and are complementary to echocardiographic cardiac imaging and serial physical examinations.

Treatment of Metabolic Acidosis

Widely debated in the critical care literature is the threshold at which to treat acidosis with bicarbonate. Many experts recommend treatment of severe acidosis, defined as a pH <7.2, with sodium bicarbonate. This is especially advantageous in patients with acute kidney injury who do not have the compensatory mechanisms to retain bicarbonate effectively.

However, use of bicarbonate to treat metabolic acidosis is controversial in patients without renal dysfunction. Firstly, exogenously infused bicarbonate will be metabolized to carbon dioxide ($HCO_3^- + H^+ \rightarrow CO_2 + H_2O$), which is indeed an acid. Of most importance, carbon dioxide must be excreted from the body via respiration. In extubated patients, this increased work of breathing may not be sustainable and may lead to fatigue and further deoxia due to increased oxygen consumption in critically ill patients. In patients who are receiving mechanical ventilation, frequent monitoring of arterial blood gas should be undertaken and minute ventilation increased accordingly.

A theoretical risk to administering exogenous bicarbonate is the potential for a paradoxical increase in intracellular acidosis. Following bicarbonate infusion, there will be an increase in CO_2 which rapidly diffuses into the cell. Once inside the cell, carbon dioxide increases the acidotic milieu. This is compared to the slower transport of HCO_3^-, resulting in the preponderance of intracellular acid compared to base.

Severe acidemia may necessitate dialysis for acid clearance. Acidotic patients on dialysis effectively receive a bicarbonate infusion through the dialysate. However, in severe acidosis, the amount of bicarbonate in the dialysate may not be adequate, and patients may require peripheral bicarbonate infusions complementing the dialysate. Of note, dialysis is poor at clearing lactic acid due to the large size of the molecule. While dialysis filter size can be adjusted in attempts at increasing the potential for lactic acid clearance, the expectation of dialysis is not to remove the lactic acid molecule. Identification and correction of the source of lactic acid production, or in some cases the lack of clearance of lactic acid, are necessary in order to adequately treat lactic acidosis.

CASE RESUMES

The metabolic acidosis for our patient started developing intraoperatively and was multifactorial in nature. The calculated anion gap, corrected for albumin for this patient, was elevated. This anion gap is most likely due to the elevation in lactate. In this case the patient was mechanically ventilated, was given fluid resuscitation and electrolyte treatments, and was on CVVHD. Therefore, calculation of the delta anion gap to delta HCO_3^- ratio is less helpful.

The patient's hematocrit had a nadir of 18%, suggesting that there may have been a component of impaired oxygen carrying capacity. When the cross-clamp was released, the myocardial function was initially reduced, requiring milrinone and epinephrine infusions. With up-titration of the epinephrine infusion, the myocardial function improved to normal and the patient was able to successfully separate from bypass.

However, while necessary for inotropy, epinephrine is associated with elevated lactate production via a beta-2 agonism mechanism in this case. Given the patient's end-stage renal disease, normal acid secretion and bicarbonate production from the kidneys were impaired; thus, her renal disease also contributed to her lactic acidosis. Even with CVVHD in place, flow rates, filter size, and a dialysate bath may need to be optimized in order to effectively clear acid when it is being rapidly produced in a dynamic state, such as in conjunction with cardiopulmonary bypass and receipt of a heart transplant.

Over the next 24 hours, the patient received modest fluid resuscitation and inotropic support optimization in the ICU while remaining on CVVHD. Her right ventricular function was closely monitored for signs of right ventricular pressure and volume overload in the newly transplanted heart, which has a propensity for right ventricular dysfunction due to the nature of the transplantation surgery. Her lactic acidosis improved, as displayed in Figure 8.1. During this time her epinephrine infusion was decreased to off, and she remained on milrinone for inotropic support. The following day, her lactate level was 2.3 mmol/L, and she was taken back to the operating room for her kidney transplant.

Lactate Values in the ICU

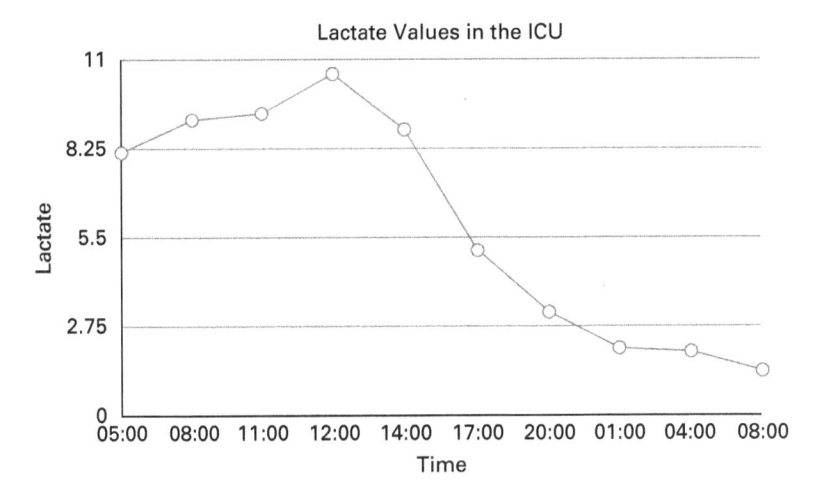

[Graph showing lactate values on y-axis (0, 2.75, 5.5, 8.25, 11) versus time on x-axis (05:00, 08:00, 11:00, 12:00, 14:00, 17:00, 20:00, 01:00, 04:00, 08:00)]

FIGURE 8.1 Lactate values trended over time. Three mechanisms that lead to metabolic acidosis and the association with anion gap presence.

KEY POINTS TO REMEMBER

1. Metabolic acidosis is caused by increased hydrogen ion production, decreased bicarbonate production, or reduced hydrogen ion clearance.
2. Lactic acidosis is common after cardiopulmonary bypass and is typically cleared, assuming adequate oxygen delivery to tissues, no impairment to liver clearance, and no hypermetabolic process is in place.
3. Epinephrine induces type B lactic acid production via a beta-2 receptor–mediated mechanism, resulting secondarily in overwhelming the glycolysis pathway.
4. Understanding Winter's formula and the serum anion gap calculation is necessary when assessing the etiology of metabolic acidosis.
5. Treatment with bicarbonate is controversial but generally warranted if pH <7.2, especially in patients with renal impairment.

Suggested Reading
1. Glasmacher SA, Stones W. Anion gap as a prognostic tool for risk stratification in critically ill patients—a systematic review and meta-analysis. *BMC Anesthesiol.* 2016;16(1):68.
2. Jansen TC, van Bommel J, Schoonderbeeke FJ, et al., Early lactate-guided therapy in intensive care unit patients: a multicenter, open-label, randomized controlled trial. *Am J Respir Crit Care Med.* 2010;182(6):752–761.
3. Pierce NF, Fedson DS, Brigham KL, Mitra RC, Sack RB, Mondal A. The ventilatory response to acute base deficit in humans. Time course during development and correction of metabolic acidosis. *Ann Intern Med.* 1970;72(5):633–640.
4. Silva JM Jr, de Oliveira AMRR, Nogueira FAM, et al. Metabolic acidosis assessment in high-risk surgeries: prognostic importance. *Anesth Analg.* 2016;123(5):1163–1171.
5. Jaber S, Paugam C, Futier E, et al. Sodium bicarbonate therapy for patients with severe metabolic acidaemia in the intensive care unit (BICAR-ICU): a multicentre, open-label, randomised controlled, phase 3 trial. *Lancet.* 2018;392(10141):31–40.

9 Rhabdomyolysis Due to Extracorporeal Membrane Oxygenation

Candice Metzinger and Aaron LacKamp

A 55-year-old woman with myocarditis and cardiogenic shock is emergently cannulated for venoarterial extracorporeal membrane oxygenation (ECMO) with percutaneous femoral access using 25Fr arterial and venous cannulae. She also received support from an intra-aortic balloon pump (IABP), for left ventricular unloading. She was limited in other advanced options by the presence of a left ventricular apical mural thrombus. She developed pulmonary edema and acute kidney failure with limited response to diuretics.

Distal pulses below the cannulation site diminished until they were no longer palpable, nor could they be obtained by Doppler assessment. The patient's urine is now cola-colored. Serum creatine phosphokinase (CK) is checked and found to be is 23,000 U/L.

What do you do now?

DISCUSSION

The patient's physical exam changes in the limb distal to the ECMO cannulation site are concerning (Figure 9.1). Lack of pulses in the affected limb is likely due to decreased or absent blood flow. There are several potential etiologies of limb ischemia during ECMO, and the cause may be multifactorial (Box 9.1). It is likely that the limb ischemia has caused rhabdomyolysis as evidenced by the dark urine and the markedly elevated CK level. The increased CK level in conjunction with the limb swelling raises the concern that muscle breakdown may have resulted in compartment syndrome, which further compounds the injury. Rhabdomyolysis and ischemic muscle injury may result in renal failure, loss of limb, and even death due to hyperkalemia and acidosis. The first step is to identify the cause of the muscle injury.

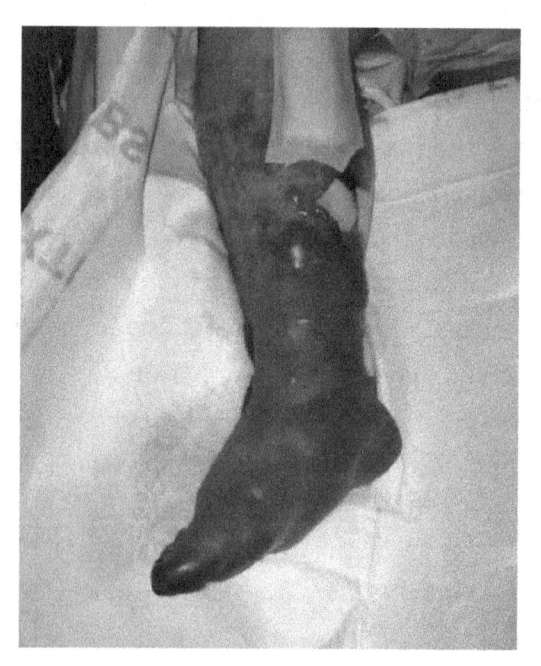

FIGURE 9.1 Image of a leg with ischemic changes secondary to hyperemia. Note the swelling and erythema leading to fasciotomy in order to avoid compartment syndrome.

> BOX 9.1 **Potential Risk Factors for Limb Ischemia with ECMO**
>
> Potential Risk Factor
>
> Peripheral arterial disease*
> Large-bore cannula
> Ischemia–reperfusion injury
> Arterial emboli
> Younger age
> Vasopressor use
> History of diabetes
> Pulmonary disease
> Lack of perfusion cannula
>
> *Of these, only peripheral arterial disease has been shown to statistically correlate with peripheral limb ischemia.

ECMO Cannulation Strategies

The sheer size of ECMO arterial cannulae can cause decreased blood flow distal to the cannula, especially in patients with small-caliber arteries. Small-caliber arteries may be due to female gender or history of peripheral arterial disease. Decreased blood flow may also be a manifestation of the technique used to cannulate the artery. Knowledge of the type of cannulation access is required in order to ascertain if ischemia is likely due to the cannulation technique and to evaluate strategies to revise or replace the cannulation site.

There are various techniques used to acquire femoral arterial cannulation for ECMO which alter the risk of peripheral ischemia. Transcutaneous femoral arterial cannulation or femoral arterial cut-down are the commonest methods of peripheral ECMO access.

The cut-down procedure also utilizes the Seldinger technique but with a surgical incision allowing for complete exposure and visualization of the femoral vessels. The advantage of the cut-down procedure is not only direct visualization but also the ability to place arterial clamps and to stop blood flow during the procedure. Additionally, during an open procedure, the cannula can be tunneled under the skin away, to exit at a convenient site. This tunneling may aid in stabilizing the cannula in case the patient should move the leg. Another advantage is the possibility of placing a small bypass cannula in the superficial femoral artery or posterior tibial artery to perfuse the leg. This would decrease the risk of distal ischemia with a large cannula to artery size ratio.

Alternatively, a vascular graft may be attached to the femoral artery in an end-to-side anastomotic manner, with the direct connection to the ECMO cannula through a connector on the graft. The goal of an end-to-side graft is to allow perfusion without obstructing arterial flow distally. An additional technique utilized to ensure adequate distal perfusion and to prevent hyperperfusion of the limb when using an end-to-side graft is the placement of a "purse-string" suture. This suture is placed around the femoral artery below the graft in order to allow for restriction or increases in distal flow as necessary by simply adjusting the tightness of the suture at the bedside.

If revision attempts at the femoral site are unable to be adequately adjusted, axillary cannulation can also be performed and the outflow cannula placed at this site with removal of the femoral cannula. However, axillary cannulation has a higher rate of bleeding complications than femoral access, and it may be difficult to apply compression due to the location below the clavicle.

Another much more invasive strategy is to replace peripheral cannulation with central cannulation. This requires a sternotomy and open chest surgery. Central cannulation will have fewer regional blood flow problems due to the large caliber of the central vessels and can provide the highest flows. Unfortunately, central cannulation may carry a higher risk of systemic events including embolic events, air embolism, or inadvertent central decannulation.

Ischemia–Reperfusion Injury

Another potential source of peripheral ischemic injury is ischemia due to reperfusion, or ischemia–reperfusion injury. Ischemia–reperfusion injury occurs after a limb, or other part of the body, is without adequate perfusion for a period of time. This can occur in an ECMO patient when blood flow to a limb is stagnant due to low cardiac output or during the ECMO cannulation procedure itself. When ECMO is flowing adequately, a relatively large amount of blood is perfused into the limb.

The mechanism behind this phenomenon is due to anoxia-induced inflammatory mediators and reactive oxygen species formed during anaerobic times. Furthermore, and likely most detrimental, the reinstituted perfusion will bring white blood cells and oxygen to these sites of injury, instigating further inflammatory responses that release interleukins and more free radicals, leading to cellular protein and DNA damage. This type of injury is often associated with microvascular injury, leading to increases in capillary permeability and reactive edema.

Arterial Emboli

This risk of embolic phenomena is greatest while artificial devices remain in arteries, such as IABP catheters and ECMO cannulae. Arterial emboli create occlusion of arterial blood flow due to embolic particles traversing the arterial blood system and eventually lodging in an arterial space. This creates tissue, organ, and/or limb ischemia. The risk of arterial emboli formation in patients with ECMO or IABP is greatly reduced with systemic anticoagulation. However, in many patients, life-threatening bleeding occurs, and cessation of the anticoagulation is necessary until hemostasis can be achieved.

A Doppler ultrasound study should be obtained to evaluate arterial emboli. If an arterial embolism is identified, therapeutic options include open surgical clot removal or minimally invasive over-wire thrombus retrieval procedures, often performed by interventional radiologists. With either open or minimally invasive techniques, finding and removing a clot is often unsuccessful due to the nature of migrating emboli, especially with mechanical support in process.

Rhabdomyolysis

Rhabdomyolysis results from the breakdown of skeletal muscle tissue with the release of toxic substances into the bloodstream. Tea- or cola-colored urine is often the first sign of rhabdomyolysis and often precedes laboratory findings. If suspected, urine myoglobin should be checked, which will provide supportive evidence in the early stages. Eventually, hyperkalemia to the point of cardiac dysrhythmia and severe acidosis will occur if untreated. Other electrolyte abnormalities, lactic acidosis, and an elevation in CK will soon ensue following the muscle injury.

Rhabdomyolysis can have many causes in critically ill patients (Table 9.1). In all patients, identifying all potential contributing factors will aid in most rapidly correcting the problem and preventing kidney injury.

TABLE 9.1 **Other Causes of Rhabdomyolysis in Critically Ill Patients**

Cause	Signs	Treatment
HMG-CoA reductase inhibition	Muscle pain, most commonly lower extremity; elevated CK	Switch statin, reduce dose, or discontinue medication
Immobility for prolonged periods	Patients often "found down" due to catastrophic event	Electrolyte and acidosis correction, renal replacement if needed
Obesity	Pallor, swelling, pain, coolness after procedure or with restrictive immobilization	Electrolyte and acidosis correction, renal replacement if needed
Seizures	Witnessed seizure and/or EEG	Anti-seizure medications
Peripheral arterial disease/emboli	Claudication pain, numbness, weakness, pallor, pain	Anti-platelet therapy, surgical clot removal, and/or arterial bypass
Autoimmune disorder: dermatomyositis polymyositis	Often associated with rheumatologic disease; presents with weakness in multiple muscle groups	Steroids, physical therapy
Metabolic myopathies	Often congenital; exacerbations often present with weakness, lab abnormalities	Replacement of necessary metabolites and supportive care
Neuroleptic malignant syndrome	Exposure to dopamine inhibitor (butyrophenones, phenothiazines, atypical antipsychotics); associated with fever, tea-colored urine, hyperdynamic state	Stop offending agent; supportive therapy for fever, hyperdynamics; dantrolene, amantadine, benzodiazepines

TABLE 9.1 **Continued**

Cause	Signs	Treatment
Hyperthermia	Fever, rigidity, tea-colored urine	Stop any offending agents, treat infection, cooling
Medications: ketamine, succinylcholine, propofol	Use of these medications; tea-colored urine, lactic acidosis with propofol infusion syndrome	Stop offending agent; fluid resuscitation
Infections	Coexisting influenza A and B; coxsackie, Epstein-Barr; human immunodeficiency virus; legionella viruses; *Salmonella*, *Streptococcus*, and *Staphylococcus* bacteremia	Supportive treatment and administration of antiviral or antimicrobial medications
Diabetic ketoacidosis	Increased anion gap acidosis, hyperglycemia, urine and serum ketones	Insulin, fluids, potassium replacement, and frequent lab monitoring
Endocrine disorders	Hypoaldosteronism, hypothyroidism supported by history and laboratory results	Correction of metabolic derangement
Electrolyte imbalances	Hypokalemia, hypophosphatemia, hypocalcemia, hypo-/hypernatremia, hyperosmotic states seen on laboratory results	Correction of electrolyte derangement(s)
Genetic defects	Impairment of glycolysis or glycogenolysis, G6PDH deficiency	Genetic testing along with correction of metabolic derangement

EEG, electroencephalogram; G6PDH, glucose-6-phosphate dehydrogenase; HMG-CoA, 3-hydroxy-3-methyl-glutaryl-coenzyme A.

A common etiology of rhabdomyolysis in patients who may not be critically ill is use of 3-hydroxy-3-methyl-glutaryl-coenzyme A reductase inhibitors, known as "statin therapy." Patients may have markedly elevated CK, especially if the statin therapy is continued in the face of acute renal failure. These medications should be switched to a less offensive statin, decreased in dose, or discontinued.

Immobility is a common cause of CK elevation but usually causes a modest elevation in CK. Rhabdomyolysis can occur in patients who are "found down" after indeterminate periods of time or after sustaining cardiac arrest or seizures. Seizures may independently elevate CK due to muscle overuse. In fact, CK alone may be used to help identify subclinical seizures. Obesity can predispose patients to rhabdomyolysis. Severe muscle breakdown can be seen after relatively brief periods of immobility, such as during an operation with very obese patients. Immobility causing elevations in CK can be seen in intensive care unit patients who cannot be readily mobilized or who have contraindications to mobilization such as tenuous groin cannulations. Indeed, it is difficult to mobilize a patient on ECMO or other mechanical circulatory support devices, patients who require substantial assistance, and patients who are neurologically injured. However, attempts at mobilization, even with passive range-of-motion exercises, should be employed.

Other considerations listed in Table 9.1 include myositis due to rheumatologic disease or viral illness, metabolic myopathies, neuroleptic malignant syndrome, hyperthermia, stimulant toxicity, diabetic ketoacidosis, hyperosmolar coma, endocrine disorders, or infections within the muscle.

With any large peripheral cannulation, attention to color, pulse presence, temperature, limb circumference, and presence of pain need to be evaluated on an hourly basis at times. Of note, pain is a late finding in ischemic limbs. Girth of extremities with large-bore cannulae should be measured regularly even if compartment syndrome is not suspected. Measurements should be documented at the same exact location by tracing the tape measure with a marker in order to assess acute changes in circumference regularly. These findings should be documented, and if changes occur, further investigation is warranted.

Monitoring Rhabdomyolysis

CK is the most important laboratory measure of rhabdomyolysis and can be used for the diagnosis. The diagnosis of rhabdomyolysis has been defined as a CK level 5-fold higher than normal values. The CK level can also be useful for risk stratification and in determining treatment. Elevations in CK less than 5000 U/L are much less likely to be associated with acute kidney injury, whereas CK levels above 20 000–30 000 U/L have markedly increased risk of kidney injury. The CK level often peaks 24–48 hours after the insult. This may help to predict the time of the injury and anticipate the course of recovery. Treatment is continued until the CK level has nearly normalized.

Myoglobin levels are less useful than CK for directing treatment as most treatment protocols have been developed to follow CK. Furthermore, detectable myoglobin elevations may be present in asymptomatic persons. Nonetheless, myoglobin is extremely injurious to renal function by binding and precipitating with Tamm-Horsfall proteins. These precipitates lead to renal tubular obstruction and injury. This precipitation occurs more readily in the setting of acidosis, which is routinely present in rhabdomyolysis. Alkalization of the urine reduces this precipitation and is one of the justifications for use of bicarbonate infusions when treating rhabdomyolysis. Some protocols suggest titrating bicarbonate infusions to a urine pH >8 in order to quell renal injury from these precipitates.

Treatment of Rhabdomyolysis

Prevention of acute kidney failure is a major treatment goal. Kidney failure increases the mortality rate with rhabdomyolysis from 15% to >50%. The majority of deaths due to rhabdomyolysis are a result of uncontrolled hyperkalemia and acidosis due to renal failure. The foundation of treatment to avoid this is hydration. Intravenous fluid therapy is the only treatment that is indisputably beneficial for rhabdomyolysis. Hydration is started early and continued aggressively unless contraindicated.

The largest source of clinical information concerning the treatment of rhabdomyolysis comes from the trauma literature, especially after crush injuries. This literature dictates that it may be reasonable to titrate fluid therapy to achieve urine output in excess of 200 mL/h or 2–3 mL/kg/h. However, in patients with cardiovascular disease and devices, this may lead to negative hemodynamic consequences. Echocardiography should be used routinely to evaluate fluid resuscitation in patients on venoarterial ECMO.

The choice of intravenous fluid is less important than the replacement of the fluid deficit. Fluid replacement can be in the form of isotonic resuscitative fluid, such as normal saline, lactated Ringer's solution, plasmalyte, or an isotonic sodium bicarbonate infusion. Early case series and reports described the use of hypotonic fluids. However, the emphasis has changed to resuscitative fluids with the recognition that rhabdomyolysis patients will be hypovolemic. Normal saline may be favored in cases where hyperkalemia becomes a concern early in order to avoid excess potassium administration. However, normal saline may actually compound the metabolic acidosis of renal failure by administering a large chloride (154 mmol/L) load and creating hyperchloremic metabolic acidosis. Patients with rhabdomyolysis are likely already acidotic due to hyperkalemia creating hydrogen ion shifts.

On the other hand, lactated Ringer's solution contains nearly the same amount of chloride as human plasma at 109 mmol/L. Likely due to this distinction, lactated Ringer's has been shown to improve outcomes in this setting. Both lactated Ringer's solution and normal saline are acidic fluids with pH 6.5 and 5, respectively. Plasmalyte is an isotonic solution that has the benefit of having a neutral pH. However, plasmalyte contains more potassium at 5 mmol/L than lactated Ringer's solution at 4 mol/L. Despite the choice of fluid for resuscitation, the important concept is to initiate fluid therapy soon and expeditiously. Laboratory values should be monitored and corrected to near normal values throughout fluid resuscitation.

Conventional treatment of rhabdomyolysis also includes forced diuresis. The osmotic diuretic mannitol has been utilized in this regard. When mannitol is utilized, it is recommended to administer 1–2 g/kg/d as an infusion or in divided doses in order to encourage diuresis. Goal urine output of 200 mL/h may already be achieved with fluid therapy alone without the use of osmotic diuresis, thus obviating the need for mannitol. Care should be taken to avoid inducing hypovolemia due to overzealous mannitol-induced diuresis. Adverse sequelae of mannitol include hypotension and pulmonary edema. Loop diuretics to aid diuresis are typically avoided in the setting of rhabdomyolysis because these may cause unwanted acidification of the urine. Loop diuretics may be used specifically to address hyperkalemia or hypervolemia.

Many clinicians routinely administer a sodium bicarbonate infusion at 50–500 mL/h while replacing fluid deficits with isotonic fluid administration. As stated earlier, alkalinization of the urine may help prevent precipitation of Tamm-Horsfall myoglobin complexes in the renal tubules and, thus, has the theoretical benefit of preventing renal failure. Urine pH >8 is often recommended for mitigation of the Tamm-Horsfall–myoglobin complex obstruction of the renal tubules. In order to avoid the complications of systemic alkalemia, urine and plasma pH should be measured often. Bicarbonate infusion should not be continued after a patient in renal failure becomes overly alkalemic or frankly hypervolemic.

It is important to avoid excess plasma alkalosis, especially in patients who are not mechanically ventilated as the bicarbonate will eventually be broken down into carbon dioxide. Increases in carbon dioxide require increased minute ventilation by the patient to exhale this acidotic molecule. This increased work of breathing may not be tolerated by the patient, leading to hypercarbia and paradoxic acidosis due to respiratory acidosis, along with the potential need for mechanical ventilation.

Bicarbonate infusion will also mitigate the effect of hyperchloremic metabolic acidosis that would occur with large volumes of normal saline. Another benefit of systemic alkalinization is the mitigation of the early effects of renal failure by alleviating hyperkalemia and acidosis. This alone may forestall the need for dialysis.

If conservative therapies are not adequate, hemodialysis may need to be employed for patients with rhabdomyolysis-induced renal failure. Indications for hemodialysis are worsening acidemia and/or hyperkalemia and decreased urine output. There is no universally accepted evidence that early initiation of hemodialysis (prior to standard indications for dialysis) alters outcomes in terms of the development of end-stage renal failure or mortality in rhabdomyolysis. This is because hemodialysis is not expected to effectively clear myoglobin due to the large size of the molecule. In fact, the myoglobin molecule is similar in size to the albumin protein. Special high-porosity filters used with continuous venovenous hemodialysis have been able to reduce myoglobin with hemofiltration in case reports; however, this may not be readily reproducible in all institutions. Thus, dialysis should be reserved for patients with renal failure who meet standard criteria for initiation of dialysis.

CASE RESUMES

The patient's extremity was in dire need of blood flow. Her kidneys were risking severe and long standing injury and her metabolic acidosis was worsening. Her heparin drip was providing systemic anticoagulation.

Attempts to wean ECMO were not successful due to ongoing hemodynamic instability. The decision was made to revise her arterial cannula to include a small caliber bypass graft to her superficial femoral artery. Fluid resuscitation continued, however her urine output ceased and she was initiated on renal replacement therapy. Her metabolic acidosis thereafter improved with renal clearance and further resuscitation. However, her extremity became gangrenous and was subsequently amputed. She remained on ECMO for several more days prior to palliative withdrawal of all heroic interventions.

> **KEY POINTS TO REMEMBER**
> 1. Treat the underlying cause of muscle breakdown.
> 2. Flush the renal tubules with fluid. Target urine output at 200 mL/h.
> 3. Bicarbonate infusions (150 mEq/L) at 250 mL/hr may be a reasonable component of your fluid choice.
> 4. Mannitol 1–2 g/kg/d may be beneficial, especially at high CK level >30 000 U/L.
> 5. Monitor for hyperkalemia, hypocalcemia, hyperphosphatemia, hyperuricemia, and acidosis.
> 6. Avoid complications of your treatment including worsening renal failure, fluid overload, and cardiac failure.

Suggested Reading
1. Avalli L, Sangalli F, Migliari M, et al. Early vascular complications after percutaneous cannulation for extracorporeal membrane oxygenation for cardiac assist. Minerva Anestesiol. 2016;82(1):36–43.
2. Brown C, Rhee P, Chan L, Evans K, Demetriades D, Velhamos G. Preventing renal failure in patients with rhabdomyolysis: do bicarbonate and mannitol make a difference? J Trauma. 2004;56(6):1191–1196.
3. Iraj N, Saeed S, Mostafa H, et al. Prophylactic fluid therapy in crushed victims of Bam earthquake. Am J Emerg Med. 2011;29(7):738–742.
4. Knottenbelt JD. Traumatic rhabdomyolysis from severe beating—experience of volume diuresis in 200 patients. J Trauma. 1994;37(2):214–219.
5. Michelsen J, Cordtz J, Liboriussen L, et al. Prevention of rhabdomyolysis-induced acute kidney injury—a DASAIM/DSIT clinical practice guideline. Acta Anaesthesiol Scand. 2019;63(5):576–586.
6. Nielsen J, Sally M, Mullins R, et al. Bicarbonate and mannitol treatment for traumatic rhabdomyolysis revisited. Am J Surg. 2017;213(1):73–79.

10 Postoperative Septic Shock

James E. Littlejohn

A 69-year-old man with hypertension presents to the cardiothoracic intensive care unit (ICU) following a 3-vessel coronary artery bypass graft. He is extubated 6 hours postoperatively. His course is uneventful until the morning of postoperative day 3 when he becomes diaphoretic and complains of acute chest pain. He has new-onset sinus tachycardia and fever to 38.9°C. Chest X-ray reveals unchanged mild pulmonary edema. Troponin levels are elevated to 4.2 ng/mL, and leukocytosis is now present. The next hour, his fever increases to 39.2°C, and he develops atrial fibrillation with a heart rate in the 130s. He is now hypotensive, requiring vasopressors to maintain his mean arterial blood pressure (MAP) goal of 65 mm Hg.

What do you do now?

DISCUSSION

Diagnosis

Sepsis is a severe systemic inflammatory response to an infection. Controversy still exists regarding the diagnostic criteria, precise pathophysiology, and best treatment of this life-threatening condition. Sepsis is particularly difficult to diagnosis in the early postoperative period because the systemic inflammatory response syndrome (SIRS) from cardiac surgery alone can mimic the early symptoms. Sepsis characterization utilizing the traditional SIRS criteria (temperature, heart rate, respiratory rate, and white blood cell count) was first described in 1992 as part of the American College of Chest Physicians/Society of Critical Care Medicine Consensus Conference. The SIRS approach has been criticized because of the low specificity for infection. Considering post–cardiac surgery patients specifically, many variables included in the SIRS criteria are modulated by common postoperative treatments such as perioperative beta-blockade, mechanical ventilation, and patient warming post-bypass. In the previous SIRS-based guidelines, the diagnosis of sepsis was only confirmed with a culture-proven, microbiologic source. This threshold runs countercurrent to the need for sepsis treatment to begin within the first hour of initial presentation.

Organ dysfunction identified using the Sequential Organ Failure Assessment (SOFA) score has been replacing the SIRS criteria as a more sensitive means by which to identify physiologic effects of infection (Table 10.1).

According to the SOFA-guided definition, also known as the Sepsis-3 recommendations, the diagnosis of sepsis only requires the suspicion of infection accompanied by organ dysfunction, defined as a SOFA score ≥2. The Sepsis-3 criteria were specifically studied in cardiac surgery patients, to determine whether the guidelines may overdiagnose sepsis in a population that frequently encounters transient, postoperative organ dysfunction. In that study the diagnosis of septic shock, according to the proposed Sepsis-3 guidelines, had a negative association with length of cardiothoracic ICU stay, 30-day mortality, and 2-year survival. This evidence supports the use of the Sepsis-3 guidelines for early identification and treatment of patients who are at high risk of adverse outcomes from sepsis and septic shock.

TABLE 10.1 SOFA Table

Organ System	SOFA Score				
	0	1	2	3	4
Respiratory, PO_2/FiO_2, mm Hg (kPa)	≥400 (53.3)	<400 (53.3)	<300 (40)	<200 (26.7) with respiratory support	<100 (13.3) with respiratory
Coagulation, platelets (× $10^3/mm^3$)	≥150	<150	<100	<50	<20
Liver, bilirubin (md/dL)	<1.2	1.2–1.9	2.0–5.9	6.0–11.9	>12.0
Cardiovascular	MAP ≥70 mm Hg	MAP <70 mm Hg	Dopamine <5 or dobutamine (any dose)	Dopamine 5.1–15 or epinephrine ≤0.1 or NE ≤0.1	Dopamine >15 or epinephrine >0.1 or NE >0.1
Central nervous system, Glasgow Coma Scale	15	13–14	10–12	6–9	<6
Renal, creatinine (mg/dL) Urine output (mL/d)	<1.2	1.2–1.9	2.0–3.4	3.5–4.9 <500	>5.0 <200

Catecholamine doses are given as micrograms per kilogram per minute for at least 1 hour.
FiO_2, fraction of inspired oxygen; PO_2, partial pressure of oxygen.

The role of biomarkers to expedite diagnosis and management of infections and/or sepsis has been explored. Procalcitonin was originally characterized as a polypeptide precursor to calcitonin synthesized in the thyroid but has since been recognized as a general inflammatory biomarker, found to be secreted by nearly all organs and tissues throughout the body in response to both endotoxin (of gram-negative bacteria) and proinflammatory cytokines such as interleukins 1 and 6 and tumor necrosis factor alpha. High serum levels of procalcitonin have been shown to strongly correlate with the extent and severity of bacterial infections, as well as other non-infection inflammatory states. Given that cardiopulmonary bypass alone can elevate procalcitonin in the first 24 hours postoperatively, the threshold at which it indicates infection and/or sepsis is unclear. A procalcitonin level >2.95 ng/mL the morning after cardiac surgery was shown in one study to be associated with complications, although not necessarily due to infection. It is reasonable to trend procalcitonin levels in any patient where sepsis is suspected, especially if some time has passed since surgery. If the diagnosis of infection is confirmed, procalcitonin may also be a useful indicator of when to stop antibiotics. It is important to note that there is insufficient evident to base decisions on initiation or discontinuation of antibiotics solely on procalcitonin (or any other biomarkers).

Treatment

The first objective in the early stages of sepsis management is to identify possible causes of infection and accomplish source control. This includes removal of any intravascular lines and consideration of any other indwelling tubes or devices that could be a potential nidus for infection and/or colonization. Occult sources of infection should also be investigated with a "total-body exam" including sites specific to the post–cardiac surgery patient like vein harvest sites, chest tube sites, the sternotomy wound, and external pacing wires. If the patient has been in the ICU for a while, consider skin breakdown and pressure ulcers in dependent areas, as well as the oral cavity and the sinuses, especially if there is a nasal gastric tube in place. It is recommended that appropriate routine microbiologic cultures be obtained before starting empiric antimicrobial therapy in patients with suspected sepsis, if doing so results in no substantial delay in the start of antimicrobials. Isolation of an infecting organism(s) allows for de-escalation of antimicrobial therapy, first at the point of identification and then again when susceptibilities are obtained. De-escalation of antimicrobial therapy is a mainstay of antibiotic stewardship programs and is associated with less resistant microorganisms, fewer side effects, and lower costs.

Once sepsis has been identified, early resuscitation interventions are pivotal to reduce morbidity and mortality. The most important tenet of addressing and treating sepsis and septic shock includes a detailed initial assessment and ongoing re-evaluation of the patient's response to treatment. The Rivers trial, published in 2001, changed the outlook and approach to sepsis with the concept of early goal-directed therapy (EGDT). The original EGDT elements included arterial blood pressure, central venous pressure (CVP), systemic central venous oxygen saturation (ScvO$_2$), and hemoglobin level. This initiated a worldwide campaign to better identify, understand, and treat septic shock, known as the Surviving Sepsis Campaign. Although the Rivers trial showed a significant mortality benefit, 3 large multicenter randomized controlled trials did not effectively reproduce those results: the Protocol-Based Care for Early Septic Shock (ProCESS) trial, the Protocolized Management in Sepsis (ProMISE) trial, and the Goal-Directed Resuscitation for Patients with Early Septic Shock (ARISE) trial. A significant amount of work and study has ensued in order to better ascertain what goals are appropriate to use and the precise timing of each intervention. The recommendations for how to approach and treat sepsis are being continually updated and promoted by the Surviving Sepsis Campaign.

Surviving Sepsis guidelines from 2016 recommend an initial resuscitation of 30 cc/kg of intravenous crystalloid for sepsis-induced hypoperfusion, within the first 3 hours. The initial fluid resuscitation gives the clinician time to gather more specific information on the patient and other measurements of the patient's hemodynamic status. This precise volume is not based on data from controlled studies; however, it is based on "usual practice" in early resuscitation and consistent with average prerandomization volumes from the ProCESS, ARISE, and ProMISe trials.

In the cardiac surgical population, with cardiac dysfunction at baseline and/or postoperatively, the administration of such high volumes of resuscitation fluid can pose a risk of volume overload and heart failure. At the moment there is no specific guidance for fluid resuscitation in patients at risk for heart failure. A reasonable approach is judicious fluid administration based on "fluid responsiveness." Fluid responsiveness is commonly defined as some increase in stroke volume (usually 10%–15%) after the patient receives a bolus of volume over time (usually ~500 mL over 10–20 minutes). Dynamic assessments of fluid responsivity include techniques such as the passive leg raise; fluid challenge with contemporary stroke volume measurements; variation in systolic pressure, pulse pressure, or stroke volume; and changes in intrathoracic pressure induced by mechanical ventilation. After the initial bolus, additional fluids may be guided by a dynamic assessment of fluid responsivity.

The EGDT initially published by Rivers, et al., advocated for the use of objective goals such as CVP and $ScvO_2$ to determine treatment endpoints. However, such an approach has failed to show a mortality advantage in the other 3 large multicenter randomized controlled trials (RCTs). Still, many of the tenets of EGDT are still utilized by intensivists. While the safety and utility of a pulmonary artery catheter (PAC) have been challenged in the general critical care population, the PAC is a useful tool in the resuscitation of patients with, or at risk for, heart failure. The PAC provides the ability to dynamically track cardiac filling pressures, plasma colloid osmotic pressure (PCOP), cardiac output, and mixed-venous oxygen saturation ($SmvO_2$). The information can also inform decisions about inotropic therapy, vasopressor selection, and fluid resuscitation. This population is at risk of both underresuscitation (for fear of causing overload) as well as heart failure from overhydration.

In patients with preexisting heart failure, if a PAC is used during the resuscitation, the direct hemodynamic and pressure measurement trends can help inform this decision. With regard to the left heart, typically, PCOP values >18–20 mm Hg are signs that the left heart has adequate volume and one might consider the addition of an inotrope. Increasing pulmonary artery (PA) pressure in the setting of low PCOP pressures would prompt the care team to consider a potential role for pulmonary vasodilators, to help offload the work of the right ventricle. Finally, a sudden increase in the CVP in conjunction with a decrease in the $SmvO_2$ is concerning for acute right heart failure, best treated with inotropy.

Other less invasive modalities, such as point-of-care ultrasound and bedside echocardiography, have become increasingly utilized by clinicians for hemodynamic assessments and re-evaluations during treatment and resuscitation. In intubated patients, respiratory variation of inferior vena cava diameter by 16% had reasonable diagnostic accuracy for predicting fluid responsiveness but is limited by the requirements of controlled ventilation with larger tidal volumes (≥8 cc/kg) and low positive end-expiratory pressure (≤5 cm H_2O). The left ventricular outflow tract velocity time integral, measured by transthoracic echocardiography, can be used as an accurate measurement of stroke volume. Serial measurements provide a dynamic monitor in the setting of fluid responsiveness, even in the context of severe, chronic heart failure.

Fluid administration beyond the initial resuscitation for sepsis requires careful assessment because a sustained positive fluid balance in the ICU can also be harmful. This is a very challenging process because the acutely septic patient is in a state of dynamic disequilibrium. Early fluid resuscitation is vital for stabilization of tissue hypoperfusion due to sepsis and septic shock. Once fluid responsivity ceases, vasopressors and inotropic support should be considered in place of additional fluid.

It is important to identify and define the endpoints of resuscitation and the hemodynamic information that will be tracked during the resuscitation. The surviving sepsis guidelines suggest an initial MAP goal of ≥65 mm Hg in patients with septic shock requiring vasopressors. Norepinephrine (NE) is the first-choice vasopressor to maintain MAP ≥65 mm Hg. After that, either epinephrine or vasopressin should be added when an additional agent is needed to maintain adequate blood pressure. Vasopressin (at 0.03 U/min) can be added to NE to either raise MAP to target or to decrease NE dose but should not be used as the initial vasopressor. Dopamine is not recommended except in highly selected circumstances, which will not be discussed here. Dobutamine administration can be considered in the presence of (1) myocardial dysfunction as suggested by elevated cardiac filling pressures and low cardiac output or (2) ongoing signs of hypoperfusion despite achieving adequate intravascular volume and adequate MAP.

Another physiologic parameter that has shown promise in guiding resuscitation in septic patients is serum lactate level. Although serum lactate is not a direct measurement of tissue perfusion, it can serve as a surrogate since increases in lactate may represent tissue hypoxia, accelerated glycolysis driven by excess beta-adrenergic stimulation, and other causes associated with poor outcomes. Importantly, RCTs have demonstrated a significant

TABLE 10.2 **Surviving Sepsis 1-Hour Bundle**

Bundle Element	Grade of Recommendation Level of Evidence
Measure lactate level; remeasure if initial lactate is >2 mmol/L	Weak recommendation, low quality of evidence
Obtain blood cultures prior to administration of antibiotics	Best practice statement
Administer broad-spectrum antibiotics	Strong recommendation, moderate quality of evidence
Rapidly administer 30 mL/kg crystalloid for hypotension or lactate ≥4 mmol/L	Strong recommendation, low quality of evidence
Apply vasopressors if patient is hypotensive during or after fluid resuscitation to maintain MAP ≥65 mm Hg	Strong recommendation, moderate quality of evidence

reduction in mortality in septic patients treated with lactate-guided resuscitation when compared to resuscitation without lactate monitoring. Two meta-analyses demonstrated moderate evidence for reduction in mortality when an early lactate clearance strategy was used compared with either usual care (non-specified) or an $ScvO_2$ normalization strategy.

Compliance with bundles has been associated with improved survival in patients with sepsis and septic shock. Sepsis is a medical emergency, and thus the initial evaluation and management in the early presentation of sepsis can have profound implications in the patient's clinical course. Members of the Surviving Sepsis Campaign published an updated "hour-1 bundle" in 2018 of critical elements that are to be initiated within the first hour of presentation (Table 10.2).

CASE RESUMES

This patient presented with fever in conjunction with his tachycardia, on postoperative day 3. This acute inflammatory change is most likely sepsis. It is important to distinguish if he has 2 primary problems occurring or if his hemodynamic instability is due entirely to septic shock. The single positive troponin value cannot be interpreted as it may represent residual troponin leak from surgery, demand ischemia, or graft dysfunction. Since there were signs of potential infection, cultures should be obtained as well as prompt, empiric antibiotics. Concurrently a cardiac evaluation should occur including echo and possibly catheterization, to rule out coronary graft dysfunction.

The patient's CVP was <10, PA pressures were 30s/10s mm Hg, pulmonary capillary wedge pressure was 10 mm Hg, and cardiac index was 3.0 L/min/m^2 despite a rising lactate. Most likely sources of the presumed sepsis in this patient at postoperative day 3 are his intravascular lines, his lungs, or his urine. His preoperative urinalysis was negative. He was not on a lot of oxygenation support, and his lines were only 72 hours old. Blood, urine, and respiratory cultures were drawn; and empiric antibiotics were administered within the first hour of presentation. The patient was fluid-resuscitated, and NE was initiated to maintain a MAP >65 mm Hg. It was eventually determined that he had pneumonia due to *Klebsiella pneumoniae* bacterium. He was treated with a 7-day course of antibiotics based on the susceptibility profile for the cultured organism and recovered without further incident.

> **KEY POINTS TO REMEMBER**
>
> 1. Sepsis is a medical emergency. Early and effective treatment can have a dramatic impact on morbidity and mortality.
> 2. Sepsis-3 guidelines allow for early and accurate identification of septic patients including post–cardiac surgery.
> 3. Lactate-guided resuscitation strategies have been shown to reduce mortality in septic patients.
> 4. Procalcitonin level is a biomarker that shows promise in predicting bacteremia, as well as lending clinical support to wean antibiotic duration in certain circumstances.
> 5. Microbiologic cultures should be obtained before starting antimicrobial therapy only if doing so results in no substantial delay in the start of antimicrobials (within 1 hour of presentation).

Suggested Reading

1. Rivers E, Nguyen B, Havstad S, Ressler J, Muzzin A, Knoblich B, et al. Early goal-directed therapy in the treatment of severe sepsis and septic shock. *N Engl J Med*. 2001;345:1368–1377.
2. Howitt SH, Herring M, Malagon I, McCollum CN, Grant SW. Incidence and outcomes of sepsis after cardiac surgery as defined by the Sepsis-3 guidelines. *Br J Anaesth*. 2018;120(3):509–516.
3. Ding X-F, Yang Z-Y, Xu Z-T, Li L-F, Yuan B, Guo L-N, et al. Early goal-directed and lactate-guided therapy in adult patients with severe sepsis and septic shock: a meta-analysis of randomized controlled trials. *J Transl Med*. 2018;16(1):331.
4. Rhodes A, Evans LE, Alhazzani W, Levy MM, Antonelli M, Ferrer R, et al. Surviving Sepsis Campaign: international guidelines for management of sepsis and septic shock: 2016. *Intensive Care Med*. 2017;43(3):304–377.
5. Levy MM, Evans LE, Rhodes A. The Surviving Sepsis Campaign Bundle: 2018 update. *Crit Care Med*. 2018;46(6):97–1000.
6. ARISE Investigators, ANZICS Clinical Trials Group; Peake SL, Delaney A, Bailey M, Bellomo R, et al. Goal-directed resuscitation for patients with early septic shock. *N Engl J Med*. 2014;371(16):1496–1506.
7. Messina A, Longhini F, Coppo C, Pagni A, Lungu R, Ronco C, et al. Use of the fluid challenge in critically ill adult patients: a systematic review. *Anesth Analg*. 2017;125(5):1532–1543.

11 Postoperative Right Ventricular Failure

Marguerite Hoyler and Natalia S. Ivascu

A 72-year-old woman with type 2 diabetes mellitus and hypertension presents for elective aortic valve replacement for severe aortic stenosis. Her preoperative transthoracic echo reveals left ventricular (LV) hypertrophy, an LV ejection fraction of 55%, impaired LV diastolic function, and a mildly dilated right ventricle (RV) with normal systolic function.

The operative course is unremarkable, and the patient is brought to the intensive care unit intubated on moderate-dose vasopressors and no inotropes. Over the next 24 hours, she receives 2 L of intravenous fluids and 2 units of packed red blood cells for a laboratory hemoglobin value that has trended from 9.0 g/dL to 7.4 g/dL without evidence of active bleeding. She is extubated and weaned off of vasopressors. The night of postoperative day 1–2, her cardiac index declines, urine output drops, and arterial lactate rises. Central venous pressure (CVP) increases from 12 to 16 mm Hg. An additional 250 cc fluid bolus yields further elevation in CVP with no hemodynamic improvements.

What do you do now?

DISCUSSION

The constellation of decreased cardiac output, elevated right-sided filling pressures, and significant post-cardiotomy volume resuscitation is most consistent with acute postoperative RV failure (RVF). The differential diagnosis includes "mimickers" of RVF, such as auto–positive end-expiratory pressure (auto-PEEP) and cardiac tamponade. Untreated, RVF leads to LV failure and cardiogenic shock. RVF is also associated with markedly worse perioperative outcomes; timely diagnosis and management are thus of the utmost importance.

Perioperative RVF Risk Factors

The early period following cardiac surgery presents particular risks for RVF. The condition may occur secondary to inadequate intraoperative cardioplegia or long aortic cross-clamp and cardiopulmonary bypass times. The RV may also fail due to increased afterload from an acutely elevated pulmonary vascular resistance (PVR). The latter may be precipitated by perioperative hypoxia, hypercarbia, and acidosis. Importantly, even moderate postoperative volume resuscitation can strain a vulnerable RV to the point of failure.

The patient in this case likely developed acute RVF on top of preexisting mild dysfunction due to intraoperative ischemia ("stunning") and a markedly positive postoperative fluid balance.

Mechanisms of RVF

A brief review of RV physiology is useful in framing our approach to RVF management (Figure 11.1). A normal RV pumps blood through the low-pressure pulmonary circuit to provide adequate LV filling. The anatomy and structure of the RV reflect these functions: it is a compliant chamber, with a thin free wall and a baseline larger volume and lower ejection fraction than the left ventricle. In contrast to concentric LV contraction, RV contraction is primarily longitudinal and depends both on the motion of the RV free wall and on LV contraction mediated by the interventricular septum (IVS). Due to relatively low intraventricular pressures, RV myocardial perfusion occurs during systole and diastole.

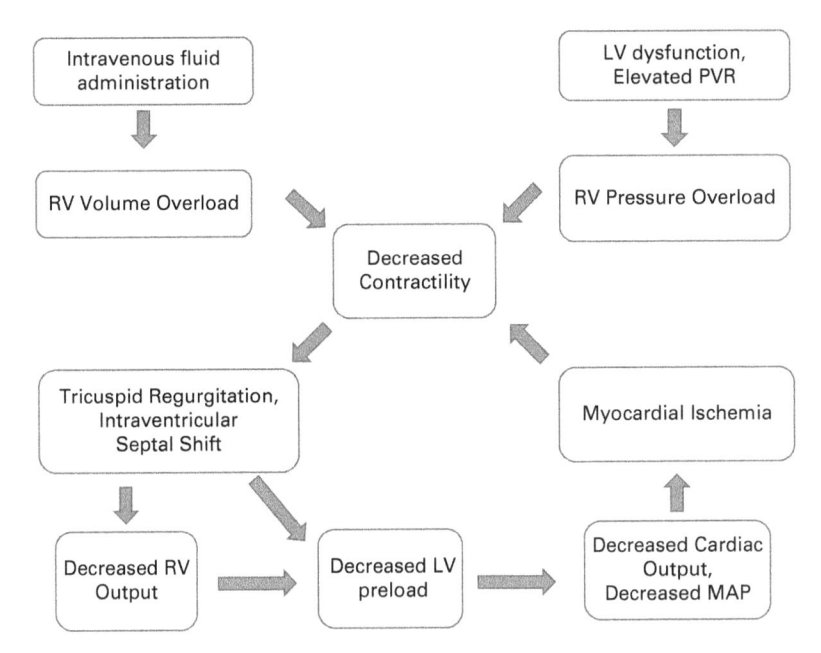

FIGURE 11.1 Postoperative RV failure: mechanisms and management strategies. MAP, mean arterial pressure.

In general, the RV tolerates increases in volume better than increases in pressure, though both can cause acute RVF. When the RV is stressed due to increased preload or afterload, the IVS shifts leftward, impairing LV filling and output, and leading to decreased systemic and coronary perfusion. This general concept is referred to as "ventricular interdependence."

In this setting, increased RV end diastolic pressure (RVEDP) further diminishes right-sided coronary perfusion pressure and impairs RV perfusion. Increased RV volume also leads to dilation of the tricuspid valve orifice and acute tricuspid regurgitation, impairing both venous return and forward flow to the LV. Each of these factors contributes to systolic dyssynchrony between the LV and RV, less efficient myocardial oxygen utilization, decreased systemic and myocardial perfusion, and even greater compromise in RV function.

RVF: Clinical Presentation and Diagnosis

Clinically, postoperative RVF presents as systemic hypotension and end-organ dysfunction, with elevated right-sided filling pressures. While non-specific, patients may demonstrate lactic acidosis and low mixed venous oxygen saturation. Depending on the degree of LV dysfunction or preexisting pulmonary arterial hypertension, pulmonary arterial and pulmonary artery occlusion pressures may be elevated.

In a patient who fits this clinical picture, the next diagnostic step is a bedside transthoracic echocardiogram (TTE) to rule out pericardial effusion and tamponade. In addition, TTE can help assess RV function and confirm the diagnosis of RVF. TTE may be challenging in post-sternotomy patients but is typically notable for dilation of the RV and a flattened interventricular septum ("D sign") on parasternal short-axis view (Figure 11.2). Longitudinally, the RV may comprise the majority of the cardiac apex, tricuspid regurgitation may be visible, and the tricuspid annular plane systolic excursion (TAPSE) is decreased. If transesophageal echocardiography is available, a calculated fractional area change can help quantify RV dysfunction. Serial TTEs, particularly the parasternal short-axis and apical 4-chamber views, are helpful to diagnose RVF and monitor the effects of our interventions.

RVF: Management

Once the diagnosis of RV dysfunction is confirmed, we employ a multipronged management strategy. We find it useful to consider, individually, the elements of preload, contractility, afterload, rate, rhythm, and perfusion. Key management points include decreasing RV volume and preload, increasing RV contractility, reducing RV afterload, and increasing

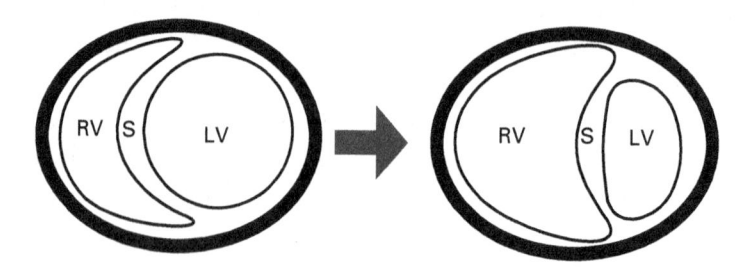

FIGURE 11.2 Interventricular septal shift, TTE parasternal short axis view. S, septum.

RV and systemic perfusion. Ultimately, the goal of these interventions is to support RV function such that the LV receives sufficient preload, adequate cardiac output can be maintained, and cardiogenic shock is avoided or resolves.

These strategies, as well as the interrelated mechanisms of RVF they target, are illustrated in Figure 11.1.

Preload
An important early maneuver in managing RVF is to determine whether or not the patient in shock is "fluid-responsive"—that is to say, whether additional preload optimizes RV (and by extension LV) function. This can be achieved through a passive leg raise or a small (i.e., no greater than 250 cc) bolus of crystalloid, with close subsequent monitoring of hemodynamic parameters. Any fluid challenge must be administered with caution as excessive volume loading will exacerbate RVF. The patient in this case clearly "failed" her fluid challenge.

Patients with RV dysfunction most often require fluid removal in order to decrease RVEDP, facilitate perfusion, and increase RV output. As a result, volume removal is frequently the mainstay of managing postoperative RVF. While actively diuresing, CVP should be followed, with a goal CVP of 8–12 mm Hg or a several-point reduction daily. Adequate diuresis can usually be achieved with loop diuretic boluses or infusions. In some patients, hemofiltration may be necessary. In this patient, an appropriate next step in management would be the initiation of an aggressive loop diuretic regimen, with careful minimization of fluid inputs.

Bear in mind, however, that volume removal in RVF is not an end unto itself: its purpose is to increase RV function, particularly RV output and LV preload, and enable adequate systemic perfusion. Underdiuresis and overdiuresis of the failing RV can be equally detrimental to these aims. Markers of systemic perfusion and LV output should therefore inform clinical decisions regarding ongoing volume removal in RVF management.

Contractility
Marked RV dysfunction frequently requires inotropic support. In patients whose systemic vascular resistance and perfusion pressure can tolerate moderate vasodilation, dobutamine or milrinone has the added benefit

of direct pulmonary arterial vasodilation. Dobutamine use may be limited by concomitant tachyarrhythmias. In profoundly hypotensive patients who are not inodilator candidates, epinephrine may be indicated, though arrhythmias are a potential side effect and may independently compromise RV output and LV preload. In the patient described here, low- to moderate-dose inodilator support would be the likely next step in management, along with ongoing diuresis and vasopressor therapy.

Afterload

Efforts should also be made to reduce RV afterload. Pulmonary hypertension triggers, such as hypoxia, hypercarbia, and acidosis, should be strictly avoided. In intubated patients, positive pressure ventilation should be minimized as much as oxygenation and ventilation parameters allow. Auto-PEEP is clearly detrimental.

Pulmonary vasoconstriction can also be pharmacologically targeted. Inhaled nitric oxide is a highly effective and localized pulmonary vasodilator and is often the next treatment for RVF that has not improved with preload optimization and inotropes. Inhaled prostaglandin analogues, such as iloprost and epoprostenol, may be introduced as adjuncts for refractory RVF; these may also facilitate weaning patients off of inhaled nitric oxide. Direct pulmonary artery (PA) pressure measurements from a Swan-Ganz catheter can facilitate titration of these medications but are not strictly necessary, particularly if a patient is felt to have relatively normal LV function.

If the patient in this case had persistent shock in the setting of aggressive diuresis and inotropy, pulmonary vasodilators such inhaled nitric oxide or inhaled prostacyclin therapy should be added for RV afterload reduction.

Rate and Rhythm

In supporting the RV, measures should be taken to ensure normal sinus rhythm and atrioventricular synchrony. As mentioned previously, arrythmogenicity may limit the use of certain medications.

Perfusion

Patients with postoperative RVF frequently require vasopressors to maintain systemic and coronary perfusion in the setting of reduced LV preload, cardiac output, and mean arterial pressure. Of note, in contrast to other shock states, RVF tends not to require vasopressors for maintenance of RV preload per se as the RV is generally already volume-overloaded.

Ideal vasopressors in RVF will support myocardial and systemic perfusion without concomitantly increasing PVR. Due to the absence of vasopressin receptors in the pulmonary vasculature, vasopressin does not cause pulmonary vasoconstriction and may in fact induce nitric oxide release and vasodilation in the lung. By contrast, norepinephrine may increase PVR through direct vasoconstriction, but the positive inotropy it provides may compensate for this. Phenylephrine is in general the least useful agent as it can increase PVR and precipitate bradycardia. Norepinephrine and vasopressin are thus the vasopressors of choice.

Monitoring and Additional Measures

Effects of the above interventions can be monitored by generic perfusion parameters (arterial lactate, mixed venous saturation, blood pressure, etc.) and by serial bedside echocardiograms. We also pay close attention to trends in CVP. Direct measurement of PA pressures, via Swan-Ganz catheter, may be a helpful adjunct but in isolation is less useful than some of the other markers of RV function described here. While many patients will respond to the mainstays of diuresis, inotropy, and afterload reduction, some patients with postoperative RVF will also require some form of mechanical support.

CASE RESUMES

The team performs bedside echocardiography and finds a dilated RV and septal shift to the left during diastole. Her TAPSE measures 1.2 cm. Intravenous furosemide is administered and the inotropic agent, dobutamine, is added. Over the next 12 hours, her urine output increases along with her cardiac index. A repeat echocardiographic exam demonstrates TAPSE of 1.8cm and with minimal septal flattening. Her dobutamine is slowly weaned to off over the next 24 hours.

CONCLUSION

RVF is not uncommon following cardiac surgery and often portends a worse clinical outcome. After establishing the diagnosis of RVF, the central goal of treatment is to increase RV function in order to achieve adequate LV preload and cardiac output. Management involves decreasing RV volume and preload, increasing RV contractility, reducing RV afterload, maintaining normal rate and rhythm, and supporting RV and systemic perfusion. Diuresis, inodilators and inopressors, and inhaled direct pulmonary vasodilators are mainstays of treatment. Serial TTEs and CVP measurements, as well as markers of cardiac output and systemic perfusion, are critical for guiding RVF management.

> **KEY POINTS TO REMEMBER**
>
> 1. Consider postoperative RVF in patients with evidence of cardiogenic shock and elevated right-sided filling pressures; "mimickers" include tamponade and auto-PEEP.
> 2. In patients with a vulnerable RV, even marginal volume overload can precipitate RVF.
> 3. Early and serial bedside TTEs can be useful for diagnosing and monitoring RV dysfunction.
> 4. Volume removal is a mainstay of RVF management, but excessive volume removal can compromise LV preload and precipitate shock. In guiding diuretic therapy, CVP trends as well as markers of LV cardiac output and systemic perfusion are more useful than fluid balance alone.

Suggested Reading
1. Vieillard-Baron A, Naeije R, Haddad F, Bogaard HJ, Bull TM, Fletcher N, et al. Diagnostic workup, etiologies and management of acute right ventricle failure: a state-of-the-art paper. *Intensive Care Med.* 2018;44(6):774–790.
2. Estrada VH, Franco DL, Moreno AA, Gambasica JA, Nunez CC. Postoperative right ventricular failure in cardiac surgery. *Cardiol Res.* 2016;7(6):185–195.
3. Ventetuolo CE, Klinger JR. Management of acute right ventricular failure in the intensive care unit. *Ann Am Thorac Soc.* 2014;11(5):811–822.
4. Haddad F, Couture P, Tousignant C, Denault AY. The right ventricle in cardiac surgery, a perioperative perspective: II. Pathophysiology, clinical importance, and management. *Anesth Analg.* 2009;108(2):422–433.

12 Postoperative Atrial Fibrillation

Liang Shen

A 72-year-old man with a history of obesity, hypertension, diabetes, and coronary artery disease (CAD) undergoes a 3-vessel coronary artery bypass graft (CABG) surgery. At the end of surgery, intraoperative transesophageal echocardiography showed a left ventricular ejection fraction (LVEF) of 45%, and the patient was started on a low dose of epinephrine infusion with improvement of LVEF to 55%. Later that night, he is extubated without difficulty, weaned off vasopressor medications, and maintained on the low dose of epinephrine. On postoperative day 2, continuous telemetry demonstrates that the patient is in atrial fibrillation, with a ventricular rate of 127 bpm. A 12-lead electrocardiogram (ECG) verifies the diagnosis of atrial fibrillation. His blood pressure (BP) is 112/62, his blood oxygen saturation is 98% on 2 L of nasal cannula, and his pulmonary artery catheter (PAC) measures a cardiac index of 2.8 L/min/m^2. The patient has no complaints and does not feel palpitations.

What do you do now?

DISCUSSION

Postoperative atrial fibrillation (POAF) is very common after cardiothoracic surgery, with an estimated incidence of approximately 30% after CABG surgery, 40% after valve replacements or repairs, and 50% after combined CABG and valve surgery. Most patients who experience POAF after cardiac surgery develop it within 4 days postoperatively. POAF is associated with a variety of worse outcomes for patients, including increased morbidity, mortality, intensive care unit and hospital length of stay, and healthcare utilization. Risk factors associated with POAF are numerous and include advanced age (≥75 years), preoperative history of atrial fibrillation (AF), renal failure, heart failure, chronic obstructive lung disease, mitral valve disease or surgery, longer cardiopulmonary bypass times, comorbidities causing cardiac restructuring such as enlarged left atria, perioperative issues such as fluid and electrolyte shifts, acute atrial distension, and both local and systemic inflammation (Table 12.1). The majority of POAF in patients without a prior history of AF is self-limited, with most patients returning to sinus rhythm by 6 to 8 weeks postoperatively.

POAF Prophylaxis

According to a recent Cochrane systematic review and meta-analysis, effective medications to prevent POAF include the use of beta-blockers, amiodarone, sotalol, and magnesium (see Table 12.2). The majority of studies on beta-blockers initiated the medication postoperatively, while roughly half of studies on amiodarone and sotalol initiated the medications postoperatively, and about half of studies on magnesium started it intraoperatively. Magnesium may have a slightly lesser effect on decreasing the rates of POAF compared to the other pharmacologic agents. The studies included in the meta-analysis were heterogeneous, and no clear conclusions

TABLE 12.1 **Risk Factors for the Development of POAF**

Age >75
History of atrial fibrillation
Renal failure
Mitral valve disease or surgery
Heart failure
Chronic obstructive lung disease

TABLE 12.2 **Summary of Strategies for POAF Prophylaxis**

Effective pharmacologic agents
    Beta-blockers
    Amiodarone
    Sotalol
    Magnesium

Effective non-pharmacologic approaches
    Atrial pacing
    Posterior pericardiotomy

Possibly effective pharmacologic agents
    Statins
    Colchicine

could be drawn about the most effective drug dose or time of initiation. The review also highlighted effective nonpharmacologic prophylactic strategies including atrial pacing and posterior pericardiotomy. The studies utilizing atrial pacing used a variety of pacing locations, including left and right atrial as well as biatrial locations. Posterior pericardiotomy was accomplished via a 4 cm longitudinal incision parallel to the phrenic nerve in the posterior pericardium and is proposed to reduce POAF through reduction of postoperative pericardial effusions.

A recent practice advisory, based on published guidelines and expert consensus, suggests that to reduce rates of POAF, patients already taking beta-blockers preoperatively should continue them throughout the perioperative period, while patients at elevated risk for POAF should be considered for preoperative initiation of amiodarone. Additionally, all patients after cardiac surgery should have beta-blockers started postoperatively for POAF prophylaxis. Other medications which have been described for POAF prophylaxis, though with mixed evidence, include statins and colchicine. Digoxin does not appear to be effective for POAF prevention.

Initial Management

In all patients, after verifying the diagnosis with 12-lead ECG, initial management of POAF should include correcting hypoxia or electrolyte abnormalities and weaning off stimulating medications such as inotrope infusions, when possible. It is important to note that the cardiac output and index may be unreliable monitors of cardiac performance at very fast heart rates. In general, with or without invasive monitoring such as a PAC, it is essential to establish whether or not the patient has adequate perfusion, and thus would be classified as hemodynamically stable or unstable. The appropriate medical treatment of patients in POAF hinges on this classification. Signs of hypoperfusion include hypotension requiring escalating doses of vasopressors or evidence of a low–cardiac output state, such as decreasing urine output, worsening mental status, and mottled or cool extremities.

Treatment of Hemodynamically Stable POAF

The patient in this case did not exhibit any signs of hypoperfusion and can be classified as hemodynamically stable. In these patients, beta-blockers are typically first-line agents for rate control of the POAF, either in oral or intravenous (IV) form, though the latter is faster-acting. No strong evidence exists for the superiority of one beta-blocker over another, though to avoid prolonged side effects such as hypotension or bradycardia, shorter-acting beta-blockers such as metoprolol may be preferred over longer-acting ones. The initial goal for heart rate control may target <100 bpm, though this may be different depending on patient-specific risk factors; for example, in a patient with a history of severe residual CAD, a lower heart rate target is reasonable to avoid myocardial ischemia.

When beta-blockers are ineffective at rate control, non-dihydropyridine calcium-channel blockers are recommended. Both diltiazem and verapamil may be used, but verapamil may have a more potent, negative effect on inotropy and should be used cautiously in patients with low LVEF. Diltiazem may also be used as an infusion if BP remains normal and can be an effective form of continuous rate control in otherwise refractory cases.

Amiodarone is an effective agent for rhythm control of POAF, and it also reliably causes slowing of the ventricular rate. Mostly because of concerns about its multitude of side effects, including QT prolongation and pulmonary or thyroid toxicity, amiodarone is often used as a second-line agent. In settings of hypotension, however, amiodarone is preferred over beta-blockers and calcium-channel blockers. Amiodarone slows the heart rate shortly after administration, though its chemical cardioversion effect takes longer—usually after 30 minutes to several hours. A common side effect of amiodarone is persistent bradycardia after patients convert to sinus rhythm,

TABLE 12.3 **Summary of POAF Treatments**

Hemodynamically stable patients
Beta-blockers
Non-dihydropyridine calcium-channel blockers
Amiodarone
Digoxin

Hemodynamically unstable patients

Direct current synchronized cardioversion

which may require temporary pacing using epicardial or transvenous pacemakers. Importantly, the multiple toxic side effects of amiodarone primarily occur in settings of chronic administration over months to years, with larger cumulative doses, rather than short perioperative courses. Various dosing regimens exist for amiodarone, depending on institutional or local practice patterns.

Digoxin is another rate control agent that can be employed in POAF. It has a relatively narrow therapeutic window and numerous potential side effects, and because of this safety concern, it is typically not a first-line agent for POAF. As digoxin does not cause hemodynamic instability and has some weak inotropic properties, it can be a better choice in hypotensive patients who have systolic heart failure, though if a patient's hemodynamics are worsening, it may be most prudent to follow the hemodynamically unstable POAF management pathways outlined in the following section (Table 12.3).

Of note, in patients who have evidence of pre-excitation syndromes such as Wolff-Parkinson-White, the use of beta-blockers, calcium-channel blockers, amiodarone, and digoxin is contraindicated as they can precipitate ventricular fibrillation. Instead, IV procainamide or ibutilide can be used for rate or rhythm control in these patients.

Treatment of Hemodynamically Unstable POAF

In the event the patient is or becomes hemodynamically unstable, emergent direct current synchronized cardioversion should be performed. If the patient is conscious, procedural sedation may be considered if time allows; but patient comfort and lack of recall should be weighed against risk of hypoventilation, hypoxia, and hypotension resulting from the sedatives. Using biphasic defibrillators, the initial energy used for cardioversion ranges from 120 to 200 joules. If starting at a lower energy, unsuccessful attempts may be followed by subsequent shocks at higher energy levels. Using a higher energy for the initial shock increases the chance of success and decreases the number of attempts, though high-energy shocks may also theoretically cause myocardial damage. The risk of embolic stroke from electrical cardioversion is considered very small if performed in the first 48 hours after new-onset AF. If patients remain in hemodynamically stable, rate controlled POAF over 48 hours postoperatively, it may be reasonable to consider a trial of electrical cardioversion to avoid starting anticoagulation.

If repeated attempts at electrical cardioversion are ineffective, the rate control strategies mentioned in the previous section using amiodarone and digoxin are likely the next best option. Use of both of these medications results in a hemodynamically stable decrease in heart rate, which can potentially improve cardiac filling time, cardiac output, and end-organ perfusion. Vasopressors should be used to correct hypotension while rate control is attained.

Refractory Cases

In rare instances, patients may be in rapid POAF, converted to sinus rhythm with cardioversion, but experience recurrence of the AF. Alternatively, some patients experience significant bradycardia with rate control agents and will require decreased dosing or discontinuation of those agents, with resultant recurrence of rapid POAF. These recurrent cases of rapid AF can be challenging to manage. Ultimately, a decision must be made about the risks of allowing the AF to persist versus the risks of aggressively pharmacologically rate-controlling the rhythm to a point of requiring either a temporary or a permanent pacemaker. In patients shortly after cardiac surgery, who have functional epicardial pacemaker wires in place, the strategy of aggressive rate control is less risky—as the ability to pace the heart already exists. In those patients whose epicardial pacemaker wires are no longer functional, such as those many days after surgery or who did not receive epicardial wires in the first place, a transvenous pacemaker wire may need to be inserted or a permanent pacemaker installed.

Atrial Flutter

Atrial flutter also occurs after cardiothoracic surgery, though at lower rates than POAF. Its management largely follows the same pathways, though atrial flutter is more amenable to electrical cardioversion than AF and typically at lower energy levels. Thus, when performing synchronized cardioversion for atrial flutter, initial energies of 50–100 joules may be sufficient to convert the patient to sinus rhythm.

CASE RESUMES

In this case of a 72-year-old man who experiences rapid POAF after CABG surgery, his initial presentation is hemodynamically stable. Appropriate management strategies would include titrating off the epinephrine infusion to decrease irritability to the heart, optimizing serum electrolyte levels, while initiating beta-blocker medications. Were beta-blockers to be ineffective at rate control, calcium-channel blockers can also be attempted. Amiodarone can also be considered, either for more rate control or for rhythm control. If at any time the patient became hemodynamically unstable, with signs of impaired end-organ perfusion, emergent synchronized cardioversion should be performed.

> **KEY POINTS TO REMEMBER**
>
> 1. POAF is very common after cardiothoracic surgery, with an estimated incidence of 30%–50% of patients.
> 2. Prevention of POAF involves continuation of preoperative beta-blockers, initiation of postoperative beta-blockers, and consideration of initiation of preoperative amiodarone in high-risk groups.
> 3. In all patients, initial management of POAF includes correcting hypoxia, electrolyte abnormalities, and consideration of weaning stimulating agents such as inotrope infusions.
> 4. Medical management of hemodynamically stable patients includes the use of rate control agents such as beta-blockers, calcium-channel blockers, and digoxin or rhythm control agents such as amiodarone.

5. When the patient is hemodynamically unstable, emergent synchronized cardioversion should be performed.
6. In refractory cases of rapid POAF, an aggressive rate control strategy may be pursued using one or more medications, but this approach must be weighed against the risk of requiring temporary or permanent pacing.
7. Postoperative atrial flutter may be managed similarly to POAF, though it is typically more amenable to electrical cardioversion.

Suggested Reading
1. Muehlschlegel JD, Burrage PS, Ngai JY, et al. Society of Cardiovascular Anesthesiologists/European Association of Cardiothoracic Anaesthetists practice advisory for the management of perioperative atrial fibrillation in patients undergoing cardiac surgery. *Anesth Analg.* 2019;128(1):33–42. doi:10.1213/ANE.0000000000003865
2. Arsenault K, Yusuf A, Crystal E, et al. Interventions for preventing post-operative atrial fibrillation in patients undergoing heart surgery. *Cochrane Database Syst Rev.* 2013;(1):CD003611. doi:10.1002/14651858.cd003611.pub3
3. Gillinov A, Bagiella E, Moskowitz A, et al. Rate control versus rhythm control for atrial fibrillation after cardiac surgery. *N Engl J Med.* 2016;374(20):1911–1921. doi:10.1056/nejmoa1602002
4. Greenberg J, Lancaster T, Schuessler R, Melby S. Postoperative atrial fibrillation following cardiac surgery: a persistent complication. *Eur J Cardiothorac Surg.* 2017;52(4):665–672. doi:10.1093/ejcts/ezx039
5. January C, Wann L, Alpert J, et al. 2014 AHA/ACC/HRS guideline for the management of patients with atrial fibrillation: executive summary. *Circulation.* 2014;130(23):2071–2104. doi:10.1161/cir.0000000000000040
6. Kirchhof P, Benussi S, Kotecha D, et al. 2016 ESC guidelines for the management of atrial fibrillation developed in collaboration with EACTS. *Eur Heart J.* 2016;37(38):2893–2962. doi:10.1093/eurheartj/ehw210

13 QTc Prolongation and Torsades de Pointes

Ankur Srivastava and James E. Littlejohn

A 70-year-old female with a past medical history of atrial fibrillation is brought to the cardiac critical care unit after a witnessed out-of-hospital cardiac arrest. The arrest team obtained return of spontaneous circulation after defibrillation. She was intubated in the field and brought to the emergency department. She is sedated and started on targeted temperature management. Her admission labs show that electrolytes were all within normal limits, but her electrocardiogram (ECG) had prolonged QTc interval (610 ms). Medical history shows she was started on sotalol for paroxysmal atrial fibrillation 2 weeks ago. After admission to the critical care unit, she experiences 2 more episodes of polymorphic ventricular tachycardia, requiring defibrillation.

What do you do now?

DISCUSSION

In cases of recurrent polymorphic ventricular tachycardia, torsades de pointes (Tdp) should be an immediate consideration. Tdp appears like a "twisting of points" of the cardiac axis, which is most often due to acquired QTc prolongation. The QT interval (measured from the start of the Q wave to the end of the T wave) is inversely related to heart rate; therefore, it is corrected (QTc) using formulas such as Bazett's, Fridericia, or Framingham. Bazett's is the most commonly used formula, where the QT interval is divided by the square root of the RR (seconds) interval. It is estimated that as many as 30% of patients admitted to cardiac critical care units have QTc prolongation, but only a small percentage of them will develop Tdp. The risk of developing this arrhythmia increases by ~5% for every 10 ms prolongation above the normal values. The normal QTc interval for men is <450 ms, and that for women is <460 ms. This patient's QTc was noted to be 610 ms.

Causes of QTc Prolongation

There are several congenital and acquired causes of QTc prolongation. The congenital long QT syndrome, Romano-Ward syndrome, and Jervell and Lange-Nielsen syndrome are commonly associated with QTc prolongation and Tdp. Congenital long QT syndrome is known to be related to mutations in genes that code for cardiac ion channels in the majority of cases. There is also growing evidence that the QT interval is an independent heritable trait and that some patients can be at intrinsically higher risk. Other risks include female gender, structural heart disease, bradycardia, and advanced age (>65 years).

Since this patient had a prior ECG with a normal QTc before starting sotalol, it is unlikely that she has an occult congenital syndrome. She is female and of advanced age (70 years), which both contribute to a prolonged interval. Drugs are the other common cause of acquired QT prolongation. Drug classes such as anti-arrhythmics, antidepressants, antipsychotics, antibiotics, anti-histamines, and others have been implicated (Table 13.1). Electrolyte disturbances like hypokalemia, hypocalcemia, and hypomagnesemia can also contribute to acquired QTc prolongation. In this case, the anti-arrhythmic sotalol that was prescribed 2 weeks prior is the likely cause. Sotalol is known to prolong the QT interval by blocking cardiac potassium channels, which are responsible for repolarization.

TABLE 13.1 **Common QTc Prolonging Medications**

Anesthetics	Sevoflurane, propofol
Anti-arrhythmic drugs	Type 1A: quinidine, procainamide Type 1C: flecainide Type 3: amiodarone, sotalol, ibulitide, dofetilide
Psychiatric drugs	Thioridazine, haloperidol, droperidol, amitriptyline, nortriptyline, lithium, ziprasidone, quetiapine, chlorpromazine
Antihistamine	Hydroxyzine, diphenhydramine, loratadine
Antibiotics	Aminoglycosides (gentamycin, tobramycin), macrolides (clarithromycin, azithromycin, erythromycin), fluoroquinolones (ciprofloxacin, moxifloxacin), sulfonamides (trimethoprim/sulfamethoxazole)
Anti-fungal	Fluconazole, voriconazole, ketoconazole
Anti-nausea	Ondansetron
Immunosuppressants	Tacrolimus
Antidepressants	Fluoxetine, escitalopram, trazodone
Others	Albuterol, terbutaline, methadone, furosemide, fosphenytoin, octreotide, famotidine

Another common setting of drug-induced QTc prolongation is antipsychotic use in the treatment of acute delirium and agitation. Typical anti-psychotics like haloperidol have had a clear association with both QTc prolongation and Tdp. However, newer atypical anti-psychotics like quetiapine and olanzapine have shown QTc prolongation but have not been linked to Tdp. Risks and benefits should be carefully evaluated on an individual basis before administering these medications.

Treatment

Primary management of QTc prolongation and Tdp consists of minimizing risk factors like alternative medications and correcting electrolyte abnormalities. Current recommendations encourage a baseline ECG before starting QTc prolonging drugs, then follow-up with repeat ECGs at some reasonable interval. In an acute care setting, an ECG should be checked more often (up to daily) as medications are being titrated quickly and multiple concomitant medications are started. Patients should also be educated to seek immediate medical help in case of palpitations, lightheadedness, dizziness, or syncope. In a hemodynamically stable patient with QTc prolongation, treatment should focus on discontinuing the possible offending medications and correcting electrolyte levels. Pro-arrhythmic situations are commonly precipitated when multiple QT prolonging drugs are combined.

Patients with Tdp and hemodynamic instability require emergent electrical cardioversion in conjunction with preventative measures. Treatment should be initiated with a bolus of magnesium sulfate (2 grams) to help stabilize the myocardium and can be repeated in case of persistent episodes. Hypomagnesemia, hypokalemia, hypocalcemia, and other electrolyte abnormalities should be corrected immediately. Medications such as isoproterenol or dobutamine can be used to help increase the heart rate, which decreases the repolarization time and decreases the QTc interval. In case of persistent Tdp, overdrive pacing using transcutaneous or transvenous pacemakers can be employed. Most Tdp cases should respond to pacing at 100–110 bpm, but case reports requiring up to 140 bpm have been noted. The next step in treatment should be to remove the offending drug, sometimes involving emergent hemodialysis. Especially in the case of an offending drug like sotalol where its half-life can range 7–18 hours, hemodialysis should be considered for refractory Tdp.

Tdp caused by QTc prolongation can be a fatal arrhythmia, and all efforts should focus on prevention and urgent treatment. Any patient requiring QTc prolonging medications should be monitored closely even in the ambulatory setting. In cases of congenital QTc prolongation, relatives of the patient should also be monitored with routine ECG. When patients do present with Tdp, they should receive immediate specialized care in order to reduce their morbidity and mortality.

CASE RESUMES

In the case presented, the patient was started on isoproterenol after the second occurrence of Tdp, while her electrolytes were optimized. She sustained a kidney injury during her out-of-hospital cardiac arrest, so when the

Tdp returned, the patient was placed on hemodialysis. After 2 hemodialysis treatments and 60 hours (approximately 5 half-lives) of sotalol, the isoproterenol was weaned and her QTc normalized. She made a full recovery and was discharged 7 days later, with plans to follow up with electrophysiology for her paroxysmal atrial fibrillation.

KEY POINTS TO REMEMBER

1. Torsades de pointes is a ventricular dysrhythmia that appears like a "twisting of points" of the cardiac axis, which is most often due to acquired QTc prolongation in the perioperative period, although numerous congenital forms exist.
2. Postoperatively, electrolyte abnormalities and drug classes such as anti-arrhythmics, antidepressants, antipsychotics, antibiotics, and antihistamines are common cause of acquired QTc prolongation.
3. Treatment includes defibrillation if unstable or 2 grams intravenous magnesium, if stable. This is followed by investigation and correction of other etiologies.

Suggested Reading
1. Yap YG, Camm AJ. Drug induced QT prolongation and torsades de pointes. *Heart*. 2003;89(11):1363–1372. doi:10.1136/heart.89.11.1363
2. Trinkley KE, Page RL, Lien H, Yamanouye K, Tisdale JE. QT interval prolongation and the risk of torsades de pointes: essentials for clinicians. *Curr Med Res Opin*. 2013;29(12):1719–1726. doi:10.1185/03007995.2013.840568
3. Isbister GK, Page CB. Drug induced QT prolongation: the measurement and assessment of the QT interval in clinical practice. *Br J Clin Pharmacol*. 2013;76(1):48–57. doi:10.1111/bcp.12040
4. Thomas SHL, Behr ER. Pharmacological treatment of acquired QT prolongation and torsades de pointes. *Br J Clin Pharmacol*. 2016;81(3):420–427. doi:10.1111/bcp.12726
5. van Uum SH, van den Merkhof LF, Lucassen AM, Wuis EW, Diemont W. Successful haemodialysis in sotalol-induced torsade de pointes in a patient with progressive renal failure. *Nephrol Dial Transplant*. 1997;12(2):331–333.
6. Glassman AH, Bigger JT. Antipsychotic drugs: prolonged QTc interval, torsade de pointes, and sudden death. *Am J Psychiatry*. 2001;158(11):1774–1782. doi:10.1176/appi.ajp.158.11.1774

14 Postoperative Ventricular Fibrillation

Gurbinder Singh and Natalia S. Ivascu

A 57-year-old woman with a long history of mitral valve prolapse and severe mitral regurgitation presents for an elective mitral valve repair. In the operating room, the surgery is uneventful except for "stunned myocardium." She requires milrinone and norepinephrine to separate from cardiopulmonary bypass. An hour after arriving in the intensive care unit the patient is awakening and appears relatively stable. She suddenly goes into ventricular fibrillation and becomes severely hypotensive. She receives a brief period of chest compressions and is defibrillated, which restores sinus rhythm. An echocardiogram (ECG) reveals a new lateral regional wall motion abnormality.

What do you do now?

DISCUSSION

Incidence

Arrhythmias are common after cardiac surgery. Atrial arrhythmias are by far the most common type of disturbance and are discussed in Chapter 12. Ventricular arrhythmias are far less frequent; however, they signify a more serious problem.

Types of Arrhythmia

Premature Ventricular Complexes

The most common ventricular arrhythmias are premature ventricular complexes (PVCs), which can occur in up to 34% of patients. Occasional PVCs are rarely harmful and may be related to tissue reperfusion or electrolyte abnormalities. High sympathetic tone and adrenergic medications are potential causes of PVCs. Frequent PVCs (>30 per hour) may be hemodynamically significant and require treatment (Figure 14.1).

Non-Sustained Ventricular Tachycardia

Non-sustained ventricular tachycardia (NSVT) is considered as 3 or more ventricular beats at a rate over 120 bpm but for a duration less than 30 seconds (Figure 14.2). In general, patients with frequent PVCs or even NSVTs do not have an increased risk of mortality. However, patients with reduced ejection fraction (<40%) and complex ventricular tachycardias (VTs) after surgery had an increased mortality rate as well as rate of sudden death .

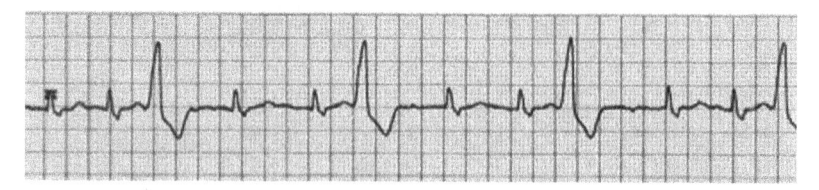

FIGURE 14.1 Example of premature ventricular complexes.

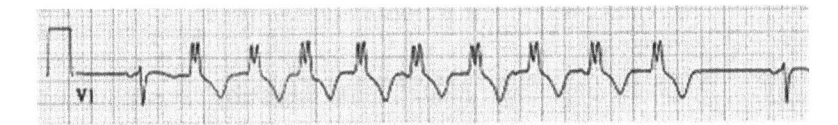

FIGURE 14.2 Example of non-sustained ventricular tachycardia (NSVT).

Ventricular Tachyarrhythmias (VT and Ventricular Fibrillation)

VT is defined as a rate >100 bpm with 3 or more ventricular complexes in a row that is sustained. Ventricular fibrillation is a form of complex ventricular arrhythmias and usually indicates a left ventricular problem (Figure 14.3). The incidence after cardiac surgery is estimated to be up to 1.4%, although this is based on relatively old data. The associated in-hospital mortality is up to 50%. It is notable that these data are mostly based on patients with coronary artery disease undergoing bypass surgery.

Mimickers of Ventricular Arrhythmias

At fast rates, VT may be difficult to distinguish from atrioventricular nodal re-entry tachycardia. The Brugada criteria describe a systematic approach to making this diagnosis as follows:

1. If all the QRS complexes are completely upward or completely downward (i.e., absence of RS complex in all precordial leads), diagnosis is VT.
2. If the R to S interval is >100 ms in any of the precordial leads, diagnosis is VT.
3. If atrioventricular dissociation is present (i.e., P waves occur at a different rate from QRS), diagnosis is VT.

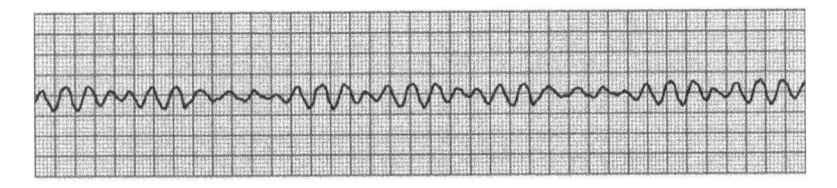

FIGURE 14.3 Example of ventricular fibrillation.

4. Morphologic criteria for QRS complexes in VT
    a. If QRS complex is upward in V1, then VT is the likely diagnosis if one of the following is present:
        i. A monophasic R or biphasic qR complex in V1
        ii. An RSR′ pattern ("bunny-ear") is present in V1, with the R peak being higher in amplitude than the R′ peak
        iii. An rS complex in lead V6
    b. If QRS complex is downward in V1, then VT is the likely diagnosis if one of the following is present:
        i. The presence of any Q or QS wave in lead V6
        ii. A wide R wave in lead V1 or V2 of 40 ms or more
        iii. Slurred or notched downstroke of the S wave in V1 or V2
        iv. Duration of onset of the QRS complex to peak of QS or S wave >60 ms

Etiology

There are many possible causes of ventricular arrhythmias in the perioperative period:

1. Ischemia
    a. Ventricular cells are extremely sensitive to changes in oxygen tension. Acute ischemia results in an immediate disturbance of the cardiac myocyte. During this time tissue excitability and automaticity are increased, and VT may be initiated. In the postoperative period, new-onset, complex ventricular arrhythmias should demand a thorough investigation for potential coronary ischemia.
2. Electrolyte abnormalities
    a. *Hypokalemia*: Potassium affects electrophysiologic properties of the heart. Hypokalemia increases resting membrane potential and increases both the duration of the action potential and the duration of the refractory period. This combination could lead to re-entrant arrhythmias. Hypokalemia also increases the threshold potential of the myocardium, which can lead to arrhythmias as well.

b. *Hyperkalemia*: Increases in the extracellular potassium concentration result in a decrease in the resting membrane potential and membrane threshold. This leads to an increased myocyte excitability by shifting the resting membrane potential to a less negative value and making the myocardium more prone to ventricular arrhythmias. However, as potassium levels continue to rise, myocyte depression occurs.

c. *Hypomagnesemia*: Magnesium depletion can manifest as tachycardia followed by severe arrhythmias and finally bradycardia. The ECG changes that can be seen are short PQ and QRS intervals, as well as shortening of the QT. In less severe magnesium depletion the ECG changes that occur are sinus tachycardia, high-peak T waves, and ST segment depression.

d. *Hypocalcemia*: Low calcium levels may lead to prolongation of the QT interval and precipitation of ventricular fibrillation. Mild hypocalcemia is generally well tolerated. Dysrhythmias are associated with severe hypocalcemia or an acute decrease in calcium.

3. Pulmonary artery catheters

   a. Several factors have been reported to lead to ventricular arrhythmias during the placement of a pulmonary artery catheter, including acidosis, hypoxia, electrolyte imbalance, and reduced ejection fraction. Long in-dwelling time has also been shown to increase incidence of arrhythmias. The development of arrhythmias during the placement might be caused by mechanical contact with the endocardium. Valvular disease is another significant risk factor for the arrhythmias during the placement. This is usually due to pulmonic valve stenosis or tricuspid valve regurgitation that can change the shape of the right ventricle. The enlargement of the right ventricle might increase the mechanical contact between the catheter and the endocardium during catheter placement and the propensity for arrhythmias to appear higher secondary to this.

4. Hypothermia and acid base abnormalities
   a. Hypothermia can lead to marked reduction in conduction velocity. If not counterbalanced by a proportional prolongation of the refractory period, this can lead to ventricular fibrillation and ventricular re-entrant tachycardia in patients who are prone to them.
   b. Metabolic acidosis makes myocardium susceptible to ventricular fibrillation by reducing the ventricular fibrillation threshold, whereas during metabolic alkalosis, the threshold for ventricular fibrillation is increased. Acidosis leads to intracellular potassium leaking out of the cells into the extracellular fluid, leading again to decreased action potential threshold and increased excitability in the myocardium.
5. Antiarrhythmic medications
   a. Antiarrhythmic therapy can paradoxically lead to ventricular tachyarrhythmias in patients who present with VT. Sudden deaths upon initiation of these medications have been reported. Decreased systolic function of the left ventricle is associated with an increased incidence of arrhythmogenicity from these medications. Therefore, patients who are being started on these antiarrhythmic medications need in-hospital cardiac monitoring during initiation of antiarrhythmic drug therapy for ventricular tachyarrhythmias.
6. Adrenergic medications and inotropes
   a. Milrinone and dobutamine are both associated with atrial and ventricular arrhythmias, due to increased intracellular calcium levels. Sympathomimetic drugs have also been associated with arrhythmias.
7. Pacing wires
   a. Temporary pacing wires are often placed during heart surgeries as these patients very frequently get blocked conduction pathways due to inflammation. The pacing wire is inserted directly into the myocardium on one end and to a temporary pacemaker on the other end. Any small electric current, which would otherwise be harmless, passing through these pacing wires could interfere with the natural electrical activity of the patient's heart and result in VT or even fibrillation. This is largely a theoretical risk as electrical

medical equipment are held to strict standards regarding the allowable leak of current, and devices in good condition should not pose a threat.

Treatment
1. Cardioversion and defibrillation
   a. Unstable arrhythmias should be treated with prompt electrical conversion or defibrillation. Cardioversion is a shock that is synchronized to the QRS complex, whereas defibrillation describes an asynchronous shock. Anterior–lateral pad placement is adequate.
   b. Biphasic defibrillators are preferred as they better compensate for thoracic impedance.
   c. For VT with a pulse, administer 120 J by a biphasic device as a *synchronized* shock (200 J by a monophasic device).
   d. For pulseless VT or ventricular fibrillation, administer 120–200 J by a biphasic device (360 J by a monophasic device).
   e. See Chapter 15 for further details.
2. Identification and treatment of ischemia
   a. Coronary artery bypass grafting:
      i. ECG should be carefully investigated for signs of ischemia. Diagnostic cardiac catheterization should be considered to determine anastomotic issues. A return to the operating room for graft revisions may be required. Alternatively, and/or additionally, intra-aortic balloon pump counterpulsation may be helpful in stabilizing coronary perfusion.
   b. Valvular surgery:
      i. Even patients with little to no preoperative coronary artery disease are at risk for air or particular embolization. Again, an emergent ECG is indicated. Discussion with the surgeon is helpful to determine other risk factors for a coronary problem. In aortic valve surgery or transcatheter aortic valve replacement, low-lying coronaries can be obstructed by the valvular apparatus. In mitral valve surgery, posterior stitches are placed within millimeters of the circumflex artery. Oversizing of the mitral prosthesis can also lead to compression of the circumflex artery.

c. Aortic root surgery:
   i. Aortic root replacement surgery requires reimplantation of the coronary ostia. These patients are at risk of coronary embolization. In addition, anatomic distortion may occur including twisting, kinking, or stretch. The latter phenomenon can occur when the artery cannot be adequately mobilized and is sewn to the aortic graft on tension. When the heart begins to beat, the artery can be stretched and narrowed. This has been described as looking like a Chinese finger trap.
3. Lidocaine
   a. Lidocaine should be administered as an intravenous push of 0.5–1 mg/kg. An infusion of 1–4 mg/min may be used for maintenance if effective. No more than 3 mg/kg/h should be administered. There is a risk of sedation and local anesthetic toxicity, particularly in high doses. If available, measurement of lidocaine level is recommended on a daily basis.
4. Amiodarone
   a. Amiodarone is often chosen for both VT and supraventricular tachycardias. In a postoperative patient a typical initial bolus is 150 mg, followed by an infusion of 1 mg/min for 18 hours and then 0.5 mg/min for 6 more hours. Additional boluses of 150 mg may be used for persistent arrhythmias.

CASE RESUMES

Ventricular arrhythmias coupled with a new regional wall motion abnormality should prompt investigation into coronary blood flow. The patient was taken to the catheter lab for coronary angiography. Decreased flow was detected in the circumflex artery. In this case the valve stiches caused narrowing of the circumflex artery, resulting in ischemia to the lateral wall. Myocardial ischemia is an important cause of ventricular arrhythmias. VT and/or ventricular fibrillation in a postoperative patient can be assumed to be due to ischemia until proven otherwise.

> **KEY POINTS TO REMEMBER**
> 1. Common causes of ventricular arrhythmias in the perioperative period include ischemia, electrolyte abnormalities, pulmonary artery catheter physical contact with bundles, hypothermia, metabolic acidosis and adrenergic medications.
> 2. Identification and treatment of ventricular ischemia should remain high priority until excluded as this is highest risk for mortality and can be correctable.
> 3. Other treatments of ventricular arrhythmias include management of identified etiologies, antiarrhythmic medications such as amiodarone and lidocaine and defibrillation.

Suggested Reading
1. Pinto RP, Romerill DB, Nasser WK, Schier JJ, Surawicz B. Prognosis of patients with frequent premature ventricular complexes and non-sustained ventricular tachycardia after coronary artery bypass graft surgery. *Clin Cardiol*. 1996;19(4):321–324.
2. Huikuri HV, Yli-Mäyry S, Korhonen UR, et al. Prevalence and prognostic significance of complex ventricular arrhythmias after coronary arterial bypass graft surgery. *Int J Cardiol*. 1990;27(3):333–339.
3. Sapin PM, Woelfel AK, Foster JR. Unexpected ventricular tachyarrhythmias soon after cardiac surgery. *Am J Cardiol*. 1991;68(10):1099–1100.
4. Verckei A. Current algorithms for the diagnosis of wide QRS complex tachycardias. *Curr Cardiol Rev*. 2014;10(3):262–276.

15 Advanced Cardiovascular Life Support Post–Cardiac Surgery

Caryl Bailey and Michael Faulkner

A 76-year-old female underwent open aortic valve replacement and 2 coronary artery bypass grafts. On arrival to the intensive care unit (ICU), she is supported with norepinephrine 3 µg/min and paced via epicardial wires in DDD mode for post-bypass complete heart block. Four hours later, the patient suddenly develops ventricular fibrillation. The pacing wires are disconnected to confirm the patient's underlying rhythm. Transcutaneous pads are placed, and an unsynchronized shock is delivered, which results in asystole. The pacemaker is reattached, but despite pacing spikes and a QRS waveform, there is no pulsatile waveform noted on the arterial or pulmonary artery tracings. The pacemaker is again paused, and ventricular fibrillation is noted on the monitor.

What do you do now?

DISCUSSION

This patient has suffered a post–cardiac surgery cardiac arrest. Annually, there are over 250 000 cardiac surgeries performed in the United States, of which the quoted incidence of post–cardiac surgery cardiac arrest varies from 0.7% to 8%. Approximately half of these patients will survive to hospital discharge, in contrast to the quoted 24.8% success rate of overall in-hospital arrest and resuscitation. The difference in outcomes is attributable to the frequency of reversible causes in the postoperative group.

The American Heart Association's advanced cardiovascular life support (ACLS) guidelines do not specifically address cardiac arrest in post–cardiac surgery patients (Figure 15.1). It has become recognized that post–cardiac surgery patients have multiple characteristics which require different resuscitation strategies from those used in other patient populations. In 2009, the European Association of Cardiothoracic Surgeons provided recommendations for the management of post–cardiac surgery arrest, which have since been augmented by publication of consensus guidelines from the European Resuscitation Council in 2015 and the Society of Thoracic Surgeons in 2017. These guidelines are preferred over traditional ACLS for cardiac arrest resuscitation of post–cardiac surgery patients.

In the immediate postoperative period, cardiac surgery patients have invasive monitors in situ including an arterial line, a central venous catheter, and/or a pulmonary artery catheter. Additionally, they have continuous electrocardiography (ECG), pulse oximetry, and often capnography monitoring. Abnormalities in these monitors often immediately trigger monitor alarms, and the loss of waveforms in multiple measurement modalities is usually sufficient to confirm cardiac arrest and rapid initiation of resuscitation. Additional confirmation by palpation of a pulse before commencing treatment is not required unless there is suspected monitor failure. As a first intervention, it is recommended that pre-arrest infusions be stopped, to prevent inadvertent administration of vasoactive medications. Special attention should be paid to stop sedative medications, which are often vasodilatory. The risk of patient awareness in this setting is low.

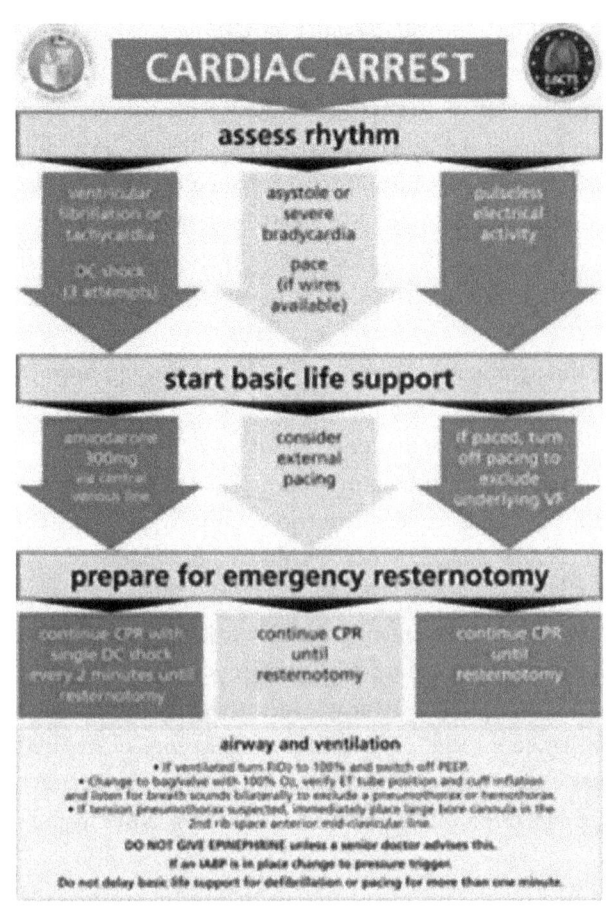

FIGURE 15.1 "Consensus Guidelines from the European Resuscitation Council in 2015 and the Society of Thoracic Surgeons in 2017."

Ventricular Fibrillation

Ventricular fibrillation is the cause of 25%–50% of cardiac arrests in post–cardiac surgery patients. Treatment of this rhythm in the post–cardiac surgery patient differs from that in standard ACLS in at least a couple of significant ways. Chest compressions in this patient are deferred until defibrillation had been attempted. Guidelines recommend up to 3 attempted shocks prior to external cardiac massage (ECM) if they can be delivered within 1 minute of arrest. Early defibrillation is often successful in this population and minimizes potential intrathoracic trauma from ECM on a fresh sternotomy. Three stacked shocks are recommended prior to resternotomy due to the decreasing efficacy with successive shocks. The chance of successful defibrillation goes from 78% to 35% and 14% for each successive shock. If return of spontaneous circulation (ROSC) cannot be achieved, then the team should prepare for resternotomy in the ICU. At this point ECM with a firm backboard in place should be instituted and continue with as little interruption as possible while reopening the chest incision.

One of the theoretical concerns of ECM is bleeding; however, massive hemorrhage is relatively uncommon. The overall risk of post-ECM injury in noncardiac surgical populations include an 8.9% risk of pericardial injury, a 15% risk of sternal fracture, and a 32% risk of rib fractures. Other types of injury occur much less frequently. Automatic external compression devices should not be used on post–cardiac surgical patients.

Another deviation from traditional ACLS is the cautious use of epinephrine in post–cardiac surgery arrest. There is little evidence that routine use of epinephrine boluses improves outcomes. In addition, at the time of ROSC, circulating epinephrine may result in significant and sudden hypertension, which could lead to bleeding or dehiscence of the fresh vascular anastomoses. Epinephrine, if used, should be limited as directed by a senior physician, preferably titrated in small 10–30 mcg doses in the peri-arrest period.

Bradycardia and Asystole

As with most post–cardiac surgery patients, this patient had epicardial pacing leads placed during surgery. In patients with severe bradycardia or asystole, the pacer should be set to emergency mode, which provides dual-chamber (when atrial and ventricular wires are present), asynchronous pacing at 80–100 bpm with maximum atrial and ventricular amperage. If pacing does not produce a pulse, it should be briefly paused to evaluate the rhythm for fine ventricular fibrillation, which may not be noticed while asynchronously pacing. In the event of mechanical failure to capture despite maximal current amplitude, all connections should carefully be checked. If any part of the metal pacing lead is in contact with another metallic surface, the circuit of electricity will not pass through the heart. Failure to capture can also be due to internal lead dislodgement or pulseless electrical activity (PEA) arrest. If a pulse cannot be restored with pacing within 1 minute of arrest, ECM should be initiated. Transcutaneous pacing can also be utilized, but due to longer setup time, it is typically commenced after ECM has been started.

PEA

This rhythm is also common in the post–cardiac surgery patient. If there is a perfusing rhythm on ECG but all waveforms are absent, then the arrest algorithm should be activated. If the patient was paced prior to the arrest and the rhythm is PEA, the pacemaker should be paused or disconnected to exclude underlying ventricular fibrillation. As with traditional ACLS, the "Hs and Ts" can serve as a guide to the potential etiology of the arrest (Table 15.1). If ROSC is not immediately restored, timely resternotomy (within 5 minutes) improves outcome. The incidence of tamponade or active bleeding as the underlying cause for arrest is obviously higher in the patient population, so resternotomy may treat the underlying etiology as well as improve perfusion during resuscitation. Non-ventricular fibrillation/ventricular tachycardia arrest portends a worse prognosis in the post–cardiac surgery patient.

Cardiac Arrest with Intra-aortic Balloon Pump In Situ

There are special considerations for PEA cardiac arrest occurring in the presence of an intra-aortic balloon pump (IABP). If the IABP is set to an ECG trigger in the presence of a pacemaker or PEA, a waveform can still be produced. Circulatory arrest is confirmed by noting loss of the cardiac

TABLE 15.1 **Causes of PEA Arrest: Hs and Ts**

Hypovolemia	Tamponade
Hypoxia	Tension pneumothorax
H+ ions (acidosis)	Thrombosis (myocardial infarction)
Hypo-/hyperkalemia	Thrombosis (massive pulmonary embolism)
Hypothermia	Toxins

component of the IABP tracing or flattening of the waveform in other monitoring modalities. It is useful to pause the IABP for confirmation. During chest compressions, the IABP should be switched to a pressure trigger with 1:1 counterpulsation and maximum augmentation so that there can be reliable diastolic inflation to improve coronary and cerebral perfusion and mean arterial pressure. In a period of no cardiac massage, the IABP can be set to an internal trigger, which will provide asynchronous pulsation without any trigger.

Resternotomy

Resternotomy within 5 minutes is recommended when resuscitation after cardiac arrest has been unsuccessful or when cardiac arrest from tamponade is highly likely. Resternotomy can directly relieve symptoms from tamponade or tension pneumothorax as well as allow for internal cardiac massage. Compared with chest compressions, internal cardiac massage has been shown to provide better coronary and organ perfusion pressure, increased rates of ROSC, a better survival rate, and the ability to reinstitute cardiopulmonary bypass if needed. Emergency resternotomy should be performed by trained personnel, and the support staff in the ICU needs to be appropriately trained for this possibility. A simple resternotomy set should be readily available. Emergency bedside resternotomy beyond postoperative day 10 should be decided on a case-by-case basis by a senior surgeon, given the increased risk of complications due to adhesions. Resternotomy is indicated in 20%–50% of post–cardiac surgery arrests, and as such, once a cardiac arrest is called, the resternotomy team should gown and glove to reduce the time to resternotomy if it becomes indicated.

Airway Considerations

As in this case, the potential for airway or respiratory compromise as the cause of cardiac arrest must be considered. A focused examination to assess airway patency, endotracheal tube position, and air entry to rule out tension pneumothorax as the cause of the arrest should be performed. Airway management is the same as for conventional ACLS guidelines: 100% oxygen via bag valve mask should be administered at a rate of 8–10 breaths per minute in the absence of an advanced airway or a ratio of 2 breaths to every 30 compressions for non-intubated patients. Confirmation of end tidal CO_2 is appropriate, with the caveat that in the setting of arrest the number may be low. Manual ventilation to assess compliance is useful. In the absence of concerns over a primary respiratory problem, the patient can be placed back on the ventilator with attention paid to increasing the fraction of inspired oxygen to 100% and removing positive end-expiratory pressure in order to promote venous return. Pneumothorax, tension or otherwise, can be addressed in the traditional fashion: needle decompression and thoracostomy tube placement.

Cardiac arrest after cardiac surgery requires specialized, protocolized care. Cardiac surgery ICUs should have policies in place to deal with these relatively frequent, potentially catastrophic scenarios. Drills and competency tests regarding these treatment protocols should be regularly practiced by personnel working in post–cardiac surgery care units.

Important modifications to the traditional American Heart Association's ACLS algorithm in the post–cardiac surgery patient are as follows:

- Ventricular fibrillation—2 stacked shocks before starting chest compressions (within 1 minute)
- Ventricular fibrillation—perform resternotomy after the third shock
- Judicious use of epinephrine due to hypertension with ROSC
- Resternotomy within 5 minutes

CASE RESUMES

The patient is given a small doses (10µg) of epinephrine intravenously while defibrillator pads are attached to the patient. ECM ensues as the patches are being placed and the defibrillator is prepared. A total of 3 separate shocks were delivered without success and the patient remained in ventricular fibrillation. The cardiac surgical team arrived and reopened the patient's sternotomy while in the intensive care unit. The patient was noted to have a kinked coronary graft that was revised at bedside with return of sinus rhythm. The patient's chest was closed and the rest of the hospital course was uneventful.

KEY POINTS TO REMEMBER

1. Defibrillation before chest compressions if can be performed within 1 minute of arrest
2. Use of epicardial pacer in asystole or symptomatic bradycardia
3. Avoidance of full dose epinephrine
4. Resternotomy and internal cardiac massage if resuscitation unsuccessful after 5 minutes

Suggested Reading
1. Society of Thoracic Surgeons Task Force on Resuscitation After Cardiac Surgery. The Society of Thoracic Surgeons Expert Consensus for the resuscitation of patients who arrest after cardiac surgery. *Ann Thorac Surg*. 2017;103:1005–1020.
2. Truhlar A, Deakin CD, Soar J, et al. European Resuscitation Council guidelines for resuscitation and emergency cardiovascular care. *Resuscitation*. 2015;95:148–201.
3. Dunning J, Fabbri A, Kolh PH, et al. Guideline for resuscitation in cardiac arrest after cardiac surgery. *Eur J Cardiothorac Surg*. 2009;36:3–28.

16 Critical Case of Aortic Stenosis

Rebecca Lee and Natalia S. Ivascu

A 91-year-old female with a past medical history of diabetes mellitus, chronic kidney disease stage II, hypertension, mild chronic obstructive pulmonary disease, mitral valve repair 12 years prior, and known aortic stenosis (AS) presents with increasing shortness of breath and dyspnea on exertion for the last several months. Transthoracic echocardiography (TTE) reveals severe AS.

Given her comorbidities, age, and history of previous cardiac surgery, she was deemed a high surgical risk but a suitable candidate for transcutaneous aortic valve replacement. She undergoes transaortic valve replacement (TAVR) under monitored anesthesia care. Intraoperative TTE shows a mild paravalvular leak. Shortly after arrival to the intensive care unit (ICU), her heart rate slows to 42. An electrocardiogram demonstrates complete heart block with a ventricular escape rhythm. Her blood pressure is 80/40, blood oxygen saturation is 92% on 4 L nasal cannula, and she feels nauseated and lightheaded.

What do you do now?

DISCUSSION

TAVR: Postoperative Management/Pitfalls

AS affects 2%–9% of the population older than 60 years, with degenerative calcification as the most common etiology. Surgical intervention is typically unnecessary in asymptomatic patients, but severe AS warrants evaluation for treatment. Traditionally, surgical aortic valve repair (SAVR) was the definitive intervention. Prior to the introduction of TAVR, balloon aortic valvuloplasty (BAV) was the minimally invasive therapeutic choice for patients who could not tolerate open replacement. BAV may improve hemodynamics but carries an unacceptably high incidence of restenosis and a risk of new aortic insufficiency. TAVR now provides a minimally invasive alternative which diminishes many of the risks associated with cardiopulmonary bypass while still providing a durable solution that BAV does not.

The patient described in the case represents many of the considerations made when a patient is considered for TAVR versus open SAVR. Her age, multiple comorbidities including chronic obstructive pulmonary disease (COPD), severe AS with worsening symptoms, and previous sternotomy make TAVR a better option than SAVR. Although the risks of cardiopulmonary bypass are avoided, there are still significant severe risks associated with this minimally invasive approach which should be considered postoperatively, as outlined in Table 16.1.

In 2013, the PARTNER (Placement of AoRTic TraNscathetER Valve Trial) 1A showed non-inferiority of TAVR to SAVR with regard to mortality, whereas the PARTNER IB trial showed significantly lower mortality rates with TAVR compared to medical treatment, 71.8% versus 93.6%. Additionally, investigators showed that SAVR had a higher incidence of major bleeding and new-onset atrial fibrillation, while TAVR showed a higher risk of vascular complications. The SURTAVI trial in 2016 demonstrated that patients who underwent TAVR had greater valve areas and lower aortic gradients up to 2 years post-intervention compared to SAVR. Additionally, they were able to show non-inferiority to SAVR in regard to the primary endpoints of death and disabling stroke.

Although the eligibility of TAVR has been broadened to intermediate- and low-risk groups, it has been suggested that relative contraindications to TAVR include myocardial infarction within the previous month,

TABLE 16.1 **Major Post-TAVR Pitfalls**

System		Comments
Cardiac	Arrhythmias (complete heart block, atrial fibrillation)	· May be asymptomatic, in some cases cause hemodynamic instability · Detected on EKG · May require PPM · May require temporary transvenous or transcutaneous pacing
	Paravalvular leak	· May require surgical intervention or valve re-expansion · Typically diagnosed intraoperative by echocardiography
	Myocardial infarction	· Rare, secondary to valve position over coronary ostia
	Aortic root rupture	· May be signs of severe arterial bleeding, tamponade, severe left ventricular myocardial failure
Neurologic	Stroke	· Can be acute or late presentation; most common embolic to MCA
Vascular	Bleeding	· Typically due to access; major vessel damage is rare but can include dissections or ruptures
Pulmonary	Minimal	· Increased with general anesthesia and transapical approach · Increased risk with COPD
Renal	Acute renal injury, renal failure	· Secondary to contrast and/or hemodynamic fluctuations. Increased risk with baseline CKD

CKD, chronic kidney disease; EKG, electrocardiogram; MCA, middle cerebral artery.

congenital unicuspid or bicuspid valve, mixed aortic stenosis with regurgitation, hypertrophic cardiomyopathy, ejection fraction <20%, native annulus size greater than manufacturer's recommended range, severe vascular disease, cerebrovascular accident in last 6 months, and emergent surgery. Preoperative considerations include computed tomographic (CT) imaging to ensure proper positioning, TTE, and vascular studies.

Intraoperatively, the provider should have blood products available, large-bore access, an arterial line, TEE if under general anesthesia (GA) to evaluate for perivalvular leak (PVL), and radiolucent defibrillator pads. Monitored anesthesia care with TTE can be performed for transfemoral TAVR, whereas GA with TEE is the typical approach for alternative access procedures.

Valve Options

The Medtronic CoreValve was a first-generation self-expanding, trileaflet, porcine pericardial tissue with a nitinol frame deployed via the transfemoral approach. Its placement did not require ventricular pacing to deploy, allowing the left ventricle to eject during deployment; however, the self-expanding nature of the valve led to arrhythmias postoperatively. The Medtronic Evolut R is a resheathable valve, which allows for repositioning, with a reduced prosthetic height while preserving the dimensions of the pericardial skirt. This design is reported to decrease the risk of permanent pacemaker (PPM) placement while also decreasing PVL and eliminating some of the bulky delivery system and need for additional sheaths. The Evolut R is available in sizes up to 34 mm, making it the largest TAVR available. The Evolut Pro is the latest valve from Medtronic, with an external pericardial wrap which decreases the risk of prosthetic valve regurgitation while retaining features of the Evolut R. Edwards' first generation of TAVR, the Sapien, is a balloon-expandable, trileaflet, bovine pericardial tissue valve attached to a stainless steel frame with either transfemoral or transapical deployment. Rapid ventricular pacing during deployment is required, to reduce cardiac output to essentially zero and to establish a motionless field. After deployment, the valve is further expanded with a balloon. Newer models from Edwards, the Sapient XT and Sapien 3, can be deployed through transapical, transfemoral, transaxillary, and transaortic approaches. The Sapien 3 design contains an outer sealing skirt to achieve better circularity, although there is an increased risk of arrhythmias postoperatively as seen with earlier Medtronic models. Boston Scientific has produced the Lotus system, which is a self-expanding, fully recapturable and repositionable valve made of trileaflet bovine pericardial tissue with an adaptive seal at the inflow segment.

Postprocedure Arrhythmias

Cardiac arrhythmias, in particular complete heart block, are not uncommon postoperatively; and risk factors include a bundle branch block baseline as well as large left atrial size. In some cases a PPM is required. The rate of PPM placement has increased as subsequent generations of valves were redesigned to lessen PVL. The original Edwards Sapien valve had a 1.8%–8.5% risk of PPM, whereas the Sapien 3, with an expanding skirt, has a reported PPM rate up to 10.2%. Medtronic's Core Valve, with the original expanding skirt design, has a reported 19.1%–42.5% risk of PPM. Although studies ultimately showed that mortality did not increase in patients with PPM post-TAVR/SAVR, they showed an increased duration of hospitalization and rehospitalization as well as an increased risk of complications from PPM such as pocket hematoma, pneumothorax, pocket erosion, lead infection, endocarditis, lead failure, and lead-induced tricuspid regurgitation and right ventricular perforation. Furthermore, PPMs require generator replacement every 10 years, making the risk less acceptable for younger patients. Atrial fibrillation was seen in up to 32% of patients after TAVR, however less than in SAVR in PARTNER 2A. Wires for rapid pacing can be left postoperatively as significant hemodynamic instability may occur intraoperatively due to rapid ventricular pacing. The patient described in this case is at an increased risk for arrhythmias and complete heart block, given her underlying right bundle branch block and implantation of an expanding valve. While she may likely require a PPM emergently, given her symptoms she can be paced with transvenous pacing wires if placed through the 6Fr introducer or transcutaneously.

PVL

The incidence of PVL with first-generation valves was up to 60% greater with TAVR than SAVR. Moderate or severe PVL is associated with increased mortality at 30 days, although rates of PVL are now much lower with the Lotus valve, Direct Flow, and Sapien 3. Predictors for PVL include valve undersizing, which is improved with left ventricular outflow measured from CT versus conventional echocardiogram. Device malpositioning can lead to PVL as there can be incomplete valve contact to native aortic annulus, as seen in cases of excessive calcification. PVL can be identified by echocardiography, although it often regresses by a significant degree in the first 5–10 minutes post-deployment. If the PVL remains significant, the valve may require re-expansion, which can be done by using the same balloon-in-valve technique to upsize and further stretch the valve's annular size. More advanced maneuvers include retrograde transcatheter PVL closure with plug or the deployment of a second TAVR. Risks of re-expansion include disruption of aortic valvular calcifications, coronary obstruction, and aortic root rupture. Aortic root rupture is a morbid complication of TAVR, seen more commonly in balloon-expanding valves, with heavy calcified device landing zones (aortic root) and overestimated sized valves. The signs of rupture include massive arterial bleeding, tamponade, left ventricular failure/rupture, and myocardial failure due to coronary artery compromise. Newer generations have less risk of PVL due to various designs, such as the Edwards Sapien 3 self-expansion and Medtronic Evolut R improved radial force.

Neurological Injuries

The major neurologic concern in TAVR is stroke. Initially, the incidence was found to be higher post-TAVR than in surgical cases. Distribution of the stroke is typically middle cerebral, posterior circulation, and embolic in nature. Acute stroke predictors after TAVR include ballooning post-dilatation and valve dislodgement, whereas late stroke predictors include advanced age, chronic atrial fibrillation, history of stroke, transient ischemic attack, and peripheral vascular disease/coronary artery disease. In the PARTNER trials, the incidence of stroke in TAVR was greater than that in SAVR (5.4% versus 2.4% at 30 days, 8.3% versus 4.3% at 1 year). Cerebral protection devices such as the Sentinel device have gained popularity, although variable study results have not shown any reduction in postoperative stroke. Some have advocated for anticoagulation, either single or dual antiplatelet therapy, on postoperative day 1 to reduce the incidence of embolic stroke.

Additional neurological complications include delirium, although this was not specifically studied in the PARTNER trials. In retrospective studies, delirium was worse with the transapical approach, with longer surgical times leading to longer ICU stays. Delirium should be treated as if present in any other postsurgical patients. Pain is also traditionally less with TAVR as it avoids sternotomy; however, patients can have significant pain after a transapical approach and may benefit from an epidural for pain control.

Many patients who would otherwise not tolerate GA for SAVR due to underlying pulmonary comorbidities are candidates for TAVR. Up to 41% had COPD in the original PARTNER trials, with these patients having an increased risk of pulmonary complications, including reintubation with the transapical approach. Avoiding sternotomy pain and prolonged anesthesia time is ideal in patients with pulmonary disease, although, as with SAVR, there could be a risk of pulmonary edema secondary to fluid resuscitation from left ventricular hypertrophy and diastolic dysfunction.

Vascular Complications

Vascular complications from TAVR include bleeding, although the risk is statistically lower compared to SAVR. Vascular injury is the most common, with a rate of up to 30% of patients in the PARTNER trials, 16% of whom had major complications often requiring surgical intervention. Most bleeding is due to access issues, and although rupture and dissection are uncommon, femoral or iliac dissection, retroperitoneal bleed, and femoral pseudoaneurysm do occur. Clinicians should suspect retroperitoneal bleed with refractory hypotension in patients with transfemoral or attempted transfemoral access. Risk factors for vascular complications are increased with a larger sheath to artery ratio, presence of circumferential calcification, severe tortuosity, and percutaneous preclosure device failure. Female gender, use of a 19Fr system, peripheral artery disease, and early stages of the learning curve are also considered increased risks. There is a significant decrease in bleeding/vascular complications with smaller delivery systems, as seen with the Sapien 3 and with accumulating operator experience and proper removal of the femoral arterial sheath with pressure.

Catastrophes from TAVR are rare but include aortic dissection or perforation, left ventricular rupture, rupture of aortic root/annulus, mitral valve apparatus injury, and cardiac tamponade. Additionally, coronary obstruction with subsequent myocardial infarction can occur due to occlusion of coronary ostia as a consequence of valve positioning. The risk of myocardial infarction is increased with valve in valve procedures (3.5% versus 0.7%)

and high implantation; however, the risk of PPM is less with valve in valve. Valve migration is a rare, but catastrophic, event.

TAVR increases the risks for acute kidney injury (AKI) and renal failure in patients with higher baseline creatinine, contrast load, and blood transfusions. Additional risk factors include low ejection fraction, age, female sex, diabetes mellitus, hypertension, and prolonged hypotension. The PROTECT-TAVI study showed a decreased incidence of AKI after furosemide-induced diuresis compared to normal saline alone (5.4% versus 25%).

The financial benefits of TAVR are not yet clear. Although supplies and education are more costly with TAVR, there is decreased length of stay and surgical time. However, if the patient requires PPM placement, the stay is increased, including ICU stay, and there is decreased reimbursement for TAVR.

TAVR, although initially approved for severe symptomatic AS, is now being broadened to intermediate- and low-risk patients. As the patient eligibility expands, clinicians will be expected to care for these patients postoperatively and should be aware of the risks of TAVR, the postoperative complications, and how to treat them.

CASE RESUMES

As the patient was having symptomatic bradycardia, an introducer and a transvenous pacing wire was urgently placed. The patient was paced at 80 beats per minute and symptoms resolved. She was evaluated for a permanent pacemaker the following morning with a turn down study of her pacemaker. She then had a junctional rhythm at 48 beats per minute and the decision to place a permanent pacemaker was made. She was discharged home following this placement.

KEY POINTS TO REMEMBER

1. Arrhythmias and high-degree heart block are not uncommon, especially with self-expanding valves. In those cases PPM may be needed.

2. Stroke is still a devastating complication of TAVR and a higher risk than in SAVR, despite the development of cerebral protection devices and advancements of valves.
3. It is important to be aware of TAVR complications as indications are being expanded to lower-risk patients.

Suggested Reading
1. Tuck BC, Townsley MM. Anesthetic management for the surgical and interventional treatment of aortic vavlular heart disease. In: Gravlee GP, Shaw AD, Bartels K, eds. *Hensley's Practical Approach to Cardiothoracic Anesthesia*. 6th ed. Philadelphia, PA: Lippincott Williams & Wilkins; 2019:345–367.
2. Mahtta D, Elgendy IY, Bavry AA. From CoreValve to Evolut PRO: Reviewing the journey of self-expanding transcatheter aortic valves. *Cardiol Ther*. 2017;6(2):183–192. doi:10.1007/s40119-017-0100-z
3. Raiten JM, Gutsche JT, Horak J, Augoustides JG. Critical care management of patients following transcatheter aortic valve replacement. *F1000Res*. 2013;2:62. doi:10.3410/f1000research.2-62.v1
4. Terré JA, George I, Smith CR. Pros and cons of transcatheter aortic valve implantation (TAVI). *Ann Cardiothorac Surg*. 2017;6(5): 444–452. doi:10.21037/acs.2017.09.15

17 Robotic Mitral Valve Surgery and Unilateral Pulmonary Edema

Cindy Cheung and Christopher W. Tam

A 51-year-old man with a history of mitral regurgitation presented with progressive dyspnea. Transesophageal echocardiogram (TEE) demonstrated severe mitral regurgitation with P2 and P3 posterior leaflet prolapse and left ventricular (LV) ejection fraction of 50%–55%. His preoperative cardiac catheterization demonstrated pulmonary hypertension with a pulmonary artery pressure of 63/24.

He subsequently underwent a robotic mitral valve repair and tricuspid valve repair. Cardiac bypass time was noted to be 196 minutes; aortic cross-clamp time was 123 minutes. Post-bypass TEE demonstrated a decreased ejection fraction by 40% with global LV hypokinesis and a cardiac index of >2.5 L/min/m^2. Shortly after arrival in the intensive care unit, the patient is noted to have copious amounts of frothy secretions in the endotracheal tube with difficulty obtaining adequate tidal volumes with mechanical ventilation. Chest X-ray immediately postoperation demonstrated new right-sided pulmonary edema.

What do you do now?

DISCUSSION

Robotic or minimally invasive mitral valve surgery was pioneered in 1998 by Carpentier and Mohr et al. to be the less invasive approach to sternotomy-based mitral valve operations. When compared to the traditional sternotomy approach, robotic mitral valve operations have known advantages of shorter hospital length of stay despite longer cross-clamp and bypass times, reduced blood loss, reduced packed red blood cell transfusions, expedited recovery for patients, and more favorable cosmetic results. It is performed with one lung ventilation with a double-lumen endotracheal tube or bronchial blocker, through a right-sided chest approach. Small working port incisions are made in the intercostal spaces, and cannulation for cardiopulmonary bypass is done peripherally, typically through the femoral vein or artery and superior vena cava. Patients undergoing robotic valve surgery carry a similar risk of complications that may occur with traditional median sternotomy surgery; however, minimally invasive valve surgeries have their own inherent complications associated with cardiac access, perfusion, and ventilation methods used in robotic surgeries. Unilateral pulmonary edema is an uncommon but potentially life-threatening complication of robotic mitral valve surgery (see Figures 17.1 and 17.2).

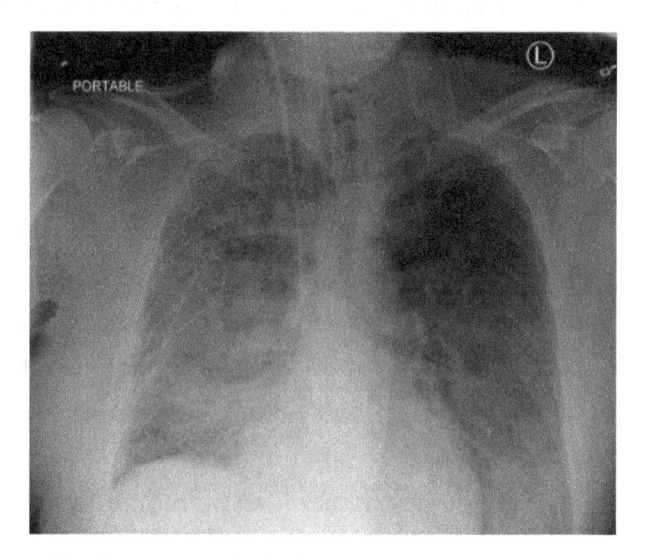

FIGURE 17.1 Chest X-ray postoperative day 0.

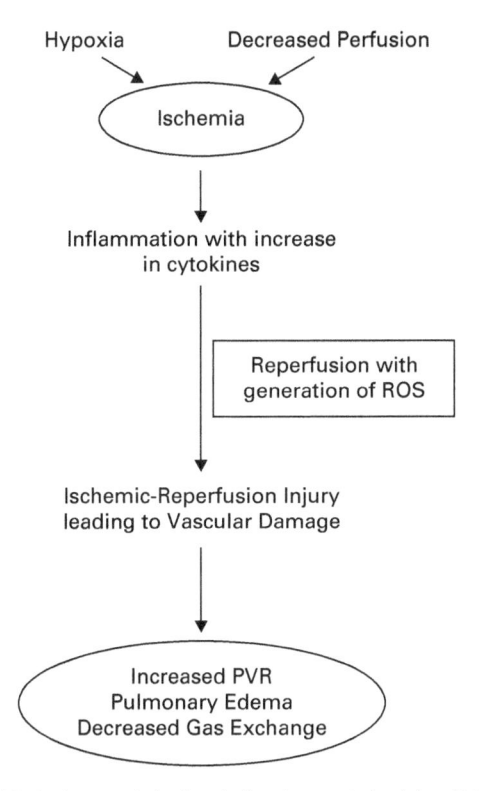

FIGURE 17.2 Physiologic changes during lung ischemia–reperfusion injury. PVR, pulmonary vascular resistance; ROS, reactive oxygen species.

Incidence

The incidence of unilateral lung injury, which commonly manifests as unilateral pulmonary edema (UPE), has been reported to be quite variable, between 2.1% and 25%. The variation in incidence could be related to the difference in patient populations, diagnostic criteria, as well management. Clinical presentation of severe right lung pulmonary edema may occur within the first several minutes to hours after prolonged periods of cardiopulmonary bypass (CPB). Common clinical manifestations that have been described include straw-colored fluid from the right main stem bronchus, hypercapnia and/or profound hypoxia from increased shunting, pulmonary hypertension, and hemodynamic instability requiring vasoactive and inotropic support.

Etiology

The pathophysiology of UPE associated with robotic mitral valve repair remains unclear. UPE can occur after re-expansion of a collapsed lung from a pleural effusion or pneumothorax but is seldom seen with video-assisted thoracoscopic surgeries where one-lung ventilation is utilized. This suggests that UPE during minimally invasive cardiac surgery cannot be singly explained by re-expansion edema from one lung ventilation. The cause of UPE is most likely multifactorial and can result from pulmonary artery venting, the temperature of insufflated CO_2, mean arterial pressure on bypass, and ischemia–reperfusion injury, although data are currently limited. Ischemic injury can occur whenever the lung parenchyma receives less oxygen supply than demand, and during CPB the lung parenchyma is largely dependent on bronchial arterial flow through collaterals. Bronchial arterial flow on CPB is dependent on systemic blood pressure, which can be influenced by anatomic and physiologic factors. If pulmonary parenchymal ischemia is severe or prolonged, subsequent reperfusion may result in the activation of multiple cellular mechanisms of injury, leading to breakdown of the alveolar capillary membrane integrity, alveolar edema, and release of humoral mediators of inflammation.

In a recent study evaluating 256 patients post–minimally invasive valve surgery, Renner and colleagues found that the 51 patients who developed right-sided pulmonary edema had a preoperative increases of C-reactive protein, suggesting an inflammatory disposition for UPE. Lung collapse and atelectasis, as seen during unilateral lung isolation, have been shown to be associated with the sequestration of polymorphonuclear leukocytes. Rapid release of reactive oxygen species, also known as *respiratory burst*, and inflammatory responses are triggered when oxygen is supplied during re-expansion and reperfusion of the lung. CPB can also contribute to the inflammatory response. Other causes of pulmonary injury, such as aspiration, barotrauma, and infection, have been largely ruled out. Notably, UPE is not seen during mitral valve repairs through the standard median sternotomy approach. Keyl and colleagues reported a reduced incidence of UPE with perioperative steroid administration, which supports the ischemia–reperfusion injury hypothesis because the administration of steroids is known to attenuate inflammatory cellular pathways after ischemia–reperfusion in animal models.

Prevention and Management

The current literature suggests that UPE can be prevented by shorter CPB times, avoiding barotrauma, limiting blood product transfusion, and minimizing lung isolation times. Lung preventive ventilation, such as low-level positive pressure and frequent alveolar recruitment, while on CPB may be beneficial. Avoiding recurrent atelectasis and reopening or lung overexpansion have been noted to reduce the inflammation. Administration of steroids to attenuate ischemia–reperfusion injury can be helpful (one study suggested dexamethasone approximately 1 mg/kg body weight), although there are limited data on optimal dosing.

In a recent study, Moss et al. implemented a modified technique during robotic valve surgeries which included targeting a lower systemic temperature while on bypass (30°C) to decrease the oxygen demand of lung parenchyma, limiting rotation of the patient with elevation of the right lung above the aorta to prevent decreases in perfusion due to gravity, discontinuation of vasodilator agents preoperatively, and targeting mean systemic blood pressure on CPB of at least >10 mm Hg higher than the standard technique (average 67 mm Hg) to maintain lung parenchyma perfusion during CPB. This modified technique ($n = 142$) group did not have any cases of UPE in comparison to the 15 cases of UPE in the standard technique group ($n = 269$), and this was shown to be statistically significant.

Treatment

Treatment for UPE is dependent on the severity of symptoms. Conservative management is recommended for mild cases, with escalation in respiratory support such as non-invasive positive pressure ventilation or mechanical ventilation with increasing symptom severity. Extracorporeal membrane oxygenation or high-frequency jet ventilation has been required for severe cases of UPE. There are reports supporting asynchronous differential lung ventilatory management with resolution of symptoms. The benefits of diuretics or continuous renal replacement therapy have not been fully established but are typically employed to treat UPE.

CASE RESUMES

The patient arrived in the intensive care unit on pressure control ventilation and 100% fraction inspired oxygen and PEEP of 12cmH$_2$O. Bedside ultrasonography demonstrated diffuse B-lines and adequate ventricular volume. Intravenous furosemide was administered with brisk response of urine output. The patient remained intubated with decreasing ventilator requirements for the next 8 hours as pulmonary compliance improved and secretions decreased. Another dose of furosemide was administered. He was extubated the next morning and was able to participate in chest physiotherapy.

> **KEY POINTS TO REMEMBER**
>
> 1. The pathophysiology of UPE associated with robotic mitral valve repair remains unclear; however, recent studies suggest ischemia–reperfusion injury as the main cause of UPE.
> 2. UPE can be prevented by shorter CPB times, avoiding barotrauma, limiting blood product transfusion, and minimizing lung isolation times.
> 3. Lung preventive ventilation, such as low-level positive pressure and frequent alveolar recruitment, while on CPB may be beneficial.
> 4. Avoiding recurrent atelectasis and reopening or lung overexpansion have been noted to reduce the inflammation.
> 5. Administration of steroids to attenuate ischemia–reperfusion injury can be helpful (one study suggested dexamethasone approximately 1 mg/kg body weight), although there are limited data on optimal dosing.

Suggested Reading
1. Fitzgerald MM, Bhatt HV, Schuessler ME, et al. Robotic cardiac surgery part i: anesthetic considerations in totally endoscopic robotic cardiac surgery (TERCS). *J Cardiothorac Vasc Anesth*. 2019;34(1):267–277. doi:10.1053/j.jvca.2019.02.039

2. Moss E, Halkos ME, Binongo JN, Murphy DA. Prevention of unilateral pulmonary edema complicating robotic mitral valve operations. *Ann Thorac Surg*. 2017;103(1):98–104. doi:10.1016/j.athoracsur.2016.05.100
3. Keyl C, Staier K, Pingpoh C, et al. Unilateral pulmonary oedema after minimally invasive cardiac surgery via right anterolateral minithoracotomy. *Eur J Cardiothorac Surg*. 2014;47(6):1097–1102. doi:10.1093/ejcts/ezu312
4. Renner J, Lorenzen U, Borzikowsky C, et al. Unilateral pulmonary oedema after minimally invasive mitral valve surgery: a single-centre experience. *Eur J Cardiothorac Surg*. 2017;53(4):764–770. doi:10.1093/ejcts/ezx399

18 Left Ventricular Assist Device Implantation and Management

Christopher W. Tam

A 45-year-old male with a past medical history significant for hypertension, hyperlipidemia, diabetes mellitus type 2, and non-ischemic cardiomyopathy secondary to amyloidosis presents to the hospital for decompensated heart failure requiring intravenous diuretics and supplemental oxygenation for the fifth time this year. The patient has a left ventricular ejection fraction (LVEF) of 10%–15% on home milrinone 0.125 mcg/kg/min, biventricular implantable cardioverter defibrillator implantation, and pulmonary hypertension due to World Health Organization (WHO) I and II classification with New York Heart Association (NYHA) class IV symptoms. The heart failure team has evaluated and medically optimized the patient for a left ventricular assist device (LVAD) implantation with a Heartmate 3 device. The patient is scheduled as the first case tomorrow, and you are briefing your resident and fellow on the anesthetic management, potential complications that may occur, as well as the understanding of the functionality of the LVAD.

What do you do now?

DISCUSSION

Preoperative Evaluation

A thorough preoperative evaluation of a patient undergoing a LVAD implantation is of utmost importance because of the confluent of associated medical problems patients can have secondary to heart failure. Knowledge of the indications and contraindications for LVAD implantation is needed to provide proper consultation.

Indications for LVAD Implantation

Bridge to transplantation (BTT):

- Provides systemic circulatory support in transplant-eligible patients until a matching donor heart is available.

Destination therapy (DT):

- Provides systemic circulatory support to patients who are ineligible for heart transplantation. DT provides increased survival compared to medical therapy.

Bridge to decision:

- Temporary treatment in patients in cardiogenic shock to reduce end-organ injury and prevent death while eligibility for heart transplantation is considered.

Bridge to recovery (BTR):

- Temporary support in patients in whom myocardial recovery is expected (e.g., myocarditis, Takotsubo cardiomyopathy).

Indications for BTT, DT, and BTR:

- NYHA IV for 60–90 days
- Pulmonary capillary wedge pressure (PCWP) ≥20 mm Hg
- LVEF <25%
- Systolic blood pressure ≤80–90 mm Hg or cardiac index ≤2 L/min/m^2
- Intrope dependence
- Maximal medical therapy

Contraindications to LVAD:

- Acute cardiogenic shock with uncertain neurologic status
- Coexisting terminal comorbidity (e.g., terminal malignancy, severe renal, pulmonary, liver, or neurological disease)
- Hematologic: active bleeding or chronic thrombocytopenia with platelets of <50 000/μL, confirmed heparin-induced thrombocytopenia
- Active systemic infection
- Body surface area <1.2 m^2
- Anatomical factors: Hypertrophic cardiomyopathy of ventricular septal defect, moderate or severe aortic insufficiency that will not be corrected or mechanical aortic valve not corrected to bioprosthetic, LV thrombus that will not be removed
- Social: Poor patient compliance to device maintenance, inability of patient or family to maintain LVAD and interpret function
- Right ventricular (RV) dysfunction (relative contraindication). RV dysfunction, whether it is primary or secondary due to the left heart, may make LVAD implantation a higher risk, and patient may end up needing right heart support (e.g., biventricular assist device)

Neurologic deficits should be evaluated and documented in order to accurately diagnose postoperative neurological changes following LVAD implantation. Furthermore, any severe irreversible neurological deficit or disorder that may prevent patients from being adequately anticoagulated or leave them too functionally impaired to operate the LVAD is a contraindication to LVAD implantation. All patients also undergo a psychiatric evaluation to investigate the patient's ability to understand and comply with care instructions. Patients who have a history of drug abuse, inability to comply with care instruction due to baseline psychiatric disorders, and/or a poor social support infrastructure may be contraindicated to have an LVAD implantation.

Pulmonary dysfunction should be thoroughly evaluated because it can impact perioperative management and outcomes of patients undergoing LVAD implantation. Elevated pulmonary arterial pressure, WHO II pulmonary hypertension, is often seen in advanced heart failure patients, as is decreased pulmonary diffusion capacity. These conditions are not contraindications for LVAD implantation and are expected to improve with time postoperatively. Severe restrictive or obstructive pulmonary disease is a contraindication for LVAD implantation because chronic hypoxia and hypercarbia will elevate pulmonary artery pressures, which will increase RV strain in patients who have RV dysfunction at baseline. Severe, chronic pulmonary conditions can also prolong mechanical ventilation time, leading to increased risk for pneumonia and other postoperative complications.

Renal dysfunction predicts higher postoperative morbidity and mortality, and therefore, the preoperative optimization of fluid balance and renal function is important. Indicators that are associated with poorer outcomes include creatinine >2.5 mg/dL and blood urea nitrogen >40 mg/dL or glomerular filtration rate of <0.5 mL/kg/min. Renal dysfunction is not an absolute contraindication to LVAD implantation; however, it can complicate postoperative care due to the fact that a negative fluid balance may be difficult to achieve, and if the patient is on hemodialysis, they are at increased risk of systemic infection that can infect the mechanical device. Renal function tends to improve after LVAD insertion and improved systemic blood flow, if the renal dysfunction was secondary to poor cardiac output. Intraoperative management is not significantly affected beyond medication dose adjustments. The presence of uremia or end-stage renal failure poses an increased risk for perioperative bleeding.

Hepatic dysfunction is commonly seen in patients undergoing LVAD evaluation and implantation secondary to hepatic congestion from RV failure. It is associated with poor outcomes and increased need for perioperative blood transfusion. The increased need for blood transfusion can worsen RV failure due to fluid overload, and in extreme cases an RV assist device (RVAD) implantation may be needed. Hepatic dysfunction can improve following LVAD implantation, as does renal dysfunction. Preoperative hepatic optimization by improving RV pressures and preload via inotropic support, mechanical support, and diuresis is recommended. Vitamin K supplementation may also be important in patients who have vitamin K–depleted coagulation factors, to minimize perioperative bleeding.

Intraoperative Management

Monitoring

Common monitors include a 5-lead electrocardiogram, pulse oximeter, arterial line, central line, pulmonary artery catheter, and transesophageal echocardiogram (TEE). Most patients have an automated implantable cardioverter-defibrillator, which should be deactivated to avoid accidental shock during cautery. External shock electrodes should be placed before surgical drape is applied. Continuous cardiac output or continuous mixed venous pulmonary artery catheters may be useful in these patients after LVAD implantation to continuously assess right heart function. The pulmonary artery catheter may also help guide volume status and changes in pulmonary arterial pressures that may affect RV function.

Echocardiography is an invaluable tool in the perioperative monitoring and diagnostic assessment of LVAD implantation. Prior to cardiopulmonary bypass (CPB), a TEE is performed to evaluate for the presence of an intracardiac thrombus, especially in the left heart because it can embolize to clot the LVAD and or lead to an embolic stroke. The baseline RV function and associated tricuspid regurgitation is evaluated prior to LVAD placement. If a patent foramen ovale (PFO) is detected, it should be closed because after LVAD implantation, right to left shunting may occur after the left heart pressure is reduced, leading to hypoxemia. An unrepaired PFO also poses a risk for paradoxical embolism. If aortic insufficiency is present, depending on the severity, it may need to be addressed with an aortic valve replacement or oversewing of the aortic valve prior to LVAD implantation. Persistent aortic insufficiency leads to a circuit of blood flow leading from the LVAD to the aorta outflow tract and back into the LV, therefore leading to insufficient systemic flow. Mitral stenosis is also of concern because it may prevent LV filling, which may affect LVAD flows and systemic perfusion.

During CPB, TEE can be used to help guide the positioning of the inflow cannula in the apex of the LV so that it is directed toward the mitral valve and away from the interventricular septum, to avoid suction events. TEE should also be used to assist during the de-airing process to minimize potential cerebral air embolus. Intracardiac shunt, specifically right to left shunting, and aortic valve insufficiency should be rechecked after the LVAD is activated.

Post-CPB, TEE is an important tool for the cardiac anesthesiologist to assess RV function and degree of tricuspid regurgitation. Inotropes and fluid management are determined based on the continuous interpretation of the TEE findings. The volume status of the LV and left atrium can also be assessed via TEE to determine if the left heart has too much volume and needs to be further decompressed or if it is too small and at risk for a suction event. The degree of LV unloading is related to the speed of the LVAD pump.

Anesthetic Induction/Maintenance

Patients with chronic cardiac failure have high levels of circulating catecholamines in order to maintain vasoconstriction and systemic perfusion. With the induction of anesthesia, the patient's sympathetic drive will be lowered, which may precipitate cardiac decompensation or cardiovascular collapse. The chronic heart failure patient is particularly sensitive to acute changes in preload, increases in afterload, elevated heart rate, and acute increases in pulmonary vascular resistance secondary to hypoxia or hypercarbia. The anesthesiologist should be mindful of these potential pitfalls during the induction of anesthesia and should continue the patient on current inotropes, vasopressors, and/or an intra-aortic balloon pump if present. A hemodynamically stable anesthetic induction can be achieved with the use of midazolam, fentanyl, ketamine, or etomidate; and anesthesia can be maintained with conventional inhaled anesthetics.

LVAD implantation is typically done via full sternotomy and on conventional CPB. Unless the patient has significant valvulopathy or an intracardiac shunt that requires surgical intervention, the heart is not arrested for the procedure. Heparinization with activated clotting time >400 seconds is necessary to prevent systemic thrombosis before going on CPB, and antifibrinolytic agents are given to minimize postoperative coagulopathy. The LVAD inflow cannula is placed at the apex of the LV, is located by the surgeon's palpation, and is confirmed via TEE in the 4-chamber or 2-chamber view. The outflow cannula is placed at the ascending aorta with a side-biting clamp. After implantation, the device is turned on, and the revolutions per minute (RPM) are gradually increased. TEE is important while weaning off CPB for de-airing purposes as well as visualizing LV decompression and RV function.

While coming off CPB, vasoplegia is common in that it occurs in up to 40% of patients post-LVAD implantation, so it is expected that the patient may need vasopressor support to maintain a mean arterial pressure (MAP) of 70 mm Hg to 80 mm Hg. RV failure occurs in 30% of these patients; therefore, the use of inotropes (e.g., epinephrine, milrinone, dobutamine) and pulmonary afterload reduction agents (i.e., inhaled nitric oxide, inhaled iloprost [prostaglandin I2 analogue]) are necessary. Furthermore, avoiding acute increases in pulmonary vascular resistance due to hypoxia, hypercarbia, hypothermia, or acidosis is important to minimize RV strain that can worsen RV function. TEE in the post-LVAD implantation period is important to evaluate RV function and tricuspid regurgitation.

LVAD recipients are at risk for significant coagulopathy post-CPB due to chronic hepatic congestion from heart failure and from fibrinolysis and qualitative platelet dysfunction following exposure to CPB. Thromboelastography may be a useful tool to guide blood product transfusion for postoperative coagulopathy. Transfusion of fresh frozen plasma, cryoprecipitate, and platelets may be needed to reverse coagulopathy.

Device Management

The perioperative management of LVADs requires an understanding of the device parameters: RPM, flow, power, and pulsatility index (PI). Echocardiography is an invaluable tool for the perioperative assessment of device function as well as native heart function.

The LVAD RPM is the only variable on the device that can be controlled by the user, and it represents the revolutions per minute of the rotor. Each device has an upper and lower recommended range of RPM to provide adequate systemic flow. In the immediate postoperative period, there is an increased risk at lower pump speeds of pump thrombosis as well as low systemic perfusion and at higher pump speeds of systemic bleeding as well as an LVAD suction event.

Power is a function of RPM and is measured in watts. Sustained elevated power may indicate LVAD thrombosis, whereas low power may indicate occlusion of the device inflow or outflow cannula or low preload.

LVAD flow represents flow from the device, and it is a variable that is dependent on the pump speed (RPM) as well as the head pressure. The head pressure is defined as the pressure difference between the LV intracavitary pressure and the afterload. Head pressure and flow are inversely proportional. The LVAD flow is not equal to cardiac output and can underestimate the true flow because it does not take into account any cardiac output from the native LV and does not consider any regurgitant flow.

Th PI represents the stroke volume contributed by the native LV. It is the equilibrium between the native cardiac function and LVAD unloading on the LV preload. Mathematically it is the difference between the maximal and minimal flow divided by the average flow per cycle. PI is dependent on multiple factors including LV preload, native myocardial function, LVAD RPM, and afterload. Increased PI can be due to recovery of native cardiac function, increase in preload, or increased afterload and can decrease with increased LVAD RPM or decreased preload. Despite LVAD implantation, the native LV still follows the Frank-Starling curve.

Early Complications

Hypovolemia

Hypovolemia presents with low MAP of <60 mm Hg and low LVAD flows with associated low central venous pressure (CVP), low jugular venous pressure (JVP), low pulmonary artery pressure, and possibly metabolic acidosis. An echocardiogram would likely reveal underfilled RV and LV. In a more serious complication of hypovolemia known as *LVAD suction event*, the inflow cannula of the LVAD may suction onto the interventricular septum when the LV cavity is extremely underfilled, causing low LVAD flow and tremendous acute RV afterload. This results in RV dysfunction. Treatment entails crystalloid or colloid resuscitation and vasopressor support as needed.

Vasoplegia

Vasoplegia syndrome was originally described in 1994 by Gomes et al. with an incidence varying between 9% and 44% of patients after cardiac surgery.

The definition of vasoplegia syndrome is variable, which accounts for the wide variability in incidence. In general, vasoplegia syndrome presents with high cardiac output and cardiac index, euvolemic filling pressures based on the CVP, and PCWP with sustained hypotension despite high vasopressor dosage. Vasoplegia syndrome is secondary to an inflammatory response activation that occurs after exposure to CPB. Treatment is supportive with vasopressors. Some patients with chronic heart failure experience vasopressin depletion and respond more effectively to exogenous vasopressin supplementation versus catecholamines. High-dose corticosteroids have not been shown to be effective for vasoplegia syndrome even though the proposed mechanism is secondary to an inflammatory response. Case reports in the literature have suggested that methylene blue and vitamin B_{12} may have some utility as rescue drugs; however, further prospective trials are needed.

RV Failure

Most patients undergoing LVAD implantation have some degree of RV dysfunction and require inotropic support and pulmonary artery vasodilators. As a result of the reduced LV pressure post-LVAD, the interventricular septum may be shifted leftward, causing increased compliance of the RV. The septal shift can lead to worsened RV function as the septum may no longer contribute to RV ejection. Occasionally, in the postoperative period these patients may develop severe RV dysfunction, leading to cardiogenic shock and malperfusion of end organs. The typical presentation of RV failure includes low LVAD flows, low PI, low MAP, high CVP, elevated pulmonary artery pressures, high JVP, and low PCWP. If an echocardiogram was performed, the right atrium and RV may be severely dilated, with the interventricular septum shifted to the left during systole and diastole, and the LV would be underfilled. The RV would also be severely dysfunctional. Management would include the use of inotropes and up-titration of inotropic therapy, utilizing vasopressors to maintain MAP at 70–90 mm Hg to maximize RV perfusion and increase LV end-diastolic pressure to maintain the septum in a midline position. Initiation of pulmonary vasodilator therapy may also augment forward flow. RV failure should be managed in conjunction with the cardiothoracic surgery and heart failure teams because other advanced mechanical support may be needed including a temporary RVAD or other temporary assist device in the right heart. If the RV fails to recover, it may be necessary to implant a total artificial heart and wait for heart transplantation, if the patient is a candidate. Acute collection of blood on or around the heart may cause tamponade physiology and mimic RV failure.

Second- and Third-Generation LVADs

Currently in the United States, there are 3 LVADs that are approved by the Food and Drug Administration for DT including the Heartmate II, Heartmate III (both St. Jude Medical, St. Paul, MN), and the Heartware (Heartware, Framingham, MA). The Heartmate II is a second-generation device, whereas the Heartmate III and the Heartware devices are third-generation devices. They are all continuous-flow devices with similar components including an inflow graft placed at the apex of the LV, where blood travels from the LV through the inflow graft into the LVAD impellar and into the outflow graft where blood is circulated systemically. A driveline is tunneled across the abdomen that connects the pump to an external controller that displays the LVAD's parameters and connects to a power source.

The main difference between the 3 pumps is that the Heartmate II is an axial pump with a larger design than the smaller centrifugal third-generation pumps. A preperitoneal pocket therefore needs to be created in order to place the Heartmate II motor, whereas the impellar in the third-generation devices is implanted directly into the apex of the LV and the device remains contained within the pericardium. Flow is more accurately measured in the third-generation devices due to the centrifugal design and the accurate assessment of blood viscosity, by inputting the current hematocrit into the LVAD monitor. The third-generation LVADs (Heartmate III and Heartware) have a feature known as "artificial pulse" or "Lavare cycle," which is depicted on the arterial waveform as pulsatile flow. This is generated by the LVAD via rapid speed modulation, where there is accelerated decrease and then increase in impellar RPM to "wash" the pump and prevent pump thrombosis. The typical parameters of these 3 LVADs can be seen in Table 18.1.

TABLE 18.1 **Typical Parameters of the Heartmate II, Heartmate III, and Heartware**

Parameters	Heartmate II	Heartmate III	Heartware
Typical speed (rpm)	8000–10 000	5000–6000	2400–3200
Flow (L/min)	4–7	4–6	4–6
Power (watts)	5–8	4.5–6.5	3–7
Pulsatility index	5–8	3.5–5.5	2.4 L/min/beat

CASE RESUMES

The patient underwent successful placement of a Heartmate III LVAD. Echocardiographic parameters demonstrated appropriate flow from the mitral valve and left ventricle into the inflow cannula of the LVAD with minimal turbulence. The patient was taken to the intensive care unit on milrinone and vasopressin with goal mean arterial pressure of 80–85 mmHg. The patient was monitored for bleeding, which was minimal. Right ventricular function was assessed with serial echocardiography exams and by trending the CVP and pulmonary artery waveform and pressures. The patient required diuretic therapy as signs of decreased RV function and dilation were demonstrated by echocardiography and by increasing CVP. Following appropriate response to diuretic, the patient was extubated. Over the course of 2 days, gentle diuresis continued, milrinone was weaned to off and the patient was discharged to the floor on postoperative day 2.

> **KEY POINTS TO REMEMBER**
>
> 1. LVAD therapy can used as a bridge to transplantation, destination therapy, bridge to decision, and bridge to recovery.
> 2. Contraindications to LVAD implantation include neurological changes following implantation, pulmonary dysfunction, renal dysfunction, and hepatic dysfunction.

3. Echocardiography is critical in identifying proper LVAD position during placement, LVAD speed, LV volume assessment and RV function in the perioperative period.
4. RV failure prior to and following LVAD placement is common.

Suggested Reading
1. Lund LH, Matthews J, Aaronson K. Patient selection for left ventricular assist devices. *Eur J Heart Fail*. 2010;12:434–443.
2. Slaughter MS, Pagani FD, Rogers JG, et al. Clinical management of continuous-flow left ventricular assist devices in advanced heart failure. *J Heart Lung Transplant*. 2010;29(4 suppl):S1–S39.
3. Mets B. Anesthesia for left ventricular assist device placement. *J Cardiothorac Vasc Anesth*. 2000;14(3):316–326.
4. Nadziakiewicz P, Niklewski T, Szygula-Jurkiewicz B, et al. Preoperative echocardiography examination of right ventricle function in patients scheduled for LVAD implantation correlates with postoperative hemodynamic examinations. *Ann Transplant*. 2016;21:500–507.
5. Sen A, Larson JS, Kashani KB, et al. Mechanical circulatory assist devices: a primer for critical care and emergency physicians. *Crit Care*. 2016;20:153.
6. Pratt AK, Shah NS, Boyce SW. Left ventricular assist device management in the ICU. *Crit Care Med*. 2014;42:158–168.
7. DeVore AD, Patel PA, Patel CB. Medical management of patients with a left ventricular assist device for the non-left ventricular assist device specialist. *JACC Heart Fail*. 2017;5(9):621–631.

19 Left Ventricular Assist Device Troubleshooting: Hypotension

Jan M. Griffin, Bushra W. Taha, and Yoshifumi Naka

A 72-year-old man with a history of familial dilated cardiomyopathy was admitted with acute decompensated heart failure. Due to his clinical trajectory, he underwent left ventricular (LV) assist device (LVAD) implantation, INTERMACS 2, as destination therapy and is now postoperative day 1. LVAD parameters are as follows: speed 5800 rpm, power 5.2 watts, flow 4.9 L/min, pulsatility index (PI) 4. He is now febrile and requiring an increase in vasopressor support. On morning rounds his drips are as follows: dobutamine 5 mcg/kg/min, epinephrine 3 mcg/min, norepinephrine 1 mcg/kg/min, vasopressin 0.04 units/min.

What do you do now?

DISCUSSION

The differential diagnosis for postoperative hypotension after LVAD implantation is broad and is defined as a MAP <60 mm Hg for continuous-flow LVADs. Etiologies to consider include vasodilatory hypotension, cardiac failure, hypovolemia or hemorrhage, and device-related complications. Clinical examination is an important component of the initial evaluation; echocardiography and placement of a pulmonary artery catheter can also be helpful. An approach to postoperative hypotension after LVAD implantation is described in Figure 19.1.

Assuming adequate preload, hypotension secondary to vasodilation leads to increased LVAD flows. Clinical examination is often notable for warm extremities. While the presence of fever and leukocytosis may be

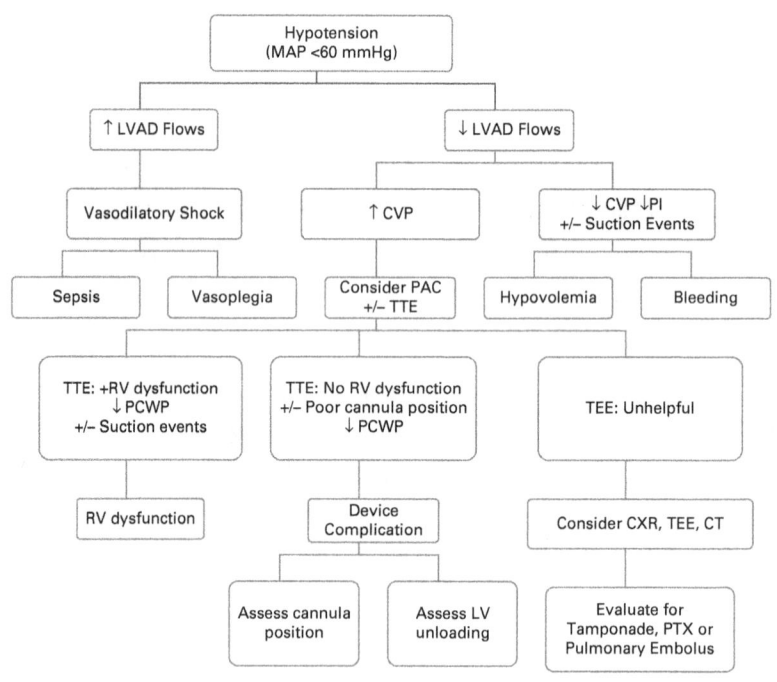

CVP = central venous pressure; LV = left ventricle; LVAD = left ventricular assist device; MAP = mean arterial pressure; PAC = pulmonary artery catheter; PCWP = pulmonary capillary wedge pressure; PI = pulsatility index; PTX = pneumothorax; RV = right ventricle; TEE = transesophageal echocardiogram; TTE = transthoracic echocardiogram.

FIGURE 19.1 Approach to post-operative hypotension after LVAD implantation.

suggestive of sepsis, both can also be observed in the systemic inflammatory response syndrome immediately after surgery. Immediate treatment with vasopressors is indicated, and evaluation of possible sources of sepsis and administration of empiric antibiotics may be warranted given the risk of seeding a newly implanted device. In contrast, hypotension associated with decreased LVAD flows necessitates evaluation of cardiac function and filling pressures and can be indicative of hypovolemia, right ventricular (RV) failure, arrhythmias, cardiac tamponade, or device-related complications.

On examination, the patient is sedated and intubated. He has mechanical breath sounds without crackles and distant heart sounds with an audible LVAD hum. His peripheries are tepid with bilateral pitting edema to the knees. His mediastinal chest tubes have had minimal output overnight, and his urine output has decreased gradually over the course of several hours. He is oxygenating adequately with oxygen saturation >95%, partial pressure of oxygen of 112, and fraction of inspired oxygen of 40% and remains ventricularly paced at 90 bpm. His MAP is 65 mm Hg with vasopressor support. LVAD parameters are as follows: speed 5800 rpm, power 2.8 watts, flow 2.1 L/min, PI 2.2.

When evaluating the possible cause of his hypotension, it is important to exclude the presence of atrial or ventricular arrhythmias. While normal sinus rhythm is not necessary for LVAD function, loss of the atrial kick can lead to decreased RV preload, RV cardiac output, and RV function. Atrial arrhythmias may require acute rate or rhythm control. Ventricular arrhythmias must similarly be addressed and are common following LVAD implantation due to either preexisting myocardial scarring, metabolic disarray, or contact between the inflow cannula and interventricular septum (i.e., suction events). Suction events occur when the LVAD flow exceeds the available LV preload, such that the walls of the LV collapse toward the LVAD inflow conduit. Suction events may incite ventricular arrhythmias and exacerbate hypotension. Management may include reduction of LVAD speed in order to promote increased LV filling, treatment of hypovolemia, intensifying vasopressor support, and administration of antiarrhythmic agents such as beta-blockers and amiodarone.

Evaluation of central venous pressure (CVP) may clarify the etiology of his hypotension. Decreased LVAD flow with a low CVP, decreased LVAD pulsatility, and suction events suggest hypovolemia. A decreased PI can be caused by factors that decompress the LV. In the case of hypovolemia, decreased preload will decompress the LV at a given speed and result in less flow variability. Treatment for hypovolemia includes administration of intravenous fluids, blood product transfusion as indicated by clinical exam and/or laboratory values, holding or reversal of anticoagulation, and identification of possible bleeding sources, including examination of chest tubes and drains.

The patient's CVP is elevated at 18 mm Hg. This elevated CVP is observed in RV failure, cardiac tamponade, and device inflow/outflow obstruction (although obstruction is often associated with solely elevated pulmonary artery [PA] pressures and pulmonary capillary wedge pressure [PCWP]). Acute post-implantation RV failure can develop in some patients and, in the setting of low LVAD flows, is characterized by elevations in CVP, reduced pressure step-up from CVP to mean PA pressures, low PCWP, and signs of RV dysfunction on echocardiogram. Following LVAD implantation, the interventricular septum shifts to the left due to LV unloading. The change in interventricular septum geometry can decrease RV function. RV preload is increased from improved cardiac output from the LVAD. RV afterload may remain high because of elevated PA pressures from chronic left-sided heart failure; however, with adequate unloading of the LV and a resultant decrease in PCWP, PA pressures may decrease. Treatment for acute RV failure includes systemic inotropes such as the phosphodiesterase-3 inhibitor milrinone, the beta-adrenergic agonist dobutamine, and selective pulmonary vasodilators including nitric oxide and prostacyclin analogues such as iloprost and epoprostenol. Reducing LVAD speed and increasing systemic pressures can counter septal shifting toward the LV. Escalation to the placement of an RV assist device is considered in a timely fashion if initial medical interventions do not restore hemodynamic stability.

His PA pressures are 36/20 with a mean of 25 mm Hg, PCWP is 14 mm Hg, Fick cardiac output is 3.7 L/min, Fick cardiac index is 2 L/min/m^2, and mixed venous oxygen is 50%. His systemic vascular resistance is normal at 1016 dynes/s/cm^5, and pulmonary vascular resistance is mildly elevated, 3 Wood units. These findings place cardiogenic shock high on the differential, though the cause is unclear. Although transthoracic echocardiography (TTE) can be challenging in the immediate postoperative period due to poor imaging windows, it can serve as a useful tool to further assess biventricular function, valvular abnormalities, pericardial effusions, and LVAD inflow cannula positioning.

The patient's TTE examination reveals a small underfilled LV cavity, poorly visualized RV, mild mitral regurgitation, trace aortic regurgitation with opening of the aortic valve on alternate beats, and a small to moderate pericardial effusion. In limited views of the inflow cannula, it appears to be well positioned with adequate inflow velocities. The placement and direction of the LVAD inflow cannula on imaging can provide information on potential obstruction to flow. If the inflow cannula is directed toward the interventricular septum or the LV free wall, it can lead to obstruction of blood flow into the device, possibly requiring surgical revision.

While his limited TTE study makes the possibility of LVAD inflow or outflow obstruction less likely, it raises the suspicion for cardiac tamponade and/or RV failure, pneumothorax, or pulmonary embolism. Chest radiograph can be a useful adjunct to TTE. His chest X-ray shows no evidence of a pneumothorax but reveals an enlarged cardiac silhouette with clear costophrenic angles and mild pulmonary congestion. These findings prompt an urgent computed tomograph (CT) of the chest, which demonstrates a focal large posterior fluid collection. In the setting of progressively increasing CVP, persistent low-flow alarms and low PI on his LVAD, and an underfilled LV cavity on TTE, these findings are suggestive of cardiac tamponade.

CASE RESUMES

The patient underwent emergent re-exploration of the chest. He receives cryoprecipitate and platelets intraoperatively and returns to the intensive care unit. Over the course of the next 48 hours, his MAP stabilizes, and vasopressors are weaned off. Dobutamine remains at 5 mcg/kg/min for RV support, and bedside TTE shows no re-accumulation of the pericardial effusion.

The incidence of cardiac tamponade post-LVAD implantation is around 24%–28%. Pericardial effusion can occur as a result of pericardial inflammation and bleeding following LVAD implantation, particularly once antiplatelet therapy and anticoagulation are initiated postoperatively. Cardiac tamponade can be associated with suction events due to low LV preload. Of note, pulsus paradoxus is often difficult to measure in this patient population. While TTE can be a diagnostic aide, in the postoperative period it may be difficult to fully visualize the pericardial space for hemopericardium, which may be focal. Transesophageal echocardiogram (TEE) and CT angiography are more sensitive tools to evaluate for tamponade after LVAD surgery, with features that include compression of the atrium or ventricle, dilation of the inferior vena cava, reflux of contrast into the azygos vein, and compression of the coronary sinus.

> **KEY POINTS TO REMEMBER**
>
> 1. Low LV afterload is associated with high LVAD flow, while low LV preload is associated with low LVAD flow.
> 2. Always consider systemic inflammatory response syndrome as a cause of postoperative hypotension, while sepsis remains as a differential diagnosis.
> 3. Although not necessary for LVAD function, loss of atrial kick can still lead to decompensation due to diminished RV cardiac output and function, and patients may therefore require rate or rhythm control for arrhythmias.
> 4. RV failure as a cause of hypotension can be inferred by a high CVP associated with a low PI, decreased LVAD flow, and decreased cardiac output.
> 5. TTE may not provide optimal imaging in the immediate postoperative period, and further assessment may require TEE or CT angiogram.

Suggested Reading
1. Chung, M. Perioperative management of the patient with a left ventricular assist device for noncardiac surgery. *Anesth Analg.* 2018;126(6):1839–1850.
2. Pratt A, Shah N, Boyce S. Left ventricular assist device management in the ICU. *Crit Care Med.* 2014;42:158–168.

20 Left Ventricular Assist Device Troubleshooting: Bleeding and Thrombosis

Jan M. Griffin, Bushra W. Taha, and Kelly M. Axsom

A 74-year-old man with non-ischemic cardiomyopathy presents for elective left ventricular assist device (LVAD) implantation. He returns to the intensive care unit post-implant on dobutamine 5 mcg/kg/min, milrinone 0.25 mcg/kg/min, norepinephrine 3 mcg/min, and inhaled nitric oxide. His central venous pressure (CVP) is 12 mm Hg, pulmonary arterial pressure is 25/14 mm Hg, pulmonary capillary wedge pressure is 15 mm Hg, and central venous saturation is 61%, with a calculated Fick cardiac index of 2.46 L/min/m^2. Over the next 4 hours, urine output drops to 30 mL/h, and 1 L of bloody fluid drains into mediastinal chest tubes. His LVAD shows a lower pulsatility index (PI) and starts to have low-flow alarms. His vasopressor requirement steadily increases to maintain MAP of 80–85 mm Hg.

What do you do now?

DISCUSSION

The most likely etiology of this worsening hemodynamic state and high chest tube output is postoperative bleeding. Postoperative bleeding following LVAD implantation is one of the most common early complications, occurring in around 48% of patients. The incidence of bleeding requiring blood product transfusion or reoperation is 31%–81%. Typically, bleeding presents with high surgical drainage and worsening hemodynamics. Postoperative bleeding can also manifest as cardiac tamponade, which can be difficult to diagnose but often presents with an elevated jugular venous pressure and can be evaluated with additional imaging such as echocardiography or computerized tomography (CT). Risk factors for perioperative bleeding include liver dysfunction, RV failure, preoperative temporary mechanical support, prolonged cardiopulmonary bypass, perioperative anticoagulation, and postoperative acidosis. Methods to minimize postoperative bleeding include cessation of all antiplatelets and anticoagulants, if possible before surgery; optimization of nutrition; and intraoperatively, minimizing coronary bypass time and administering tranexamic acid.

It is important to differentiate between postoperative surgical bleeding and bleeding due to coagulopathy (Figure 20.1a). His hemoglobin (Hb) is 7.8 g/dL (10.6 g/dL preoperatively), prothrombin time (PT) is 30 seconds, partial thromboplastin time (PTT) is 89 seconds, and fibrinogen is 76 mg/dL. Elevated PT/PTT and low fibrinogen levels indicate coagulopathy, which should be corrected with administration of blood and blood products. Cryoprecipitate is a source of fibrinogen and von Willebrand factor, while fresh frozen plasma provides the necessary clotting factors. It is prudent to avoid unnecessary massive transfusions, which can cause right heart failure post-LVAD implantation from volume overload. The use of prothrombin complex concentrate could be considered but has the potential to clot the pump from a prothrombotic effect.

An important contributor to bleeding in continuous-flow LVAD patients is acquired von Willebrand's syndrome. This has been shown to occur within 30 days of implant and can lead to increased non-surgical bleeding. The exact mechanism is unclear, though it is thought to involve the destruction of von Willebrand's factor (VWF), which is a large multimeric protein (205 kDa). When this protein is exposed to shear stress during its

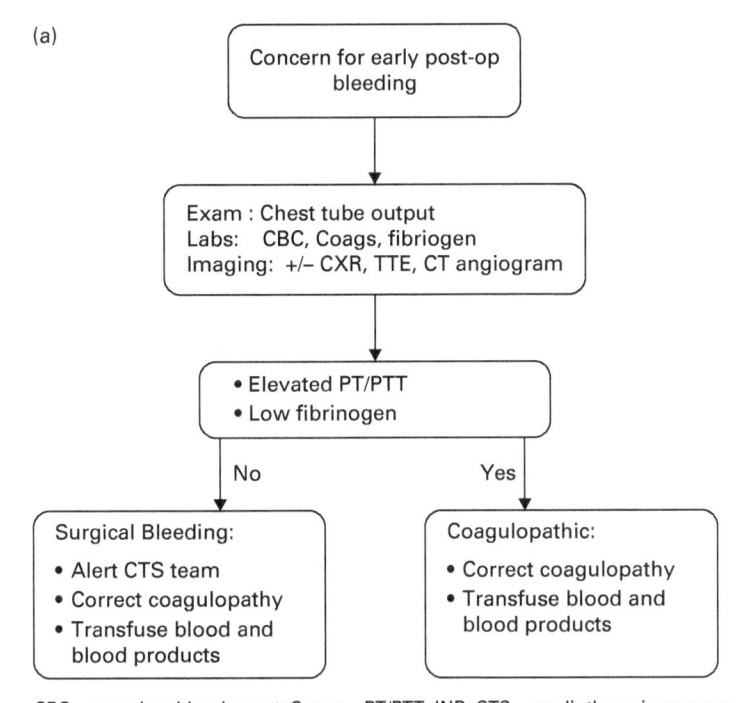

(a)

```
┌─────────────────────────┐
│ Concern for early post-op│
│ bleeding                │
└─────────────────────────┘
             │
             ▼
┌─────────────────────────────────────┐
│ Exam : Chest tube output            │
│ Labs:   CBC, Coags, fibriogen       │
│ Imaging:  +/– CXR, TTE, CT angiogram│
└─────────────────────────────────────┘
             │
             ▼
┌─────────────────────────┐
│ • Elevated PT/PTT       │
│ • Low fibrinogen        │
└─────────────────────────┘
       No         Yes
       │           │
       ▼           ▼
```

Surgical Bleeding:
- Alert CTS team
- Correct coagulopathy
- Transfuse blood and blood products

Coagulopathic:
- Correct coagulopathy
- Transfuse blood and blood products

CBC = complete blood count; Coags = PT/PTT, INR; CTS = cardiothoracic surgery; CXR = chest X-ray; TTE = transthoracic echocardiogram

FIGURE 20.1A. Flow-chart for evaluation of suspected Post-Op Bleeding.

passage through the pump, the conformation of the protein is altered and cleaved, causing a loss of the highest-weight multimers. This process effectively produces a functional deficiency in VWF, which impairs platelet plugging and occurs in patients with HeartMate II and HeartWare HVAD, similar to what occurs in Heyde's syndrome in severe aortic stenosis. The severity of acquired von Willebrand's syndrome is milder with HeartMate III compared to the HeartMate II and HVAD.

His coagulopathy is corrected, and Hb is 9 g/dL; but chest tube output remains high. Chest X-ray (CXR) shows a worsening left-sided pleural effusion. CVP, LVAD flows, and PI remain low. In this context, it is important to evaluate for periprocedural bleeding. His surgical team is notified, and he returns to the operating room for re-exploration, where 800 mL of bloody fluid and clot is removed from the pleural space. He remains

(b)

```
┌─────────────────────────────────┐
│ Exam: Signs of heart failure,   │
│ neurologic deficits, distal embolism │
└─────────────────────────────────┘
              ↓
┌─────────────────────────────────┐
│ Check Labs: Coags, Hemolysis labs │
│ Interrogate LVAD                │
└─────────────────────────────────┘
              ↓
┌─────────────────────────────────┐
│ INR < 2                         │
│ LDH > 1.5 baseline              │
│ LVAD power spikes/alarms        │
└─────────────────────────────────┘
              ↓
┌─────────────────────────────────┐
│ Assess Hemodynamics:            │
│ • HR, MAP.                      │
└─────────────────────────────────┘
       Stable ↙        ↘ Unstable
```

Imaging:
- CXR: cannula position,
- TTE: LV dimensions, valvular regurgitation, clot
- Ramp study
- +/– CT angiogram: cannula position, outflow graft
- +/– Cardiac Cath: inflow and outflow cannula evaluation

- Emergent CTS consult for LVAD exchange
- Supportive care

Coags = PT/PTT, INR; CTS = cardiothoracic surgery; CXR = chest X-ray; Hemolysis labs = Total bilirubin, fibrinogen, haptoglobin; LDH = lactate dehydrogenase; TTE = transthoracic echocardiogram

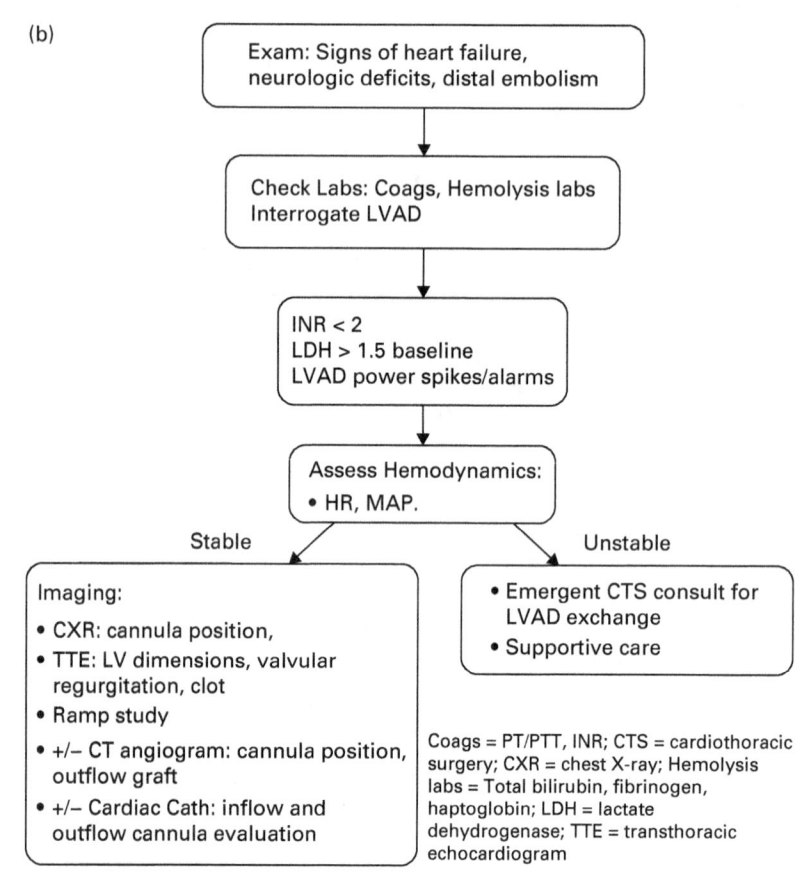

FIGURE 20.1B. Flow-chart for evaluation of suspected thrombosis.

hemodynamically stable and is initiated on unfractionated heparin as a bridge to warfarin on postoperative day 7.

Current recommendations for anticoagulation in LVAD patients include treatment with an antiplatelet agent (aspirin 81–325 mg), heparin, and anticoagulation with a vitamin K antagonist to reduce the risk of thrombosis. Initiation of intravenous heparin begins once chest tube output has stabilized, usually postoperative days 1–3. Heparin is initiated cautiously without a bolus and with a low target PTT, gradually increasing to a more therapeutic PTT as clinically tolerated. Vitamin K antagonists are usually initiated closer to postoperative days 4–7 once there are no clinical signs of bleeding. International normalized ratio (INR) goals differ between devices, and current protocols differ between institution and device, though typically INR goals are between 2 and 3.

The patient presents to the emergency room 3 months after discharge. He reports that approximately 4 hours prior to arrival he developed right hand weakness. He also notes that he has had worsening shortness of breath, new lower extremity edema, and 2-pillow orthopnea for the past month, which he attributed to dietary indiscretions. On physical exam he is afebrile, normotensive, in a regular rhythm, and saturating 98% on room air. He has bilateral pitting lower extremity edema to his knees, jugular venous pulsation is elevated, clear lung fields, and an audible LVAD hum. On interrogation of his LVAD, his power is higher and PI is lower. His neurologic exam is notable for three-fifths strength in his right upper extremity and normal sensation and is otherwise unremarkable.

Based on his presentation, the immediate concern is for a thromboembolic event, the most likely source being his LVAD. LVAD-supported patients who experience a cerebrovascular accident (CVA) have a 2-fold higher risk of death compared to those without CVA. Independent predictors for CVA post-LVAD implantation include diabetes mellitus, prior history of stroke, aortic cross-clamping, and INR values. Thrombosis can occur within areas of slow or stagnant flow such as the left atrium or LV, the device inflow or outflow cannula, on the rotor itself, or on the aortic valve. Depending on the location of the device thrombus, the LVAD parameters may differ (Table 20.1). Inflow or outflow cannula thrombus leads to lower powers and flows, and rotor thrombus leads to higher power and flows. In the most serious of cases it can result in complete obstruction to flow through the device and pump failure, but more commonly patients will develop worsening heart failure symptoms or evidence of thromboembolism.

Notable laboratory results are Hb 10.2 g/dL, platelet count 150×10^9/L, INR 1.4, and creatinine 2.5 mg/dL. He has evidence of hemolysis with a lactate dehydrogenase (LDH) of 1600 U/L, plasma-free Hb 20 mg/dL, undetectable haptoglobin, and total bilirubin 5.4 mg/dL, with an indirect fraction of 4.8 mg/dL. Inspection of urine is important as tea-colored or black urine occurs due to the presence of heme pigment and can be an early and non-invasive indicator of hemolysis. On interrogation of his LVAD, there is a notable increase in power from a baseline of 5.2 W to 7.4 W. LVAD flows

TABLE 20.1 **Hemodynamics and Left Ventricular Assist Device Parameters**

	CVP	mPAP	PCWP	LVAD Power	LVAD Flow
Sepsis	↓	↓	↓	↑	↑
RV Failure	↑	↑ or ↔	↓	↓	↓
Tamponade	↑	↓	↓	↓	↓
Massive PE	↑	↓	↓	↓	↓
Hypovolemia/ Bleeding	↓	↓	↓	↓	↓
Inflow/Outflow Thrombus	↑	↑	↑	↓	↓
Rotor Thrombus	↓	↑	↑	↑	↑ (erroneous)

CVP = central venous pressure; LVAD = left ventricular assist device; mPAP = mean pulmonary arterial pressure; PE = pulmonary embolism; RV = right ventricle; SVR = systemic vascular resistance.

and PI are similarly increased. His CXR shows cardiomegaly, small bilateral pleural effusions, and increased vascularity of the lung fields. Non-contrast CT of his head shows old infarcts with no hemorrhage or midline shift.

Neurology is consulted, and repeat neurological exam shows resolution of prior right upper extremity weakness. He cannot undergo brain magnetic resonance imaging due to the presence of the LVAD, and thrombolysis is not indicated. Due to concern for current or impending pump thrombosis, he is started on unfractionated heparin. He has a bedside transthoracic echocardiogram, which shows LVEF 10%–15%, LVED is now 8.1 cm (from 5.4 cm at the time of speed optimization echocardiogram), the aortic valve opens with each beat, and there is septal bowing into the RV. The inflow and outflow cannulae cannot be visualized.

Risk factors for pump thrombosis include poor surgical implant technique, lower pump speeds, concurrent infection, and subtherapeutic INR. It has been shown that only 20% of LVAD patients achieve their target INR range 60% of the time. Prior to the introduction of the HeartMate III LVAD, rates of pump thrombosis were approximately 8% for the HeartWare LVAD (HVAD; HeartWare, Framingham, MA) and 5%–7%

for HeartMate II at 6 months. More recently, the 6-month outcomes in the Momentum 3 trial reported no pump thrombosis events for the HeartMate III LVAD.

Non-invasive studies can be helpful in detecting pump thrombosis (Figure 20.1b). CXR can allow for evaluation of changes in pump position, cardiomegaly, and pulmonary edema. Ideally, the inflow cannula should be parallel to the long axis of the LV and directed toward the mitral inflow.

As LVAD thrombosis progresses, more cardiac output is dependent on the native heart, and heart failure ensues. Transthoracic echo can be used to visualize LV thrombus, identify increase in LV size, measure diastolic flow velocity across the inflow cannula, determine the systolic to diastolic flow ratio, visualize aortic valve opening, and visualize any worsening mitral regurgitation. If a patient has had a Parks' stitch where the aortic valve has been surgically closed, the patient will be dependent on LVAD output. An echocardiographic ramp study can be performed in axial flow pumps and has been proven to be highly sensitive and specific for detection of pump thrombosis. The patient has a ramp study performed, and the slope is calculated as –0.12, which is consistent with pump thrombosis.

CT angiogram of the chest can be performed to visualize pump position, specifically inflow and outflow cannulae, though care must be taken to limit the risk of contrast nephropathy. It may also be useful to rule out outflow graft thrombosis. CT imaging can also help assess if inflow cannula malposition has led to a risk of device thrombosis. Cardiac catheterization may be used to measure the pressure gradient in the outflow graft if kinking or stenosis is suspected based on echocardiography or CT imaging.

A crude way to help differentiate between inflow/outflow or rotor thrombosis is the trend in power, which is a direct measurement of pump motor voltage and current. Typically, pump flow is linearly related to power. In the setting of inflow/outflow cannula thrombosis, the blood flow through the device is obstructed to some degree, and there is a resultant decrease in the power required to drive the pump in addition to estimated flow. Conversely, rotor thrombosis causes an increase in device power required to drive the pump and erroneously increased flow. This displayed flow is discordant with the actual decrease in blood flow through the device since this is an estimate based on the speed and power of the device (Table 20.1).

CASE RESUMES

Given his developing acute kidney injury and presentation with heart failure, he is taken emergently to the operating room for device exchange. In cases of hemodynamic instability, emergent pump exchange or urgent heart transplantation is recommended once the patient has been stabilized. However, early medical management of clinically stable patients or patients with a prohibitively high operative risk may be effective using intravenous systemic heparin and/or thrombolysis. Studies have shown a 48%–57% success rate using medical therapy for treatment of device thrombosis in HeartWare HVAD, though with significant risk including hemorrhagic stroke (21%) and death (10%). A patient presenting with clinical and laboratory evidence of hemolysis and suspected pump thrombosis should be immediately anticoagulated with intravenous heparin, and warfarin should be discontinued because device replacement may be necessary. With the introduction of third-generation fully magnetically levitated pumps, the rate of pump thrombosis appears to have declined. These pumps have larger passages for blood flow and lack the bearings present in the older models, with a resultant reduction in shear stress. In addition, there is rapid change in rotor speed, which creates an artificial pulse with a goal to wash the impeller and limit blood stasis. Regardless, it is important to optimize practice to minimize the risk of pump thrombosis. Recommendations include focusing on implantation technique (to maximize flow through the pump), anticoagulation (initiation of heparin bridge to warfarin and aspirin as soon as possible postoperatively), optimal speed management, and maintaining a MAP <90 mm Hg.

> **KEY POINTS TO REMEMBER**
>
> 1. It is important to differentiate between surgical bleeding and bleeding due to coagulopathy.
> 2. Once perioperative bleeding has stopped, initiate unfractionated heparin at low and gradually escalating doses.
> 3. Current recommendations for anticoagulation in LVAD patients include treatment with an antiplatelet agent (aspirin 81–325 mg) and anticoagulation with a vitamin K antagonist.

4. Interrogation of LVAD power trends is important in the evaluation of suspected pump thrombosis.
5. LDH should be measured at baseline and at regular intervals to screen for impending pump thrombosis.
6. If pump thrombosis is suspected, vitamin K antagonist should be discontinued and unfractionated heparin initiated.
7. Hemodynamically unstable patients or LVAD malfunction warrants an emergent cardiothoracic surgery consult for potential LVAD exchange.
8. In some cases, tissue plasminogen activator should be administered for pump thrombosis.

Suggested Reading

1. Tchantchaleishvili V, Sagebin F, Ross R. Evaluation and treatment of pump thrombosis and hemolysis. *Ann Cardiothorac Surg.* 2014;3(5):490–495.
2. Uriel N, Morrison KA, Garan AR, et al. Development of a novel echocardiography ramp test for speed optimization and diagnosis of device thrombosis in continuous-flow left ventricular assist devices: the Columbia Ramp Study. *J Am Coll Cardiol.* 2012;60:1764–1775.
3. Boehme AK, Pamboukian SV, George JF, et al. Anticoagulation control in patients with ventricular assist devices. *ASAIO J.* 2017;63(6)759–765.
4. Meyer AL, Malehsa D, Budde U, et al. Acquired von Willebrand syndrome in patients with a centrifugal or axial continuous flow left ventricular assist device. *JACC Heart Fail.* 2014;2:141–145.
5. Uriel N, Han J, Morrison KA, et al. Device thrombosis in HeartMate II continuous-flow left ventricular assist devices: a multifactorial phenomenon. *J Heart Lung Transplant.* 2014;33:51–59.

21 Gastrointestinal Bleeding in the Setting of Left Ventricular Assist Device Support

Michael E. Kiyatkin, Adam S. Faye, and Tamas A. Gonda

A 71-year-old man with ischemic cardiomyopathy and a HeartMate II (HM II) left ventricular assist device (LVAD) on home warfarin and aspirin presents to the emergency room with 4 days of melena and 2 days of worsening lightheadedness. He is hypotensive, is tachycardic, and has guaiac-positive stool. A complete blood cell count reveals anemia (hemoglobin 5.0), and a coagulation panel reveals a therapeutic international normalized ratio (INR) of 2.6. He is transfused 2 units of packed red blood cells by the emergency department team, with subsequent normalization of his hemodynamics. An infusion of intravenous esomeprazole is started, and the gastroenterology service is consulted for workup of a suspected gastrointestinal bleed (GIB).

What do you do now?

DISCUSSION

LVAD surgery has become an essential therapy for advanced heart failure. Numerous advances in LVAD design, implantation, and postoperative care have contributed to enhanced survival of approximately 80% and 60% at 1 and 3 years post-implantation, respectively. However, even the newest LVADs continue to be plagued with a high incidence of GIB, ranging from 12% to 30% by 1 year. Although typically not fatal, LVAD-related GIB is associated with extended hospital stays and poor overall outcomes and is a leading cause for hospital readmission. Importantly, it also complicates future heart transplant candidacy because blood transfusions may lead to the development of transplant-limiting antibodies.

Risk Factors for LVAD-Related GIB

Numerous risk factors have been identified for LVAD-related GIB. The strongest is age >65 years, with a roughly 20-fold higher odds of GIB compared to those <65 years of age. Other independent risk factors include lower creatinine clearance, active tobacco smoking, and frequent infections. Interestingly, the use of selective serotonin reuptake inhibitors, which have anti-platelet properties, has also been identified as a risk factor. Surprisingly, a history of pre-LVAD GIB has not consistently been noted as a risk factor for GIB post-implantation.

Multifactorial Pathogenesis of GIB after LVAD Surgery

The pathophysiology of GIB in patients requiring LVAD support is largely unknown and likely multifactorial. One contributor may be the antithrombotic and antiplatelet therapy frequently utilized to reduce the risk of pump thrombosis and thromboembolic events such as stroke. An interesting observation, however, is that GIB occurs more frequently after implantation of LVADs compared to mechanical heart valves (18% vs. 4%) despite similar INR targets.

Another contributory mechanism may be pump-enhanced shearing of high–molecular weight multimers of von Willebrand Factor (vWF), effectively causing acquired von Willebrand Disease (aVWD). This phenomenon is seen with both axial and centrifugal continuous-flow pumps but not in now-obsolete pulsatile LVADs, where coincidently the incidence of

GIB was 3 times lower. Moreover, patients who undergo LVAD explanation for transplantation or myocardial recovery exhibit near universal recovery of aVWD. As with anticoagulation, this cannot wholly account for LVAD-related GIB as aVWD is nearly universal, while GIB is not.

One other major contributor to LVAD-related GIB is angiodysplasia, in particular the formation of gastrointestinal arteriovenous malformations (AVMs). Supporting this, AVMs are the most frequently identified lesions in this group of patients. This angiodysplasia is unique from age-related angiodysplasia and predominantly occurs in the small intestine. Driving this process is endothelial and vascular smooth muscle dysfunction due to abnormal mechanical strain transmitted from the minimally pulsatile, continuous-flow LVAD.

Presentation and Diagnosis of GIB during LVAD Support

The presentation and diagnosis of LVAD-related GIB are similar to any other GIB. Patients typically present >3 months after implantation with melena, similar to our case patient, although they may also present, less commonly, with hematemesis, coffee-ground emesis, frank rectal bleeding, heme-positive stools, or anemia with no other clear source. While most are hemodynamically stable, the threshold for prompt inpatient admission and workup should be low given that LVAD patients generally have severe comorbidities. In the initial history and physical exam, it is important to perform a thorough medication review, particularly antithrombotic and antiplatelet drugs as well as over-the-counter non-steroidal anti-inflammatory drugs, which patients often overlook and do not disclose.

If a GIB is suspected, it is imperative to consult a gastroenterologist, as was done in our case. Bleeding can occur anywhere along the GI tract, although it is most frequent in the upper GI tract (~50%), followed by the colon (~20%) and small intestine beyond the duodenum (~15%). As mentioned, AVMs are the most frequently identified lesion (up to 60%), with ulcerative lesions being the next most common (up to 30%). The next step in evaluation will depend upon whether the source of the GIB is suspected to be upper or lower. Prior data and practice had been to perform an upper endoscopy as the first diagnostic modality for a suspected upper GIB, though more recent data from our institution and others have shown push enteroscopy to have higher diagnostic and therapeutic yield as the first modality. For initial presentations with stable hematochezia, colonoscopy should be the first diagnostic modality pursued. Please refer to Figure 21.1 for the diagnostic algorithm used at our institution.

Regarding ongoing or residual antithrombotic and antiplatelet therapy, we may briefly hold anticoagulation but typically do not recommend reversal unless the patient is having hemodynamically significant bleeding. In our case, the GI consult service recommended and performed an urgent push enteroscopy on the day of admission, with no lesions noted. The patient continued to have a decreasing hemoglobin concentration, prompting a colonoscopy 2 days later, which also failed to localize any source of bleeding.

In a case like this, where the initial endoscopic exams are negative and the patient has clear signs of GIB, additional studies are warranted. One such study is device-assisted enteroscopy (DAE; single balloon, double balloon, or spiral enteroscopy), which allows evaluation deeper into the small bowel. Other modalities include video capsule endoscopy (VCE), nuclear tagged red blood cell scintigraphy, and angiography. Although VCE is most effective at discovering the source of bleeding in cases of occult and inactive

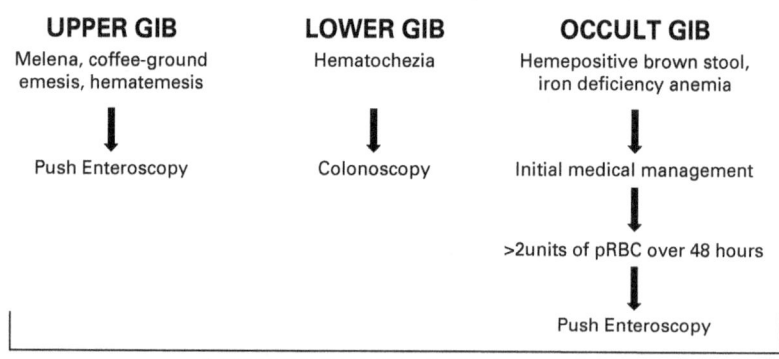

UPPER GIB	**LOWER GIB**	**OCCULT GIB**
Melena, coffee-ground emesis, hematemesis	Hematochezia	Hemepositive brown stool, iron deficiency anemia
↓	↓	↓
Push Enteroscopy	Colonoscopy	Initial medical management
		↓
		>2units of pRBC over 48 hours
		↓
		Push Enteroscopy

Additional endoscopic evaluation in cases of:
- Hemodynamic instability despite administration of blood products
- Persistent GIB despite withholding or after resumption of lower-dose antithrombotic treatment
- Age-appropriate colon cancer screening

GIB= Gastrointestinal bleed;pRBC = Packed red blood cells

FIGURE 21.1 Diagnostic and management algorithm for LVAD-related GIB at Columbia University Irving Medical Center.

GIB as it permits evaluation of the entire GI tract, in immobile hospitalized patients the feasibility and yield may be lower than in published series. Scintigraphy and angiography are better suited for active bleeding. In some instances, especially when prior small bowel AVMs have been documented, proceeding directly to DAE may be reasonable. VCE was performed in our patient, but no source was identified. This occurs in approximately 20% of patients.

Treatment and Secondary Prophylaxis of GIB with LVAD

Management of LVAD-related GIB is challenging and requires a multi-modal and multidisciplinary approach including teams from gastroenterology and cardiology as well as critical care medicine and anesthesiology in cases where resuscitation and airway protection are needed. With respect to non-pharmacologic treatment, endoscopy is the mainstay of management and is successful in 80%–90% of patients, although rebleeding is still common. Specific endoscopic treatments include argon plasma coagulation, contact coagulation, hemostatic clips, and epinephrine injection. There has been no definitive evaluation of the superiority of one endoscopic technique over another, and the choice of modality should be driven by the etiology of bleeding. Other non-pharmacologic treatments are limited. Given the association of GIB with reduced pulsatility, an LVAD pump speed reduction strategy may be considered. However, this has not been prospectively validated, and the risks of inadequate LV unloading precipitating heart failure as well as device thrombosis must be considered. Ultimately, as able, LVAD removal for myocardial recovery or transplantation is the best treatment.

With respect to medical management, if there is ongoing or hemodynamically significant bleeding, the initial treatment should be a temporary hold of antithrombotic and antiplatelet therapy. This, however, is not without risk. A multicenter study of LVAD patients noted a roughly 7-fold greater likelihood of thromboembolic events in patients with a prior GIB, which the authors attributed to reduced anticoagulation post-GIB. Moreover, a recent multicenter study called TRACE (STudy of Reduced Anti-Coagulation/Anti-platelEt Therapy in Patients with the HeartMate II LVAS) in HM II LVAD patients with a history of GIB showed that rates of rebleeding were high regardless of reduced anticoagulation strategies. While this trial has many limitations, it does not support prolonged discontinuation of anticoagulation, which is still advocated in many centers. Thus, in the acute period a temporary hold of anticoagulation can be considered, but full anticoagulation should be resumed after the GIB has resolved. This is what was done in our case.

Other pharmacotherapeutic options are available, although data surrounding their efficacy and safety are limited. The best-supported medical therapy is angiotensin-converting enzyme inhibitors (ACEIs) and angiotensin II receptor blockers (ARBs). These drugs can limit angiotensin II–induced angiogenesis and thereby reduce bleeding episodes. Conveniently, ACEI/ARB therapy is already widely used in LVAD patients. This therapy is low-cost, and the adverse effect profile is minimal. If an LVAD patient with a GIB is not already taking an ACEI/ARB, it should be strongly considered. On the other hand, antisecretory agents like proton pump inhibitors, although widely used including in our case, have no benefit unless the cause of GIB is ulcer-related. Ulcers account for only 20%–25% of LVAD-related bleeds. A novel agent for LVAD-related GIB is octreotide, a synthetic somatostatin analogue that is used to treat GIB due to angiodysplastic lesions and portal hypertension in non-LVAD patients. Octreotide reduces intestinal blood flow due to splanchnic artery vasoconstriction, improves platelet aggregation, and inhibits angiogenesis. The data supporting its use for primary and secondary prophylaxis of LVAD-associated GIB are scarce though, with most evidence coming from case reports and series. While additional prospective trials are needed to validate the utility of octreotide in this setting, it is a safe and well-tolerated option for patients with bleeding refractory to conventional therapy. This was utilized in our case patient. Possibly related to this, the patient had a stable hemoglobin and did not require further transfusion soon after initiation of octreotide.

There are many other second- and third-line pharmacotherapies that are supported only weakly by the current literature and should only be used by experienced practitioners after other treatments have failed. One such medication is thalidomide, which has anti-angiogenic properties. Another medication is danzol, a weak androgen with procoagulant properties that has been effectively used in cases of refractory GIB caused by aVWD.

Desmopressin, a synthetic analogic of vasopressin that stimulates release of vWF and dramatically increases factor VIII levels, is another potential medication. Similarly, doxycycline is now known to inhibit ADAMTS-13-mediated cleavage of vWF. Other promising pharmacotherapies for GIB that are currently untested in the setting of LVADs include lenalidomide, a second-generation immunomodulatory compound that was derived from thalidomide; high-dose 3-hydroxy-3-methylglutaryl–coenzyme A reductase inhibitors, which exhibit antiangiogenic properties; and antifibrinolytic agents like tranexamic acid.

At the time of hospital discharge, the focus should be on secondary prevention using the strategies discussed. As previously mentioned, a multidisciplinary approach involving cardiology, hematology, and gastroenterology services is key for evaluating anticoagulation targets, adjusting LVAD pump speed, and considering additional medications.

Future Developments

In addition to the need for more prospective clinical trials and the continued advancement of LVAD design driven by a growing understanding of continuous-flow physiology, a more personalized approach to the management of anticoagulation is needed as each patient has different risk factors that fluctuate over time. A more comprehensive assessment of hematologic activity may be facilitated by modern tests such as thromboelastography. This may provide a unique fingerprint of each patient's hemostasis pathways and can lead to the development of new pharmacologic strategies.

CASE RESUMES

The patient was resuscitated with volume and packed red blood cells with close monitoring of his LVAD flow and pulsatility indices. Bedside echocardiography was serially obtained to assess right ventricular volume overload and function. He was given clotting factors to partially reverse his INR. Once bleeding had subsided, he underwent a colonoscopy and was found to several areas of AVMs. After multidisciplinary consultation, the decision to maintain a lower INR goal of 1.5 and was initiated on an ACEI for hopeful recession of angiodyplasia.

KEY POINTS TO REMEMBER

1. GIB is a frequent and troublesome long-term complication of LVAD surgery.
2. The pathophysiology of LVAD-related GIB is unclear but likely results from aVWD, angiodysplasia, and abnormal vascular loading from minimally pulsatile, continuous blood flow.
3. The primary and best-supported diagnostic and treatment modality is enteroscopy, with obligatory gastroenterology consultation.
4. Other diagnostic strategies include colonoscopy, video capsule endoscopy, nuclear tagged red blood cell scintigraphy, and angiography.
5. Other pharmacologic treatments include ACEIs, proton pump inhibitors, and octreotide.

Suggested Reading
1. Axelrad JE, Pinsino A, Trinh PN, et al. Limited usefulness of endoscopic evaluation in patients with continuous-flow left ventricular assist devices and gastrointestinal bleeding. *J Heart Lung Transplant.* 2018;37(6):723–732.
2. Converse M, Sobhanian M, Mardis A, et al. Impact of angiotensin II inhibitors on the incidence of gastrointestinal bleeds after left ventricular assist device placement. *J Heart Lung Transplant.* 2017;36(4 suppl):S150.
3. Cushing K, Kushnir V. Gastrointestinal bleeding following LVAD placement from top to bottom. *Dig Dis Sci.* 2016;61(6):1440–1447.
4. Demirozu ZT, Radovancevic R, Hochman LF, et al. Arteriovenous malformation and gastrointestinal bleeding in patients with the HeartMate II left ventricular assist device. *J Heart Lung Transplant.* 2011;30(8):849–853.
5. Kim JH, Brophy DF, Shah KB. Continuous-flow left ventricular assist device-related gastrointestinal bleeding. *Cardiol Clin.* 2018;36(4):519–529.
6. Patel SR, Oh KT, Ogriki T, et al. Cessation of continuous flow left ventricular assist device-related gastrointestinal bleeding after heart transplantation. *ASAIO J.* 2018;64(2):191–195.
7. Sieg AC, Moretz JD, Horn E, Jennings DL. Pharmacotherapeutic management of gastrointestinal bleeding in patients with continuous-flow left ventricular assist devices. *Pharmacotherapy.* 2017;37(11):1432–1448.

22 Right Ventricular Assist Device Therapies

Adrian Alexis-Ruiz and Marisa Cevasco

A 60-year-old female with a past medical history of non-ischemic cardiomyopathy with an ejection fraction of 10% is admitted to the intensive care unit for hypotension and shortness of breath. She eventually undergoes implantation of a HeartMate 3 left ventricular (LV) assist device (LVAD). Her postoperative course is notable for escalating doses of vasopressors and inotropes, minimal urine output, and a rising central venous pressure (CVP). Her lactic acid is 7 mmol/L, her liver function tests are elevated, and her mixed venous oxygen saturation is 47%. You are concerned for postoperative right ventricular (RV) failure.

What do you do now?

DISCUSSION

RV Failure

RV failure after LVAD placement can occur from volume overload to the RV from increased LVAD flow and septal bowing into the LV cavity with LV decompression and increased RV volume. These changes in RV geometry reduce cardiac output and can be life-threatening. Clinical signs of acute RV failure include elevated CVP, decreased urine output, elevated liver function tests, peripheral vasodilation (warm on exam), and low mixed venous oxygen saturation. Echocardiography findings can reveal a dilated and hypocontractile RV, septal flattening or bowing into the LV cavity, and tricuspid annular plane systolic excursion <14 mm. Pulmonary artery pressures may be normal in patients with pulmonary hypertension due to long-standing left heart dysfunction also known as postcapillary pulmonary hypertension. It is important to make the correct diagnosis as these patients will benefit from medical or surgical management of LV failure. Patients with isolated RV failure due to increased afterload in the setting of pulmonary hypertension or cor pulmonale will have increased pulmonary artery pressures. Right heart catheterization and cardiac magnetic resonance imaging are useful diagnostic modalities as well but not suitable for patients in the acute postoperative period.

Management of this complex patient requires a multidisciplinary approach in a high-volume center with cardiologists, cardiac surgeons, and intensivists experienced in the management of refractory cardiogenic shock and mechanical circulatory support.

Fluid management optimizes preload and considers both RV function and RV afterload. Excessive fluid may increase free wall tension and cause and reduce myocardial perfusion. A volume-overloaded RV after LVAD placement often requires ventricular offloading with diuretics or renal replacement therapy in the acute perioperative period. Echocardiography can be helpful in managing fluid administration and removal via assessments of the both RV function and septal position.

Reducing RV afterload can enhance RV performance. Correcting hypoxemia, hypercapnia, and acidosis can reduce pulmonary vascular resistance. Additional therapies may include pulmonary vasodilators such as nitric oxide, prostacyclin derivatives, and phosphodiesterase 5 inhibitors. Administration of inotropic medications can also manage RV dysfunction.

Despite initiation of medical therapies, the patient develops multisystem organ failure, and RV assist device (RVAD) therapies are considered.

RVADs

Current RVAD options include the Impella Right Peripheral (RP), the Tandem Heart (TH), the Protek Duo system, and a surgically placed CentriMag RVAD. Important considerations when choosing a device include operator familiarity, the need for an oxygenator, the availability of a surgeon, and specific contraindications such as severe tricuspid regurgitation, an occluded internal jugular vein, and the presence of an inferior vena cava filter (Figure 22.1 and Table 22.1).

The Impella RP is a catheter-based microaxial pump designed to support the RV for up to 14 days. It is placed percutaneously through the femoral vein and positioned with transesophageal echocardiography and fluoroscopic guidance. The inflow portion of the catheter is in the inferior vena cava, and the outflow portion lies in the pulmonary artery. The Impella RP can provide flows up to 5 L/min and theoretically unloads the RV. Complications of the Impella RP include bleeding around the cannula site, which is typically remedied with a purse-string stitch.

The TH RVAD is similar to the Impella RP because it directs blood flow from the right atrium to the pulmonary artery. Unlike the Impella RP that

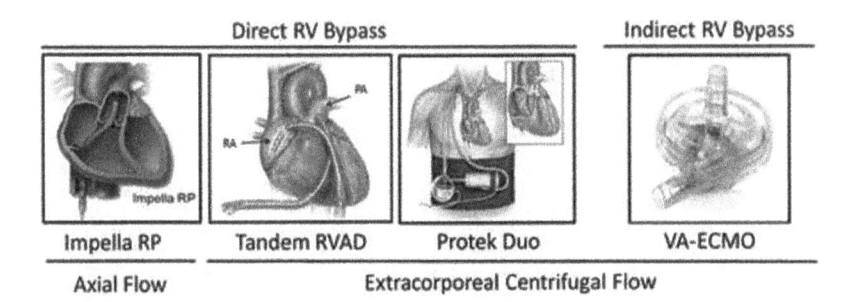

FIGURE 22.1 Classifications of acute mechanical circulatory support devices for right ventricular (RV) failure. Device options include direct and indirect RV bypass, as well as intracorporeal (Impella RP) and extracorporeal (Tandem RV assist device [RVAD], Protek Duo, venoarterial extracorporeal membrane oxygenation [VA-ECMO]) options.

TABLE 22.1 **Different Types of RVADs and Their Associated Characteristics**

Device	Major Advantages	Complications	Relative Contraindications	Disadvantages
Impella RP	Catheter lab placement via femoral vein	Bleeding, retroperitoneal hematoma, thrombus formation on the cannula	Tricuspid regurgitation/ tricuspid valve prosthesis	Inability to ambulate or sit upright in bed
Protek Duo	Inserted similar to an internal jugular Swan, increased mobility	Thrombus formation on the cannula, rare superior vena cava syndrome	Small right internal jugular or deep vein thrombosis in internal jugular	Distal cannula tip can migrate backward into the RV and not remain across the pulmonary valve
Centrimag	Significant cardiac output; maximize support, oxygenator can be added	Wound or mediastinal infection, surgical bleeding, cannula dislodgement	Patient should be considered bridge to recovery or transplant	Requires placement and removal in the operating room
Tandem Heart	Relatively simple placement	Bleeding, retroperitoneal hematoma, thrombus formation on the cannula	Inferior vena cava filter	Inability to ambulate

has an axial pump that lies within the circulation, the TH RVAD uses an extracorporeal centrifugal-flow pump and 2 venous cannulas. This device typically requires accessing both femoral veins for outflow and inflow and provides a flow between 2 and 4 L/min. Placement of this type of RVAD is generally well tolerated, and most complications are related to vascular injury.

The Protek Duo is a percutaneously placed dual-lumen cannula inserted through the right internal jugular vein over a guidewire under fluoroscopic guidance. Its proximal port lies in the right atrium, and its distal outflow port lies distal to the pulmonary valve in the main pulmonary artery. It is available in 2 different sizes and should be tailored depending on the patient's cardiac output needs. An oxygenator can be spliced in as needed.

A surgically placed Centrimag requires a sternotomy and placement of the inflow cannula in either the right atrium or femoral vein and placement of the outflow cannula in the pulmonary artery. Flows can be maximized to provide full cardiac output. Similar to the ProTek duo, an oxygenator can be spliced in.

It is important to consider the hemodynamic effects on the LV after placement of an RVAD. Identifying biventricular failure early is critical when RVAD implantation is considered. RVADs reduce right atrial pressure, increase flow through the pulmonary arteries, and increase LV preload and wedge pressure. This change in preload may worsen LV function and cause pulmonary edema in patients with LV failure. LVAD revolutions per minute may need to increase after placement of an RVAD to manage increased flow to the LV. Assessing changes in oxygen saturation, blood pressure, and echocardiographic indices can guide hemodynamic management of RVAD therapy.

Weaning from RVAD support can be accomplished after reductions in inotropic and vasopressor support, normalization of the CVP, and recovery of kidney and liver function. Of note, there are data suggesting that elevated preoperative white blood cell counts and creatinine levels are predictors of unsuccessful RVAD wean. RVAD wean is typically performed with progressive reduction of flow and monitoring of the CVP. Echocardiography can be used as an adjunct, as needed. If there is no significant impact on cardiac function, filling pressures, and RV imaging on echocardiogram, the RVAD can be removed percutaneously or surgically.

CASE RESUMES

The patient undergoes an emergent Centrimag RVAD placement with hemisternotomy and right atrial and pulmonary artery cannulation. She stabilizes with this support and inotropes and vasopressors are optimized for blood pressure and mixed venous saturation goals. She is aggressively diuresed on postoperative days 1-2 with decrease in her CVP to 7mmHg.

On postoperative day 3, her Centrimag flows are decreased while undergoing an echocardiographic exam and monitoring of her CVP and pulmonary artery pressures. Later that day, her Centrimag RVAD is removed and she continued to recover in the intensive care unit.

> **KEY POINTS TO REMEMBER**
>
> 1. RV failure after LVAD placement is an emergency.
> 2. RVAD insertion should be directed by institutional protocols, proceduralist experience, and comfort level.
> 3. RVAD therapies reduce right atrial pressure and increase LV preload.
> 4. Management of patients with an RVAD should be guided by monitoring CVP, kidney and other end-organ recovery, and echocardiography as needed.

Suggested Reading
1. Patil NP, Mohite PN, Sabashnikov A, et al. Preoperative predictors and outcomes of right ventricular assist device implantation after continuous-flow left ventricular assist device implantation. *J Thorac Cardiovasc Surg.* 2015;150(6):1651–1658.
2. Ventetuolo CE, Klinger JR. Management of acute right ventricular failure in the intensive care unit. *Ann Am Thorac Soc.* 2014;11(5):811–822. doi:10.1513/AnnalsATS.201312-446FR.
3. Takayama H, Naka Y, Kodali SK, et al. A novel approach to percutaneous right-ventricular mechanical support. *Eur J Cardiothorac Surg.* 2012;41(2):423–426. doi:10.1016/j.ejcts.2011.05.041.
4. Haneya A, Philipp A, Puehler T, et al. Temporary percutaneous right ventricular support using a centrifugal pump in patients with postoperative acute refractory right ventricular failure after left ventricular assist device implantation. *Eur J Cardiothorac Surg.* 2012;41(1):219–223. doi:10.1016/j.ejcts.2011.04.029.
5. Kapur NK, Esposito ML, Bader Y, et al. Mechanical circulatory support devices for acute right ventricular failure. *Circulation.* 2017;136(3):314–326. doi:10.1161/CIRCULATIONAHA.116.025290.

23 A Failure to Oxygenate: A Case for Venovenous Extracorporeal Membrane Oxygenation

Cara Agerstrand and Andrew Pellet

A previously healthy 32-year-old woman presents with 5 days of fever, cough, and progressive shortness of breath. Her room air oxygen saturation is 82%. A chest radiograph shows bilateral opacities, and a bedside echocardiogram demonstrates normal biventricular function. She receives empiric coverage for influenza and bacterial pneumonia and requires endotracheal intubation, after which she is managed with low–tidal volume, low-pressure ventilation; moderate positive end-expiratory pressure; and a fraction of inspired oxygen (FiO_2) of 1. Because her partial pressure of arterial oxygen (PaO_2) is 110 mm Hg, she receives neuromuscular blockade and is placed in the prone position. Despite these strategies, her oxygenation worsens and her PaO_2 to FiO_2 ratio is 69 mm Hg the following day.

What do you do now?

DISCUSSION

Diagnosis and Management of Acute Respiratory Distress Syndrome

This patient is suffering from severe acute lung injury from pneumonia and complicated by the acute respiratory distress syndrome (ARDS). The following criteria must be fulfilled to diagnose ARDS :

1. Onset or clinical worsening of respiratory symptoms within 1 week of a known insult (such as infection, trauma, transfusion)
2. Presence of bilateral pulmonary infiltrates on radiographic imaging (not fully explained by masses, nodules, effusions, or atelectasis)
3. Respiratory failure not fully attributable to cardiac failure or volume overload
4. Impairment in oxygenation, based on a PaO_2 to FiO_2 ratio ≤300 mm Hg

After ARDS is diagnosed, it is critical to characterize its severity because severity influences medical management and predicts mortality (Table 23.1). The severity of ARDS is determined by the degree of impairment in the PaO_2 to FiO_2 ratio:

The hallmark of ARDS management is a lung-protective ventilation strategy, which utilizes low tidal volumes and low airway pressures by targeting tidal volumes ≤6 cc/kg of ideal body weight and an end-inspiratory plateau pressure (Pplat) of ≤30 cm H_2O. This strategy targets a PaO_2 of 55-80 mm Hg or peripheral oxygen saturation of 88%–95%.

If a patient has moderate to severe ARDS, neuromuscular blockade may facilitate patient–ventilator synchrony, increase chest wall compliance, and improve survival, particularly in severely hypoxemic patients with a PaO_2 to

TABLE 23.1 **ARDS Severity**

ARDS Severity	PaO_2 to FiO_2	Predicted Mortality
Mild	200–≤300 mm Hg	27%
Moderate	100–≤200 mm Hg	32%
Severe	<100 mm Hg	45%

FiO_2 ration <120 mm Hg. In patients with a PaO_2 to FiO_2 ratio <150 mm Hg, prone positioning has been shown to reduce mortality, recruit lung, and improve ventilation to perfusion (V/Q) matching. Inhaled nitric oxide may also improve oxygenation by improving V/Q matching, although no survival benefit has been demonstrated in the setting of ARDS.

The clinician in this vignette has exhausted other evidenced-based approaches to manage this patient's severe ARDS. Given these circumstances, this patient should be considered for venovenous extracorporeal membrane oxygenation (ECMO).

Evidence for ECMO

ECMO has been used to support patients with severe respiratory failure since the early 1970s, but widespread application was limited by the complexity of the technology as well as a high-risk profile. Since 2009, driven by the development of safer and more biocompatible ECMO technology, the encouraging outcomes reported during the 2009 influenza A (H1N1) pandemic, and the publication of the Conventional Ventilatory Support versus Extracorporeal Membrane Oxygenation for Severe Adult Respiratory Failure (CESAR) trial, ECMO use has skyrocketed.

CESAR was a multicenter trial that randomized 180 adults with severe hypoxemic respiratory failure to conventional ventilation or transfer to an ECMO referral center for consideration of ECMO. An improvement in survival without severe disability was reported in the group referred for ECMO. However, the strength of conclusions is limited by several factors: a number of patients randomized for consideration of ECMO did not actually receive ECMO, and significantly more patients in the ECMO-referred group were managed with lung-protective ventilation. A conservative interpretation of the CESAR trial is that it demonstrated clinical benefit of treatment at an ECMO-capable center, highly experienced in the management of patients with severe respiratory failure.

The multicenter Extracorporeal Membrane Oxygenation for Severe Acute Respiratory Distress Syndrome (EOLIA) trial sought to address the limitations of CESAR by randomizing patients with severe ARDS to venovenous ECMO with an ultra-lung-protective ventilator strategy (Pplat ≤24 cm H_2O) versus a protocolized strategy of lung-protective ventilation, in which use of neuromuscular blockade and prone positioning were encouraged. The primary outcome was 60-day mortality. Based on trial design, after the fourth interim analysis and enrollment of 249 of a maximum 331 patients, the trial was stopped for being unable to reach a predicted reduction in mortality of 20% in the ECMO group. Though a 20% mortality reduction was not achieved, a still impressive 11% reduction in 60-day morality in the ECMO group was demonstrated. The key secondary outcome of treatment failure (which was defined as death in the ECMO group and death or crossover to ECMO in the control group after meeting stringent criteria) favored the ECMO group with a relative risk of mortality of 0.62 (95% confidence interval [CI] 0.47–0.82, $p < 0.001$). Other secondary endpoints, including days free of renal and other organ failure, also favored the group supported with ECMO. A notable limitation of EOLIA was the high rate of crossover from the control to the ECMO group (28% of control group patients), which diluted the benefit of ECMO in the intention-to-treat analysis. Given this high percentage of crossover, a post hoc sensitivity analysis was performed which demonstrated a hazard ratio for mortality in the ECMO group of 0.51 (95% CI 0.24–1.02, $p = 0.055$). Although EOLIA was not positive by traditional interpretation, all 3 major analyses and secondary endpoints suggest some degree of benefit of ECMO in severe ARDS.

Patient Selection
Patient selection is of the utmost importance for successful use of ECMO. Patients being considered for venovenous ECMO for ARDS should meet criteria for severe ARDS. Best guidance can be taken from the Extracorporeal Life Support Organization's recommendations and the EOLIA trial, using inclusion criteria of a PaO_2 to FiO_2 ratio <80 mm Hg or uncompensated hypercapnic acidosis with a pH <7.25 in the setting of CO_2 >60 mm Hg, despite optimized ventilator settings (low tidal volume, lung-protective ventilation targeting Pplat ≤30 cm H_2O, moderate to high positive end-expiratory pressure [PEEP]) and use of appropriate adjunctive therapies, such as neuromuscular blockade and prone positioning. ECMO should be used early in the course of illness, before the development of fibroproliferative or fibrotic ARDS.

The main contraindication to ECMO is any condition or organ dysfunction that would limit the overall benefit of ECMO, such as severe brain injury, metastatic cancer, or decompensated cirrhosis. Of note, it is generally not recommended that patients with chronic lung disease who experience decompensation be placed on ECMO unless intended as a bridge to lung transplantation. Additional relative contraindications to ECMO include advanced age, poor baseline functional status, prolonged mechanical ventilation, inability to tolerate anticoagulation, and limited vascular access.

The patient in the vignette meets criteria for severe ARDS despite optimized medical management, has been endotracheally intubated less than 7 days, and has no other contraindication to ECMO. She is placed on venovenous ECMO via cannulae placed in her right femoral and right internal jugular veins with notable improvement in her oxygenation (Figure 23.1).

How ECMO Works

Venovenous ECMO provides respiratory support and is the most common ECMO configuration used during ARDS. In venovenous ECMO, blood is pulled into a large venous cannula and pumped into an oxygenator. The oxygenator is composed of 2 chambers separated by

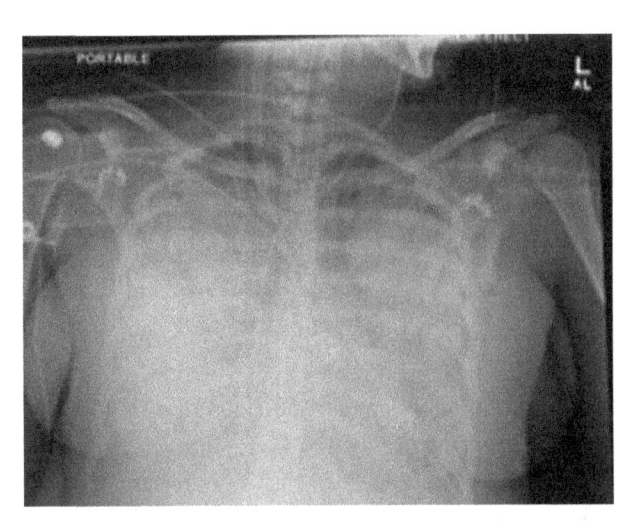

FIGURE 23.1 Chest radiograph following ECMO cannulation with a right femoral venous drainage cannula and a right internal jugular venous reinfusion cannula.

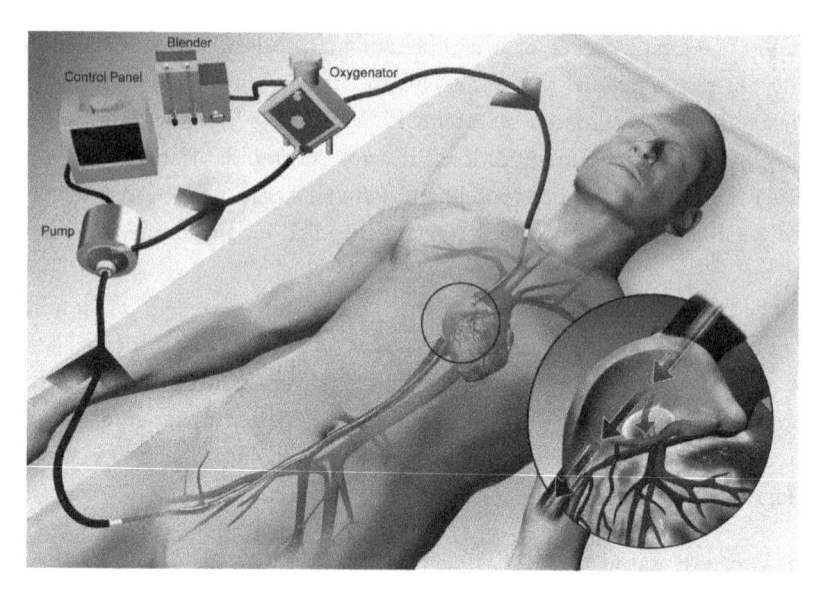

FIGURE 23.2 Venovenous ECMO. Mixing of poorly oxygenated blood traversing the lungs and ejected by the heart with well-oxygenated blood retrogradely infused from the ECMO. Location of the resultant mixing zone (purple arrows) along the aorta will determine the adequacy of brain oxygenation.

a semipermeable membrane, across which the diffusion-mediated gas exchange of oxygen and carbon dioxide occurs (Figure 23.2). While venous blood flows through one chamber, a continuous supply of sweep gas (typically comprised of 100% oxygen) flows through the other so that blood exiting the oxygenator is low in carbon dioxide and rich in oxygen. The oxygenated blood is then returned to the patient via a cannula inserted into the venous system. As venovenous ECMO is arranged in series with the lungs, it does not provide direct cardiac support but may indirectly improve hemodynamics by improving oxygen delivery to the coronary arteries and reducing hypoxemia-mediated pulmonary hypertension.

The amount of respiratory support obtained from venovenous ECMO is primarily determined by the blood flow rate through the ECMO circuit, which is largely limited by the size of the drainage cannula. Cannula size should be chosen to accommodate the patient's predicted cardiac output (based on body surface area and a cardiac index of 2.4 L/min/m^2), being mindful of the fact that actual cardiac output will likely be much higher in the critically ill state. An ECMO blood flow rate >60% of actual cardiac output has been shown to achieve an oxygen saturation >90%. More important than oxygen saturation, however, is maintaining adequate oxygen delivery, which may be possible to achieve with a significantly lower oxygen saturation.

While oxygenation is primarily dependent on blood flow rate, CO_2 clearance is primarily determined by the sweep gas flow rate. Since CO_2 more easily diffuses across the membrane oxygenator, even at a low blood flow rate, provided a continuous supply of sweep gas is present, efficient CO_2 clearance can occur.

Management During ECMO

Once the ECMO circuit is operational, ventilator settings must be optimized to protect the injured lungs by adhering to an ultra-lung-protective "lung rest" strategy. Mechanical ventilation settings consistent with this approach would be a respiratory rate <10 breaths per minute, PEEP of 10–12 cm H_2O, FiO_2 <50%, and Pplat ≤24 cm H_2O in a volume-controlled mode (or peak inspiratory pressure ≤25 cm H_2O in a pressure-controlled mode). Select patients may be able to be liberated from the ventilator altogether during ECMO and managed with ECMO-supported gas exchange alone. However, this approach should be reserved for highly selected patients at experienced ECMO centers. Maintaining a net negative volume status (in patients without severely impaired hemodynamics or other indications for fluid resuscitation) is favored to reduce pulmonary edema and improve native gas exchange.

While receiving ECMO support, patients are typically anticoagulated with a continuous infusion of intravenous heparin targeting a low-level anticoagulated state (for example, activated partial thromboplastin time of 40–60 seconds) in order to prevent thrombus within the circuit and oxygenator. Bleeding is the most common complication reported during ECMO because of anticoagulation and circuit-related consumptive coagulopathy. Though the frequency and severity of bleeding have decreased with modern, more biocompatible ECMO circuitry and reduced-dose anticoagulation, clinicians must be mindful of the delicate balance between thrombosis and bleeding.

Weaning from ECMO

On ECMO day 7, the patient has improved radiographic appearance of her infiltrates. She has been diuresed, and her oxygenation has substantially improved. Your resident asks how you know if the patient is ready to wean from ECMO.

There are several appropriate ways to wean venovenous ECMO, but all include decreasing ECMO support once the patient's clinical condition has improved in order to assess physiologic readiness for decannulation. Typically, the fraction of delivered oxygen (FdO_2) in the sweep gas and the sweep gas flow rate are incrementally decreased while the blood flow is maintained. Ventilator settings should be adjusted to a level that would be tolerated in the absence of ECMO, ensuring that there is an adequate oxygenation and ventilatory buffer should the patient decompensate after decannulation. During the weaning process, the patient should be monitored for tachypnea, and arterial blood gasses should be followed to ensure acceptable acid–base status. Once ECMO is weaned to minimal settings (FdO_2 0.21 and sweep gas flow of 0.8 L/min) but prior to decannulation, a trial run "off sweep" is in order. With the sweep gas turned off, gas exchange is eliminated in the membrane oxygenator even though blood continues to circulate. If the patient is able to maintain adequate arterial oxygenation and CO_2 clearance, the patient may be prepared for decannulation. Prior to decannulation, heparin should be held for approximately 1 hour. Cannulae placed percutaneously can be removed at bedside with hemostasis achieved by applying direct pressure.

CASE RESUMES

After reviewing the patient's current ECMO and ventilator settings, as well as her most recent arterial blood gas, you both agree that the patient is ready for a trial off ECMO support. The patient's ventilator is adjusted to a respiratory rate of 14 breaths per minute, tidal volume is increased to 6 cc/kg ideal body weight with a Pplat of 24 cm H_2O, PEEP of 10 cm H_2O, and FiO_2 of 0.5. After an incremental decrease in FdO_2 and sweep gas flow in 1 L/min increments, a trial "off sweep" is performed for 30 minutes. Her respiratory rate has not markedly increased off sweep, she appears comfortable, and her arterial blood gas shows a pH of 7.41, partial pressure of carbon dioxide ($PaCO_2$) of 38 mm Hg, and PaO_2 of 105 mm Hg. She is successfully decannulated from ECMO and extubated to nasal cannula oxygen 3 days later. After a 14-day hospital stay, she is successfully discharged to home.

KEY POINTS TO REMEMBER

1. Venovenous ECMO is an important rescue strategy for patients meeting criteria for severe ARDS (PaO_2 to FiO_2 ratio <80 mm Hg or pH <7.25 with $PaCO_2$ >60 mm Hg) despite optimized ventilator and medical management.
2. Patients should have a reversible condition and be early in the course of ARDS.
3. ECMO blood flow rate is the primary determinant of oxygen during ECMO.
4. ECMO sweep gas flow rate is the primary determinant of CO_2 clearance during ECMO.
5. Patients receiving ECMO for ARDS should be ventilated with a "lung rest" strategy.

Suggested Reading

1. Ranieri VM, Rubenfeld GD, Thompson BT, et al. Acute respiratory distress syndrome: the Berlin definition. *JAMA*. 2012;307(23):2526–2533.
2. Paden ML, Conrad SA, Rycus PT, et al. Extracorporeal life support organization registry report 2012. *ASAIO J*. 2013;59:202–210.
3. Peek GJ, Mugford M, Tiruvoipati R, et al. Efficacy and economic assessment of conventional ventilatory support versus extracorporeal membrane oxygenation for severe adult respiratory failure (CESAR): a multicentre randomised controlled trial. *Lancet* 2009;374(9698):1351–1363.
4. Combes A, Hajage D, Capellier G, et al. Extracorporeal membrane oxygenation for severe acute respiratory distress syndrome. *N Engl J Med*. 2018;378(21):1965–1975.
5. Schmidt M, Tachon G, Devilliers C, et al. Blood oxygenation and decarboxylation determinants during venovenous ECMO for respiratory failure in adults. *Intensive Care Med*. 2013;39(5):838–846.

6. Agerstrand CL, Burkart KM, Abrams DC, et al. Blood conservation in extracorporeal membrane oxygenation for acute respiratory distress syndrome. *Ann Thorac Surg*. 2015;99(2):590–595.
7. Agerstrand C, Bacchetta MD, Brodie D. ECMO for adult respiratory failure: current use and evolving applications. *ASAIO J*. 2014;60(3):255–262.

24 Critical Concepts in Extracorporeal Life Support for Cardiogenic Shock

Juan C. Diaz Soto, Justin A. Fried, and A. Reshad Garan

A 62-year-old man presents for coronary artery bypass surgery with a left ventricular (LV) ejection fraction of 30% and severe mitral regurgitation. During weaning from cardiopulmonary bypass, he is hypotensive, and venoarterial extracorporeal life support (ECLS) via his femoral vein and artery is initiated. His arterial pulse pressure measured via a right radial artery catheter is 8 mm Hg, and his partial pressure of oxygen (PaO_2) measured from that catheter is 180 mm Hg. Over the next 2 days, the patient's hemodynamics improve, but he becomes progressively hypoxemic and the arterial pulse pressure is now 30 mm Hg.

What do you do now?

DISCUSSION

Venoarterial extracorporeal membrane oxygenation (VA-ECMO), also known as ECLS, is increasingly used to support patients with refractory cardiogenic shock and cardiopulmonary collapse. VA-ECMO is a simplified form of cardiopulmonary bypass which provides both circulatory support and gas exchange. The basic components of a VA-ECMO circuit include the following: a venous drainage cannula, a centrifugal flow pump, a membrane oxygenator, a heat exchanger, and an arterial reinfusion cannula. The venous inflow cannula, typically 19F to 25F in size, drains deoxygenated venous blood from the superior vena cava, right atrium, and inferior vena cava, often via the femoral vein, right internal jugular vein, or subclavian vein. Blood then passes through an extracorporeal pump and across an oxygenator, where gas exchange occurs. A heat exchanger is used to prevent heat loss with extracorporeal transit of blood. Oxygenated blood is then reinfused to the patient's arterial system through the arterial cannula, typically 15F to 19F in size. Cannulation may be central (typically right atrial–aorta) or peripheral. Peripheral cannulation is often via the femoral vein and artery, though variations in cannulation vessels may be tailored to specific patient scenarios.

VA-ECMO has several distinct advantages over other forms of temporary mechanical circulatory support such as percutaneous ventricular assist devices (VADs). VA-ECMO is able to provide robust hemodynamic support (up to 6 L/min of blood flow depending on cannula size) and can be rapidly deployed in a variety of clinical settings including cardiac arrest because neither fluoroscopy nor echocardiographic guidance is required for its successful insertion. Furthermore, VA-ECMO provides gas exchange to support the patient with concomitant respiratory failure. Compared to other circulatory support devices, vascular complications may be more frequent because of ECMO cannula size. Another major limitation is the potential for an increase in LV afterload, which can compromise circulatory and respiratory function.

Indications and Contraindications for VA-ECMO

VA-ECMO may stabilize patients with cardiogenic shock. The underlying etiology of that shock state, however, is critical to determine the optimal use of this therapy and prognosis. Primary ischemic etiologies such as acute myocardial infarction and non-ischemic etiologies including fulminant myocarditis, peripartum cardiomyopathy, decompensated pulmonary hypertension, and primary graft failure following cardiac transplant causing cardiogenic shock are frequent indications for VA-ECMO and represent a heterogenous postoperative patient population. VA-ECMO also supports patients with massive pulmonary embolism as a bridge to more definitive therapy. In selected cases, VA-ECMO with advanced cardiac life support is initiated emergently to restore circulation during cardiac arrest in addition, a use known as extracorporeal cardiopulmonary resuscitation.

Despite VA-ECMO's broad applicability, a number of contraindications exist: severe irreversible non-cardiac organ failure limiting survival (i.e., severe anoxic brain injury), irreversible cardiac failure if transplantation or long-term VAD will not be considered, severe aortic insufficiency, and aortic dissection. Before initiation of VA-ECMO support, clinicians should identify the intended goals of support and the likelihood of myocardial recovery. VA-ECMO is not intended for patients with a low likelihood of myocardial recovery or who are not candidates for durable VAD or cardiac transplant given the lack of an exit strategy. Relative contraindications include severe coagulopathy or contraindication to anticoagulation and severe peripheral arterial disease.

Patient Selection for VA-ECMO Support

Appropriate patient selection is paramount to optimize outcomes with VA-ECMO support. Outcome data of patients supported with VA-ECMO are largely limited to retrospective, registry, and large single-center studies. Despite these limitations, several common themes have emerged. The indication for device support or the underlying etiology of shock is a major driver of outcomes. In-hospital survival has been reported to exceed 80% for patients who are supported with VA-ECMO for severe primary graft failure following cardiac transplantation, while survival is approximately 50% for those with acute myocardial infarction and acute decompensated heart failure and 30% for patients supported with VA-ECMO for post-cardiotomy shock. Increasing age, diabetes mellitus, chronic renal disease, and chronic obstructive pulmonary disease have been associated with increased risk of device complications and early mortality on VA-ECMO.

Higher lactate and markers of renal and hepatic dysfunction at the time of initiation of VA-ECMO support have been identified as strong predictors of increased mortality on device support. Prognostic scores such as the Survival After Venoarterial ECMO score have been developed, which incorporate many variables in an effort to guide clinicians in selecting appropriate candidates for VA-ECMO. Given the high mortality, morbidity, cost, and resource utilization associated with VA-ECMO support, appropriate patient selection requires careful consideration of all of the aforementioned factors.

Management of Patients on VA-ECMO

Understanding the potential complications and the hemodynamic consequences of VA ECMO support is critical to recognizing and mitigating some of the risks associated with this therapy and to avoiding some common pitfalls with its use.

An Arterial Cannula Can Compromise Perfusion to the Cannulated Extremity

If the diameter of the reinfusion cannula is too large in relationship to the size of the cannulated artery, it may reduce flow distally, resulting in extremity ischemia. Placement of an additional distally directed perfusion catheter (i.e., in the superficial femoral artery when the common femoral artery is cannulated for reinfusion) can help prevent this complication.

VA-ECMO Runs in Parallel to the Heart and Lungs

Venous blood flows from the body to the ECMO circuit via the drainage cannula, which (for peripheral cannulation) is most commonly advanced into the intrahepatic portion of the inferior vena cava via a femoral vein. After blood is oxygenated and decarboxylated by the ECMO circuit, it is returned to the body via the reinfusion cannula located in the femoral artery. This configuration results in the ECMO circuit running in parallel to the heart and lungs (see Figure 24.1). Blood that flows through the ECMO circuit will bypass the cardiopulmonary circulation, and total cardiac output will hence be the summation of the blood flow through the extracorporeal circuit and the output from the heart. Increasing VA-ECMO

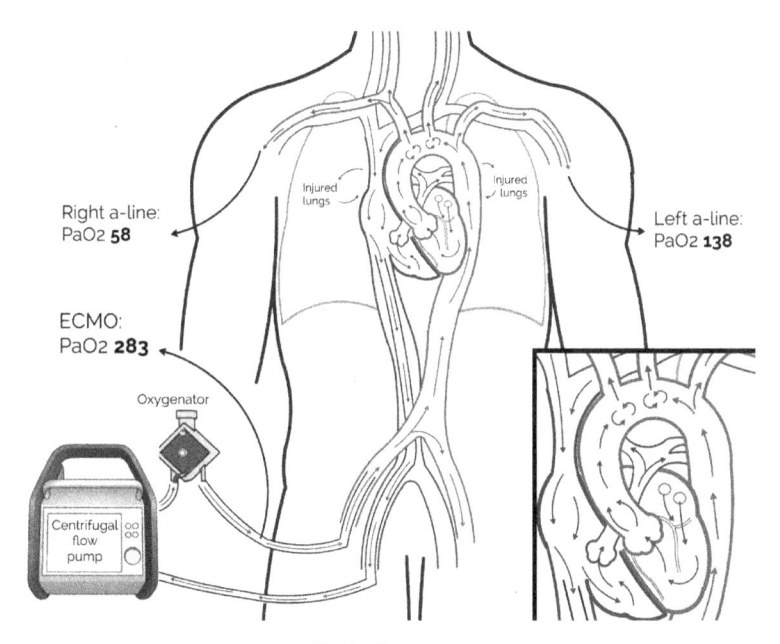

FIGURE 24.1 Peripherally cannulated VA-ECMO.

blood flow will result in less blood transiting the native cardiopulmonary circulation and vice versa.

Peripheral VA-ECMO Increases LV Afterload

Oxygenated blood returning from the ECMO circuit is reinfused under high pressure into the femoral artery (for lower extremity cannulation) and, in a retrograde manner, into the aorta, while the heart continues to pump blood in the opposite direction (i.e., antegrade). In order to eject, the LV has to overcome the increased resistance (afterload) generated by the retrograde flow of blood coming from the circuit. This causes an increase in cardiac work and afterload.

LV Venting Might Be Required in Cases of Severe LV Dysfunction

In situations of severe LV dysfunction, the ventricle might not be able to overcome the increased afterload generated by the ECMO. This will result in reduced LV ejection and, in extreme cases, can result in complete closure of the aortic valve. Assessment of ejection can be done by serial echocardiography, looking for opening of the aortic valve or by observing pulsatility of the arterial line waveform. Failure to eject may lead to elevation in the LV end-diastolic pressure and can cause frank pulmonary congestion. It can also cause LV distention, compromising coronary perfusion and hindering myocardial recovery. Furthermore, resultant stasis in the LV or at the aortic root might promote thrombus formation. This undesirable situation can be prevented by adding inotropic therapy (at the expense of increased myocardial oxygen demand) and/or by periodically adjusting ECMO blood flow to facilitate ejection from the LV. Reducing ECMO blood flow will decrease afterload to the LV and divert blood from the ECMO circuit to the cardiopulmonary circulation, increasing LV preload. In instances where reducing ECMO flow is not a feasible alternative (i.e., persistent, severe hemodynamic instability), interventions to facilitate LV emptying (known as venting) may be instituted in an effort to reduce the risks associated with LV pressure overload. Options include placement of an intra-aortic balloon pump to promote ejection by decreasing afterload during LV systole or placement of either a percutaneous LV assist device (e.g., Impella, Danvers, MA) or a ventricular cannula to directly drain the LV.

Concomitant Respiratory Failure Can Cause Upper Body Hypoxemia (i.e., Differential Hypoxemia)

There is a point along the aorta where blood that traverses the pulmonary circulation and is ejected in a natural anterograde fashion by the LV will encounter and mix with the blood that returns retrograde from the ECMO circuit via the femoral artery. The location where this occurs will depend on the relative contribution of the ECMO circuit and the patient's heart to the total cardiac output. It is important to recognize that vascular beds on either side of this location may have vastly different oxygen saturations. In cases of poor cardiac function and high ECMO flows, this zone will be located closer to the heart (i.e., ascending aorta or aortic arch), while with higher native cardiac output this will occur more distally (i.e., distal aortic arch or descending aorta).

An understanding of the presence and location of a mixing zone is essential to manage VA-ECMO in the presence of respiratory failure. In cases of lung pathology (acute or chronic), blood ejected by the heart may be poorly oxygenated. If this mixing zone is located distal to the take-off of the brachiocephalic artery, blood ejected by the heart will perfuse the head vessels, risking potential hypoxemic brain injury. The exact location of the mixing zone in the aorta will determine the relative contribution of the native cardiopulmonary and ECMO circuits in perfusing the brain. While the determination of the mixing zone's exact location is challenging, the presence of adequate oxygen saturation in blood sampled from the right upper extremity ensures that blood perfusing the brain is adequately oxygenated. If this is not the case (as is the concern for the case vignette), increasing ECMO flows will push the location of the mixing zone closer to the heart, allowing for oxygenated blood from the ECMO circuit to reach more proximally into the aortic arch (at the expense of increasing LV afterload). In refractory cases where satisfactory oxygenation to the upper body cannot be achieved, a reconfiguration of the ECMO cannulation (i.e., adding a second venous limb to reinfuse oxygenated blood) should be considered to prevent anoxic brain injury.

Weaning from Peripheral VA-ECMO

Weaning from VA-ECMO begins by determining that cardiac and/or pulmonary function have improved. Useful signs of recovery are the ability to wean vasopressor and inotropic medications and improved arterial pulse pressure. Cardiac recovery can be confirmed by echocardiography. Once the decision to wean VA-ECMO support has been made, the ECMO blood flow rate is slowly decreased as hemodynamics and blood gas parameters are monitored. Serial echocardiographic assessment is useful to identify early signs of failure to wean. It is important to note that since VA-ECMO runs in parallel to the cardiopulmonary circulation, any attempt to wean ECMO FiO_2 should be avoided to prevent an iatrogenic right to left shunting, resulting in hypoxemia. Since blood delivered to the arterial circulation by the ECMO circuit will not first pass through the patient's pulmonary circulation, reduction of ECMO FiO_2 risks delivery of oxygen-poor blood to the arterial system. Finally, if myocardial recovery occurs before respiratory recovery, transition from VA-ECMO to venovenous ECMO may be considered to reduce the risks associated with arterial cannulation.

CASE RESUMES

The patient is now hemodynamically stabilized. He is on dual inotropic support with minimal vasopressor requirement. Importantly, serial echocardiography reveals improved biventricular function during weaning of VA-ECMO flow weaning. However, his oxygen requirements remain high and his lung compliance is poor. The decision to decannulate his arterial cannulation and to convert to VV-ECMO (veno-venous ECMO) with an additional femoral venous cannula is made. The patient tolerated this with minimal increases in inotropic support. His lungs improved with meticulous medical management over the next week and was able to be liberated from VV-ECMO.

KEY POINTS TO REMEMBER

1. VA-ECMO does not cure the underlying cardiovascular disease; it merely provides end-organ perfusion during periods of cardiopulmonary failure.
2. VA-ECMO produces blood flow in a parallel circuit to the native cardiopulmonary circulation and in some ways may actually have detrimental hemodynamic effects on the heart.
3. When inserted peripherally, VA-ECMO can create differential hypoxemia, with vascular beds having widely differing oxygen content.
4. In order to minimize the risk of vascular complication, patients should be weaned from VA-ECMO as soon as safely possible.

Suggested Reading
1. Schmidt M, Burrell A, Roberts L, et al. Predicting survival after ECMO for refractory cardiogenic shock: the survival after veno-arterial-ECMO (SAVE)-score. *Eur Heart J*. 2015;36:2246–2256.
2. Muller G, Flecher E, Lebreton G, et al. The ENCOURAGE mortality risk score and analysis of long-term outcomes after VA-ECMO for acute myocardial infarction with cardiogenic shock. *Intensive Care Med*. 2016;42:370–378.
3. Khorsandi M, Dougherty S, Bouamra O, et al. Extra-corporeal membrane oxygenation for refractory cardiogenic shock after adult cardiac surgery: a systematic review and meta-analysis. *J Cardiothorac Surg*. 2017;12:55.

4. Cheng R, Hachamovitch R, Kittleson M, et al. Complications of extracorporeal membrane oxygenation for treatment of cardiogenic shock and cardiac arrest: a meta-analysis of 1,866 adult patients. *Ann Thorac Surg.* 2014;*97*:610–616.
5. Meani P, Gelsomino S, Natour E, et al. Modalities and effects of left ventricle unloading on extracorporeal life support: a review of the current literature. *Eur J Heart Fail.* 2017;19(suppl 2):84–91.
6. Hoeper MM, Tudorache I, Kühn C, et al. Extracorporeal membrane oxygenation watershed. *Circulation.* 2014;130:864–865.
7. Jayaraman AL, Cormican D, Shah P, Ramakrishna H. Cannulation strategies in adult veno-arterial and veno-venous extracorporeal membrane oxygenation: techniques, limitations, and special considerations. *Ann Card Anaesth.* 2017;20(suppl):S11–S18.

25 Orthotopic Heart Transplant Management

Artem Emple and Kelly M. Axsom

A 55-year-old male with ischemic cardiomyopathy with a left ventricular assist device (LVAD) presents for an orthotopic heart transplant (OHT). He received vitamin K and prothrombin complex concentrate to reverse his coagulopathy. Prior to separating from cardiopulmonary bypass, the patient is empirically placed on inhaled nitric oxide, norepinephrine, dobutamine, and milrinone to enhance right ventricular (RV) contractility. His heart rate is sinus tachycardia at 105 bpm, central venous pressure (CVP) is 6 mm Hg, pulmonary artery pressure (PAP) is 32/12 mm Hg, and mixed venous oxygen saturation is 72%, giving him a Fick cardiac index of 2.8 L/min/m^2.

Three hours later, the nurse notifies you that the patient has increasing vasopressor requirements. His CVP is 20 mm Hg, and his PAPs are elevated. The patient is dyssynchronous with the ventilator.

What do you do now?

DISCUSSION

OHT and LVADs are treatments for end-stage heart failure, with heart transplant considered the "gold standard" therapy. Many patients present for OHT after placement of a durable LVAD as bridge to transplantation (BTT). These patients are at increased risk of intraoperative bleeding from repeat sternotomy, preoperative use of vitamin K antagonists and antiplatelet agents, and the development of acquired von Willebrand disease from continuous-flow ventricular assist devices (VADs). Many recipients have a vasoconstricted and congested pulmonary vascular bed, which increases the afterload of the newly transplanted and fragile RV. For this reason, patients are often empirically prescribed inhaled pulmonary vasodilators. Patients receive inotropes before separating from cardiopulmonary bypass to support RV function.

New hypotension after heart transplant prompts consideration of hypovolemia from hemorrhage, post-bypass vasoplegia, cardiac tamponade, pulmonary hypertensive crisis, primary graft failure, and acute RV failure. Immediate management of this patient begins with a clinical exam of incisions, chest tube output, urine output, and assessment of invasive monitors. A bedside transthoracic echocardiogram is an invaluable tool to rule out immediate life-threatening pathology such as tamponade, RV failure, and pneumothorax and to diagnose hypovolemia and biventricular dysfunction. Echocardiographic windows may be limited from bandages and chest tubes, and a TEE may be required to assess the patient's hemodynamic condition (see Table 25.1).

CASE RESUMES

At the bedside, you notice that the patient is agitated; his CVP increases to 14 mm Hg, and his PAPs have increased to 45/20 mm Hg. His lactate has decreased from 5 mmol/L to 3 mmol/L without an increase in vasopressor doses. You increase his sedation and place the patient on a lung-protective ventilatory strategy with a higher minute ventilation. Within minutes, you observe resolution of the hypotension and normalization of his CVP and PAP. However, a few hours later, you are notified of recurrent hemodynamic instability.

TABLE 25.1 **Bedside Hemodynamic and Echocardiographic Parameters of Life-Threatening Physiology**

	Echocardiography Findings	CVP	CO/CI	Pulmonary Artery Pressure
Tamponade	End-diastolic RA collapse, RV collapse, IVC dilation, circumferential fluid accumulation in pericardium	↑	↓	Varies
Pulmonary hypertension, RV failure	D-shaped LV, RV >0.5 LV in PLAX	↑	↓	↑
Hemorrhage	Hyperdynamic LV, "kissing" papillary muscles	↓	↓	↓

CO/CI, cardiac output/cardiac index; IVC, inferior vena cava; PLAX, parasternal long axis; RA, right atrium.

Hypotension with an elevated CVP and PAP localizes pathology to the RV or pulmonary vascular bed. Given that RV dysfunction in the post-transplant patient is a disease with high morbidity and mortality, it should be quickly identified and managed. The etiology of RV dysfunction in the transplanted patient can be divided into primary and secondary causes of graft dysfunction. Secondary causes of graft dysfunction include hyperacute rejection (see Chapter 26), volume or pressure overload of the RV, prolonged cold ischemic time, reperfusion injury, and mechanical obstruction at the pulmonary artery anastomosis.

It is important to appreciate the fragility of the RV to both volume and pressure stress, avoid perturbations that elevate pulmonary vascular resistance, and judiciously manage preload to the RV. Acute changes in RV volume and pressure can cause RV dilation, decreased contractility, RV ischemia, and tricuspid regurgitation. In this scenario, hypercarbia and acidosis from ventilator dyssynchrony elevate the pulmonary vascular resistance, increase RV afterload, and cause RV failure. Figure 25.1 shows the cascade of events that lead to hypotension in this case.

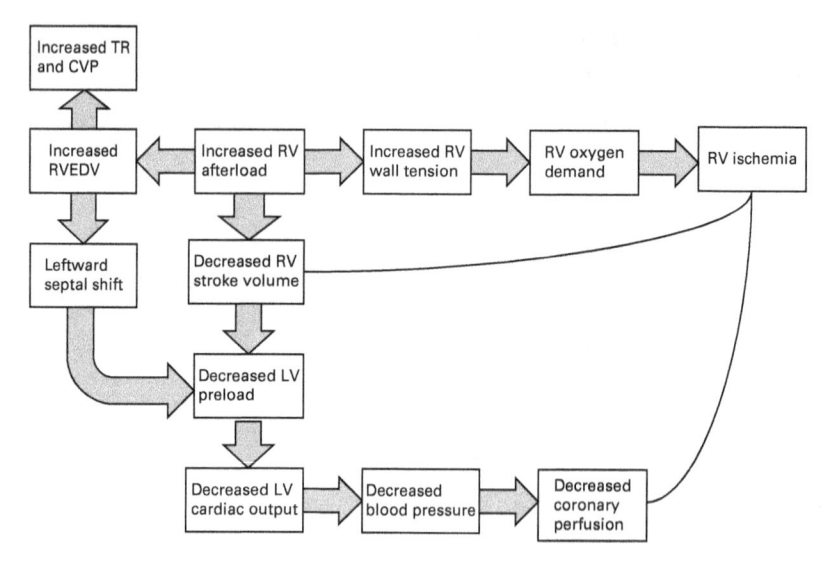

```
                    Increased TR
                    and CVP
                         ▲
                         │
  Increased    ◄──   Increased RV  ──►  Increased RV  ──►  RV oxygen  ──►  RV ischemia
   RVEDV             afterload           wall tension       demand
      │                  │                                                      │
      │                  ▼                                                      │
  Leftward          Decreased RV                                                │
  septal shift      stroke volume                                               │
      │                  │                                                      │
      │                  ▼                                                      │
      └──────────►  Decreased LV                                                │
                    preload                                                     │
                         │                                                      │
                         ▼                                                      │
                    Decreased LV   ──►  Decreased    ──►  Decreased  ◄──────────┘
                    cardiac output      blood pressure    coronary
                                                          perfusion
```

FIGURE 25.1 Pathogenesis of RV failure. RVEDV, RV end-diastolic volume; TR, tricuspid regurgitation.

As previously mentioned, initial evaluation should focus on a bedside evaluation, followed by laboratory data. Markers of end-organ perfusion should be assessed with clinical findings. Mental status, urine output, and capillary refill are sensitive but not specific markers of perfusion. An elevated or rising lactate is a marker of decreased perfusion, if impaired clearance from hepatic failure is not present. Lactate can be produced when cells convert from aerobic to anaerobic metabolism in the setting of ischemia. Mixed venous oxygen saturation quantifies the extraction of oxygen in peripheral tissues and is an indirect measure of cardiac output using the Fick equation. Marked increases in lactate or decreases in mixed venous oxygen saturation can be an indicator of circulatory failure. Treatment should entail optimization of inotropic support and pulmonary vasodilation. If there is continued escalation of medical therapy, concern for primary graft dysfunction needs to prompt a discussion with the surgical team about institution of mechanical circulatory support (i.e., intra-aortic balloon pump, Impella, extracorporeal membrane oxygenation [ECMO], or temporary VAD).

His chest tube output is minimal. His CVP has increased to 22 mm Hg, PAP is 48/32 mm Hg, estimated Fick cardiac index has decreased to 1.8 L/

min/m², lactate has increased to 7 mmol/L, his vasopressor requirement is increasing, and urine output is minimal. An echocardiogram does not support tamponade. The surgical team quickly arrives to the bedside. The decision is made to place the patient on venoarterial (VA) ECMO for primary graft dysfunction (PGD).

PGD is defined as LV, RV, or biventricular dysfunction that occurs within 24 hours after surgery and is not associated with a discernible cause. Although the etiology of PGD is poorly understood, donor-related, recipient-related, and procedure-related factors all play a role. Observational data suggest that continuous-flow LVAD as BTT with prolonged time on device support, preexisting RV dysfunction, and pretransplant use of amiodarone may identify patients at higher risk for PGD. Alternatively, the RADIAL score assists in identifying patients at risk for PGD. It assigns one point for each of the following criteria: right atrial pressure ≥10 mm Hg, recipient age ≥60, diabetes, inotrope dependence, donor age ≥30, and ischemic time ≥240 minutes. Mortality increases with increasing scores.

Once PGD is diagnosed, pharmacotherapy with vasopressors, inotropes, and pulmonary vasodilators should be instituted and maximized while consulting the surgical team for early initiation of mechanical circulatory support. The pillars of management include intra-aortic balloon pump, ECMO, or temporary VAD (LVAD, RV assist device, biventricular assist device). For primary RV PGD, peripherally cannulated VA-ECMO has shown promising results after failure of pharmacologic support. PGD is associated with increased risk of 30-day mortality. Long-term survival of patients who recover from PGD is comparable to that of OHT recipients without a history of PGD.

> **KEY POINTS TO REMEMBER**
> 1. Early and intensive hemodynamic monitoring after heart transplant is critical for management.
> 2. PGD should be distinguished from secondary graft failure.
> 3. If PGD is suspected, consult the surgical team for placement of mechanical circulatory support.

4. Risk factors for PGD include the following:
   a. Right atrial pressure ≥10 mm Hg
   b. Recipient age ≥60 years
   c. Recipient history of diabetes
   d. Recipient history of inotrope dependence
   e. Donor age ≥30 years
   f. Ischemic time ≥240 minutes
   g. Prolonged continuous-flow LVAD support
   h. Preoperative RV dysfunction
   i. Preoperative amiodarone use
5. The RV in general, and specifically in a transplanted heart, is exquisitely sensitive to volume and pressure loads. Preload and afterload should be judiciously managed.

Suggested Reading
1. Kobashigawa J, Zuckermann A, Macdonald P, et al. Report from a consensus conference on primary graft dysfunction after cardiac transplantation. *J Heart Lung Transplant*. 2014;33(4):327–340.
2. Ha YR, Toh HC. Clinically integrated multi-organ point-of-care ultrasound for undifferentiated respiratory difficulty, chest pain, or shock: a critical analytic review. *J Intensive Care*. 2016;4(1):54.
3. Vega E, Schroder J, Nicoara A. Postoperative management of heart transplant patients. *Best Pract Res Clin Anaesthesiol*. 2017;31(2):201–213.
4. Konstam MA, Kiernan MS, Bernstein D, et al. Evaluation and management of right-sided heart failure: a scientific statement from the American Heart Association. *Circulation*. 2018;137(20):e578–e622.
5. Truby LK, Takeda K, Topkara VK, et al. Risk of severe primary graft dysfunction in patients bridged to heart transplantation with continuous-flow left ventricular assist devices. *J Heart Lung Transplant*. 2018;37(12):1433–1442.

26 Orthotopic Heart Transplant Rejection and Immunosuppression

Kevin J. Clerkin and Maryjane A. Farr

A 54-year-old man who underwent heart transplantation 14 months earlier due to a non-ischemic dilated cardiomyopathy and minimal coronary vasculopathy (International Society for Heart & Lung Transplantation [ISHLT] cardiac allograft vasculopathy [CAV] 1) presented to the hospital with 4 days of shortness of breath. He was seen in clinic 2 weeks prior with no complaints and a therapeutic tacrolimus level; however, his electrocardiogram (ECG) was notable for a marked first-degree atrioventricular (AV) block (120 ms longer than his prior ECG) and transaminase elevation to 2 times the upper limit of normal. In the subsequent 2 weeks, he developed worsening dyspnea on exertion, 3-pillow orthopnea, and paroxysmal nocturnal dyspnea. On arrival to the emergency department, he was normotensive with a heart rate in the 50s, and his physical exam demonstrated jugular venous distension, an S3 gallop, bibasilar pulmonary crackles, and 1+ bilateral lower extremity edema. An ECG demonstrated atrial flutter with a ventricular escape rhythm in the 50s.

What do you do now?

DISCUSSION

Hyperacute Rejection

Hyperacute rejection is a catastrophic complication that occurs early post-transplantation. This type of rejection is most often due to pre-formed donor-specific anti–human leukocyte antigen antibodies or an ABO blood type mismatch and is rarely seen in the current era because pre-transplant virtual and prospective crossmatch has become routine practice. Evidence of hyperacute rejection typically manifests soon after donor heart reperfusion and is caused by pan-vascular endothelial injury and thrombosis.

Acute Cellular Rejection

Immune activation of recipient T cells against the cardiac allograft causes acute cellular rejection (ACR). In the 1990s about 40% of patients would experience ACR requiring hospitalization within the first year of transplantation; however, with improved monitoring and immunosuppression in the current era, less than 13% of patients experience treatment rejection during the first year. The risk of ACR is greatest in the first 6 months post-transplant. The diagnosis of ACR is made through endomyocardial biopsy and is pathologically graded as 0, 1R, 2R, or 3R for increasing severity. Biopsies in the first year after transplant are usually protocolized (e.g., weekly for the first month, biweekly for 1 month, monthly for 4 months, and bimonthly for 6 months). A biopsy may also be performed if the patient is symptomatic or rejection is clinically suspected.

Clinical manifestations of ACR can vary among patients and can be asymptomatic. Symptomatic patients represent <10% of all rejection episodes and are marked by the symptoms of heart failure: decreased exercise tolerance, orthopnea, paroxysmal nocturnal dyspnea, palpitations, pre-syncope, and abdominal fullness/congestion. Physical exam is notable for findings associated with decompensated heart failure: elevated jugular venous pressure, an S3 gallop, pulmonary edema, palpable liver edge, peripheral edema, and cool extremities. Patients may also present with atrial arrhythmias (atrial fibrillation, flutter, or premature contractions), low QRS voltage, or conduction abnormalities on ECG. Echocardiography can reveal a depressed ejection fraction but may also show impaired diastolic function and increased wall thickness that suggests myocardial edema. Right heart catheterization is also often useful to further identify hemodynamic compromise and monitor cardiac filling pressures and cardiac output.

Treatment of ACR will vary depending on the grade of rejection, symptoms, and hemodynamic significance. Mild ACR (grade 1R or 2R without hemodynamic compromise) may be treated with an oral pulse prednisone (1–3 mg/kg/d for 3–5 days).

Symptomatic ACR of any grade (1R, 2R, or 3R) is treated with intravenous pulse dose steroids (e.g., methylprednisolone 1000 mg daily for 3 days), followed by oral conversion and dose tapering. In ACR with hemodynamic compromise (see Table 26.1), anti-thymocyte globulin (ATG) is recommended. Because of the subsequent cytokine release, there can be a systemic inflammatory response in addition to serum sickness (fevers, chills, myalgia, rash) and leukopenia and thrombocytopenia that may necessitate a dose reduction. Typical dosing is 1–1.5 mg/kg/d for 5–14 days, with administration of acetaminophen, diphenhydramine, and glucocorticoids before each dose to limit side effects. The effect of ATG can be monitored by checking cluster of differentiation 3–positive ($CD3^+$) T-lymphocyte levels. During treatment for rejection, maintenance immunosuppression is continued, with consideration of changing cyclosporine to tacrolimus and azathioprine to mycophenolate mofetil if applicable. Typically, patients will undergo repeat biopsy 1 week afterward to assess response to therapy.

Antibody-Mediated Rejection

Antibody-mediated rejection (AMR), previously known as *humoral* or *vascular rejection*, is primarily mediated by antibodies and not T cells, as in ACR. AMR is most common during the early period following heart transplantation but may occur at any time. It also may occur concomitantly with ACR, representing about 10% of cases. There is a strong association between the presence of donor-specific antibodies (DSAs) and AMR, though DSAs are not required for AMR. Other predisposing risk factors are cytomegalovirus and other infections and pre-transplant sensitization. The diagnosis of AMR is pathologic (pAMR), graded as pAMR 0, 1i or 1h, 2, and 3, each representing increasing severity. The clinical presentation of AMR ranges from asymptomatic to cardiogenic shock. Similar to ACR, an echocardiogram will often show systolic and diastolic dysfunction,

TABLE 26.1 **Hemodynamic Compromise in Acute Cellular Rejection**

Cardiac index	Decreased, <2.0 L/min/m^2
Pulmonary capillary wedge pressure	Increased, >15 mm Hg
Hypotension	Need for inotropic, vasopressor, or mechanical circulatory support

and right heart catheterization can be useful in those with hemodynamic compromise.

AMR is difficult to treat because it may persist or be recurrent and is associated with an increased risk of CAV and mortality. Treatment focuses on antibody neutralization, elimination, and inhibition of further production. There is no standardized treatment protocol, though most regimens include pulse dose steroids (1000 mg/d for 3 days), plasmapheresis (3–7 sessions of 1–2 plasma exchanges), and intravenous immunoglobulin (0.5–1 gm/kg for 3–5 doses following plasmapheresis if possible). ATG dosing is similar to what is used in ACR. Adjunctive therapies targeting antibodies include rituximab (375 mg/m^2 weekly for 4 weeks), a monoclonal antibody against CD20, which is present on all B cells except the terminal plasma cell. Bortezomib, a proteasome inhibitor that targets and causes apoptosis of antibody-producing plasma cells, is another therapeutic target that is given at a dose of 1.3 mg/m^2 for 4 doses every 3–5 days. Less commonly used is eculizumab, an anti-C5 monoclonal antibody that prevents formation of the complement membrane attack complex, the final step in complement cascade leading to endothelial damage.

Management of Acute Rejection

The patient's presentation of shortness of breath, conduction abnormalities, and transaminase elevation suggests rejection and graft dysfunction.

Initial Assessment of the Patient

Important immediate considerations include the following: What are the presenting symptoms? Is the patient hemodynamically stable? Does the patient have evidence of cardiac dysfunction or symptoms of heart failure?

Does the patient have any arrhythmias or conduction abnormalities? Is monitoring in an intensive care unit warranted?

CASE RESUMES

Our patient was hemodynamically stable with an unstable rhythm. AV block (in any form) is present in about 10% of patients following transplantation. When associated with a concomitant atrial arrhythmia nearly 90% of patients will have rejection, compared to 36% without an atrial arrhythmia. Patients with high-grade AV block, in the absence of recent endomyocardial biopsy or cardiac surgery, may have an increased risk of asystole and sudden cardiac death. Consequently, pacing pads were placed on our patient, and he was triaged to the cardiac intensive care unit for further treatment and a higher level of monitoring.

Initial Management of the Patient

In the cardiac intensive care unit, he received pulse dose steroids (methylprednisolone 1000 mg/d for 3 days) due to the clinical suspicion of rejection. It is important that there is prompt treatment with steroids when rejection is suspected, without waiting for confirmatory diagnostic tests. The patient underwent a bedside transthoracic echocardiogram that demonstrated reduced biventricular function. He was started on dobutamine for both inotropic and chronotropic support. Despite this intervention, he remained in atrial flutter with a slow ventricular response that was concerning for a high-grade AV block. Temporary pacing was initiated.

He underwent right heart catheterization, endomyocardial biopsy, and temporary transvenous pacemaker insertion. His right heart catheterization demonstrated hemodynamic compromise (pulmonary capillary wedge pressure 23 mm Hg, cardiac index 1.9 on 5 mcg/kg/min of dobutamine). ATG (1 mg/kg for 5 days) was started in addition to pulse dose steroids. Treatment with ATG requires pre-treatment with acetaminophen, diphenhydramine, and corticosteroids to mitigate side effects, in addition to close monitoring for leukopenia and thrombocytopenia. While protocols vary by institution, leukopenia (white blood cell count [WBC] 2000–3000 or absolute neutrophil count [ANC] 1000–1400) or thrombocytopenia (platelets 50 000–70 000) requires a 50% dose reduction, and severe leukopenia (WBC <2000 or ANC <1000) or thrombocytopenia (platelets <50 000) requires holding the next dose. Additionally, after receiving high-dose steroid and anti-lymphocyte therapy, he was started on infection prophylaxis: nystatin (oral candidiasis), trimethoprim-sulfamethoxazole (*Pneumocystis jirovecii* or *carinii* pneumonia), and acyclovir or valacyclovir (herpesvirus infections). Valganciclovir may replace acyclovir in patients with a history of cytomegalovirus infection or those with a cytomegalovirus mismatch who are early post-transplant.

Subsequent Management

His biopsy demonstrated ISHLT grade 3R cellular rejection with no evidence of AMR by histology, though complement stains (C4d) remained pending. Therapy was continued, and he clinically improved. Although he remained in atrial flutter, his ventricular rate increased, and he no longer required transvenous pacing. After receiving diuretics, there was reduction in his cardiac filling pressures and improvement of his cardiac index. Hemodynamics may not improve with initial therapy, and an escalation of cardiac and circulatory support (e.g., intra-aortic balloon pump, percutaneous ventricular assist device, or venoarterial extracorporeal membrane oxygenation) to maintain end-organ perfusion should be considered.

The biopsy did not demonstrate evidence of AMR by immunohistochemistry (pAMR 0), but it was found that the patient had a new DSA. The decision was made to start 5 sessions of plasmapheresis in addition to ATG and steroids. Plasmapheresis requires monitoring of ionized calcium (citrate chelation) and fibrinogen levels. Often, intravenous immunoglobulin (0.5–1 gm/kg for 3–5 doses) is given following each session of plasmapheresis.

He continued to improve with therapy, and follow-up right heart catheterization and biopsy demonstrated normalization of his hemodynamics and resolution of his rejection.

Immunosuppression

Induction therapy is augmented immunosuppression in the early period following heart transplantation, when the recipient is at the greatest risk of rejection. There is no consensus on the use of induction, with about 50% of heart recipients receiving induction therapy. Neither registry data nor meta-analyses of trials have demonstrated a survival benefit associated with induction therapy. Moreover, while there is a reduction in early rejection, that does not translate into long-term differences in the incidence of rejection. The greatest benefit may be in patients with renal dysfunction as induction can allow for delayed introduction of calcineurin inhibitor (CNI) therapy.

There are 2 main strategies with induction, cytostatic therapy (interleukin [IL]-2 receptor antagonists) and cytolytic therapy (polyclonal antithymocyte antibodies [e.g., ATG] or alemtuzumab). Basiliximab, the only commercially available IL-2 receptor antagonist, is dosed at 20 mg at the time of transplantation and on postoperative day 4 and lasts for about 1 month. ATG is also used for induction, given at a dose of 1–1.5 mg/kg/d for 5–7 days. Induction with ATG has been associated with improved survival, less rejection, and less CAV when compared to IL-2 receptor antagonists.

Maintenance Immunosuppression

CNIs

CNIs are the backbone of immunosuppression for heart transplantation. The introduction of cyclosporine in the early 1980s revolutionized solid organ transplantation, increasing 1-year survival by 20%. Tacrolimus has taken over as the principal CNI, with >95% of heart transplant recipients receiving tacrolimus in the current era. Outcomes are similar between the 2 agents, though some studies have shown less rejection and possible improved survival with tacrolimus. Both drugs carry a number of side effects (neurotoxicity [posterior reversible encephalopathy syndrome], increased risk of infection, hypertension, nephrotoxicity, hyperkalemia, and hypomagnesemia). Tacrolimus has a more attractive side effect profile with less associated hypertension and dyslipidemia but may have an increased incidence of diabetes mellitus.

Both drugs are hepatically metabolized, primarily through cytochrome P450 3A4 (CYP3A4) and can cause a number of drug interactions. Amiodarone, azole anti-fungals, macrolide antibiotics (except azithromycin), calcium channel blockers (non-dihydropyridines, nicardipine), metoclopramide (weakly), and protease inhibitors (human immunodeficiency virus and hepatitis C virus treatment) can increase drug levels. Drugs that inhibit CYP3A4 will decrease levels and include anti-epileptic drugs (carbamazepine, phenobarbital, phenytoin), nafcillin, and rifampin. Tacrolimus is available as a capsule, liquid, and intravenous solution.

Tacrolimus is best initiated with weight-based dosing, 0.075 mg/kg/d initially orally. The oral and liquid doses are equivalent; however, the dose of the intravenous solution is about one-fourth the daily oral dose, and the sublingual dose is 50% of the oral dose. Tacrolimus is monitored with trough levels, with target levels typically 10–15 ng/mL in the early post-transplant period and 4–10 ng/mL later post-transplant.

Anti-Metabolites

Anti-metabolites include azathioprine and mycophenolate mofetil (MMF) or mycophenolic acid (MPA). MMF is the preferred anti-metabolite as it has been associated with decreased rejection and improved survival compared with azathioprine. MMF is available as a capsule, liquid, and intravenous formulation (1:1 conversion) with typical dosing beginning at 1500 mg every 12 hours. Routine monitoring of MMF levels is discouraged, though trough levels can be considered in select patients (renal dysfunction, rejection, malnutrition) to identify supra-therapeutic (plasma MPA >4 mg/L) or sub-therapeutic (plasma MPA <1.5 mg/L) levels. The most common dose limiting side effects are bone marrow toxicity (leukopenia) and gastrointestinal (GI) distress (nausea, abdominal pain, and diarrhea). In patients with GI distress, conversion to MPA can be considered; this has been associated with less GI symptoms compared with MMF, though more leukopenia and similar outcomes. Equivalent doses are 250 mg MMF = 180 mg MPA, 1000 mg MMF = 720 mg MPA, and 1500 mg MMF = 1080 mg MPA.

Glucocorticoids

Glucocorticoids are the original immunosuppressive agent and affect nearly every immune cell. These medications are highly efficacious agents and are a mainstay of therapy in the first year. Most patients receive high-dose (e.g., 1000 mg) methylprednisolone at the time of transplantation, which is weaned down with time and with each successive negative biopsy to doses <5 mg/d.

Proliferation Signal Inhibitors

Proliferation signal inhibitors, which include everolimus and sirolimus, target the mammalian target of rapamycin, which inhibits signaling through the IL-2 pathway and a blockage in the progression of cells from G_1 into S phase of the cell cycle, thereby affecting both B- and T-cell proliferation. These drugs are not indicated in the early post-transplant period (first 3 months) as they have been associated with an increased risk of pericardial effusion and poor surgical wound healing.

KEY POINTS TO REMEMBER

1. Rejection (cellular and antibody-mediated) is most common in the early period post-transplant, though it can occur at any time.
2. Suspicion for rejection, early recognition, and prompt, often empiric, treatment are essential.
3. Tacrolimus is the main CNI and carries a number of interactions with medications commonly used in the intensive care unit.

Suggested Reading

1. Berry GJ, Burke MM, Andersen C, et al. The 2013 International Society for Heart and Lung Transplantation working formulation for the standardization of nomenclature in the pathologic diagnosis of antibody-mediated rejection in heart transplantation. *J Heart Lung Transplant*. 2013;32:1147–1162.
2. Kobashigawa J. Clinical trials in heart transplantation: the evolution of evidence in immunosuppression. *J Heart Lung Transplant*. 2017;36:1286–1290.
3. Colvin MM, Cook JL, Chang P, et al. Antibody-mediated rejection in cardiac transplantation: emerging knowledge in diagnosis and management: a scientific statement from the American Heart Association. *Circulation*. 2015;131:1608–1639.
4. Everly JJ, Walsh RC, Alloway RR, Woodle ES. Proteasome inhibition for antibody-mediated rejection. *Curr Opin Organ Transplant*. 2009;14(6):662–666.
5. Khush KK, Cherikh WS, Chambers DC, et al. The International Thoracic Organ Transplant Registry of the International Society for Heart and Lung Transplantation: thirty-fifth adult heart transplantation report-2018; focus theme: multiorgan transplantation. *J Heart Lung Transplant*. 2018;37:1155–1168.

6. Kobashigawa J, Crespo-Leiro MG, Ensminger SM, et al. Report from a consensus conference on antibody-mediated rejection in heart transplantation. *J Heart Lung Transplant*. 2011;30(3):252–269.
7. Stewart S, Winters GL, Fishbein MC, et al. Revision of the 1990 working formulation for the standardization of nomenclature in the diagnosis of heart rejection. *J Heart Lung Transplant*. 2005;24:1710–1720.

27 Pulmonary Infiltrates and Hypoxemia After Lung Transplantation

Lauren D. Sutherland and Teresa A. Mulaikal

A 45-year-old man with idiopathic pulmonary fibrosis, severe restrictive lung disease, and moderate pulmonary hypertension presents to the cardiothoracic intensive care unit (ICU) after bilateral lung transplantation. The operative course was significant for moderate bleeding requiring transfusion of 2 units of packed red blood cells. Intraoperative transesophageal echocardiography (TEE) revealed moderately reduced right ventricular function with normal left ventricular and valvular function. He arrives to the ICU intubated, on low-dose vasopressors, and with good pulmonary compliance, oxygenation, and low pulmonary arterial pressures. Over the next 24 hours, he remains intubated and sedated but becomes increasingly hypoxemic with worsening pulmonary compliance. A chest X-ray demonstrates bilateral pulmonary infiltrates, worse on the right lung than the left, with no obvious pleural effusions. He is otherwise hemodynamically stable with minimal chest tube output.

What do you do now?

DISCUSSION

Primary Graft Dysfunction

This patient developed worsening respiratory failure shortly after lung transplantation. The presentation is suspicious for primary graft dysfunction (PGD), a syndrome of acute lung injury occurring within the first 72 hours of lung transplantation characterized by diffuse pulmonary infiltrates and hypoxemia; however, PGD is a diagnosis of exclusion. Other causes of early respiratory failure with pulmonary infiltrates including volume overload, infection, acute antibody-mediated rejection, and vascular complications must first be considered to ensure proper treatment. Early evaluation should include bronchoscopy to assess airway anastomoses and obtain culture samples, evaluation of cardiac filling pressures through use of a pulmonary artery catheter, TEE to evaluate cardiac function and vascular anastomoses, and a computed tomography (CT) angiogram to better visualize lung parenchyma and assess for thrombosis.

Pulmonary edema from volume overload is one of the most common causes of early pulmonary infiltrates after lung transplant, especially in cases of significant fluid administration intraoperatively. Blood product transfusions can result in transfusion-related acute lung injury (TRALI), though this by definition occurs within 6 hours of transfusion, specifically with high-plasma volume blood components, which this patient did not receive. In cases of elevated left atrial filling pressures or left ventricular dysfunction, diuresis should be considered, to optimize volume status. Especially in patients with preexisting infections, worsening pneumonia may develop in the setting of high levels of immunosuppressive medications. An early infectious workup is prudent, and attention should be paid to ensuring proper antimicrobial coverage of any known resistant organisms that the recipient has cultured in the past.

Antibody-mediated rejection occurs following lung transplant due to donor-specific antibodies against human leukocyte antigens (HLA). While hyperacute rejection is exceedingly rare due to preoperative HLA antibody screening and donor-specific crossmatching, a new antibody screen should be sent to evaluate for presence of higher antibody titers. Treatment of hyperacute rejection involves intensive immunosuppressive therapy, so the diagnosis should be confirmed or highly suspected prior to initiating therapy.

Early vascular anastomotic complications include pulmonary artery (PA) or pulmonary vein (PV) kinking, stenosis, thrombosis, or embolism. Obstruction to PA blood flow generally presents as worsening pulmonary hypertension and right ventricular failure with hemodynamic instability and hypoxemia, less consistent with the patient's current clinical picture. Kinking or thrombosis of a PV anastomosis typically occurs very early in the postoperative course and can result in severe unilateral pulmonary edema (unless occurring in anastomoses in both transplanted lungs), leading to hypoxemia and decreased pulmonary compliance (Table 27.1). These patients are at high risk for systemic embolization, leading to stroke, limb or bowel ischemia, or other embolic complications. With the time course and presentation of unequal pulmonary infiltrates in this patient, PV thrombosis should be seriously considered and either a TEE or CT angiography should be performed. If PV thrombosis is diagnosed, unstable patients may require emergent thrombectomy and surgical revision of the anastomosis, while more stable patients benefit from systemic anticoagulation.

Workup of this patient reveals no evidence of volume overload, infection, or vascular anastomotic complications; and the patient is diagnosed with PGD. PGD is thought to be caused by ischemia–reperfusion injury that alters the alveolar and vascular endothelium, leading to pulmonary edema, reduced lung compliance, and poor gas exchange. PGD occurs following 30% of lung transplantation procedures and is the leading cause of early mortality after lung transplantation; it is associated with longer mechanical ventilation time, longer ICU length of stay, and longer hospital length of stay. PGD is classified into different grades depending on the severity of radiographic findings and hypoxemia (Table 27.2), and grade 3 PGD is associated with the worst outcomes (Figure 27.1). Risk factors for grade 3 PGD include donor factors, such as smoking history or lung contusion, recipient diagnoses of idiopathic pulmonary fibrosis, sarcoidosis, PA hypertension, or obesity, and surgical factors, such as prolonged ischemic time, use of cardiopulmonary bypass, large-volume blood product transfusion, high fraction of inspired oxygen during reperfusion, and single lung transplant.

TABLE 27.1 **Differential Diagnosis of Hypoxemia Immediately Following Lung Transplantation**

Diagnosis	Key Features	Evaluation	Treatment
Volume overload or transfusion-associated circulatory overload	- High fluid or blood product administration - LV dysfunction or high LA pressure - Possible pleural effusions	- Evaluation of pulmonary capillary wedge pressure - Echocardiography - BNP, troponin	- Diuresis - Inotropic support for poor LV function
TRALI	- Occurs during or within 6 h of a transfusion - More common with high-plasma volume blood products (e.g., FFP) - May also present with fever and hypotension	- Evaluation of pulmonary capillary wedge pressure - Echocardiography - BNP, troponin	- Stop transfusion if still in progress - Report to blood bank for transfusion reaction workup
Pneumonia or aspiration	- History of recent infection (e.g., cystic fibrosis patients) - Witnessed aspiration event - Fevers, elevated white blood cell count, hypotension	- Bronchoscopy with bronchoalveolar lavage culture - Culture for bloodstream infection - Viral respiratory PCR - CMV PCR - Fungal culture/PCR	Broad-spectrum antibiotic antiviral, or antifungal coverage targeted to prior culture data or patient/donor risk factors

Diagnosis	Key Features	Evaluation	Treatment
Hyperacute antibody-mediated rejection	- Rapid onset, within minutes to 24 h of lung reperfusion	- Review pre-transplant HLA antibody testing and crossmatch - New HLA antibody screen - Consider transbronchial biopsy	- Plasmapheresis - IVIG - Rituximab, bortezomib
PA flow obstruction (e.g., kinking, stenosis, thrombosis, embolism)	- Hypotension, hemodynamic instability - RV dysfunction	- CT angiography - TEE to evaluate for clot or high velocities by pulse wave doppler	- Surgical repair (e.g., lung repositioning, thrombectomy, anastomosis revision) - Anticoagulation
PV flow obstruction (e.g., kinking, stenosis, thrombosis, embolism)	- Often unilateral - Decreased lung compliance - LA thrombus or systemic embolism	- CT angiography - TEE to evaluate for clot or high velocities by pulse wave Doppler	- Surgical repair (e.g., repositioning, thrombectomy, anastomosis revision) - Anticoagulation
Primary graft dysfunction	- Diffuse infiltrates - Decreased lung compliance	Exclusion of other diagnoses	- Lung-protective ventilation - Empiric antibiotics - Inhaled vasodilators - ECMO

BNP, brain natriuretic peptide; FFP, fresh frozen plasma; IVIG, intravenous immunoglobulin; LA, left atrial; LV, left ventricular; RV, right ventricular.

TABLE 27.2 **PGD Grading System**

Grade	Chest X-Ray Findings	PaO$_2$/FiO$_2$ Ratio
Grade 0	Normal	Any
Grade 1	Diffuse infiltrates	>300
Grade 2	Diffuse infiltrates	200–300
Grade 3	Diffuse infiltrates	<200

FiO$_2$, fraction of inspired oxygen; PaO$_2$, partial pressure of oxygen.

The patient becomes more hypoxemic and acidotic with worsening pulmonary compliance, and vasopressors are escalated for worsening hypotension. At this point, the hemodynamic instability may be a result of worsening hypoxemia and poor end-organ perfusion, but other causes of hypotension

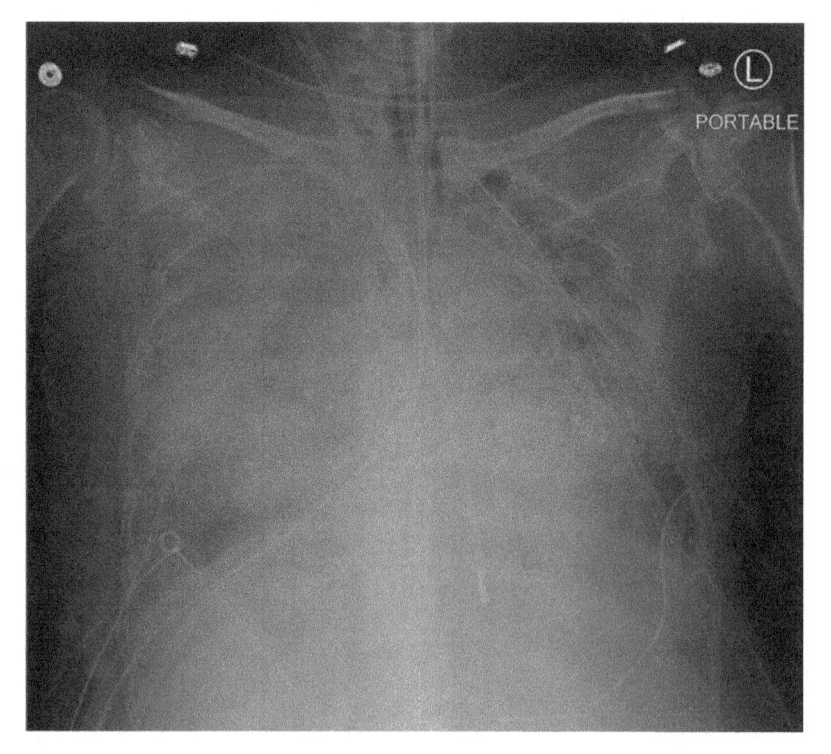

FIGURE 27.1 Chest X-ray demonstrating grade 3 PGD following bilateral lung transplant.

such as pneumothorax, cardiac pathology including arrhythmias, myocardial infarction, or left-sided heart failure, infection, or pulmonary embolism should be considered. Patients with severe pulmonary hypertension preoperatively may develop severe left ventricular failure postoperatively; they previously lived with a chronically lower left ventricular preload, and correction of pulmonary hypertension with a new, low pulmonary vascular resistance in the transplanted lungs can lead to excessive left ventricular volume and failure. TEE may be useful in diagnosing enlarging pleural or pericardial effusions, right or left ventricular failure, or previously undiagnosed vascular anastomotic complications. TEE can also guide fluid management and initiation of inotropic support. Empiric antibiotics targeting opportunistic organisms or known preoperative infections should be universally started at this point, and fluid management should aim at minimizing lung congestion while maintaining cardiac output.

While considering a differential diagnosis and pursuing a diagnostic workup, supportive care following acute respiratory distress syndrome treatment recommendations should occur concurrently. Low–tidal volume ventilation (4–6 cc/kg of ideal body weight) with positive end-expiratory pressure targeting plateau pressures <30 cm H_2O may prevent ventilator-associated lung injury, though in cases of small donor lung size, ventilation volumes should target the donor's, rather than the recipient's, ideal body weight to prevent volutrauma. Ventilation should be targeted to achieve a normal pH as many patients preoperatively have chronic carbon dioxide retention and a compensatory metabolic alkalosis. Inhaled pulmonary vasodilators such as nitric oxide or prostaglandins should be trialed for treatment of hypoxemia by improving ventilation–perfusion matching in areas that are effectively ventilated. Additionally, pulmonary vasodilation may decrease right ventricular afterload and improve cardiac function in patients with elevated pulmonary pressures and a failing right ventricle. In cases of refractory, life-threatening PGD, extracorporeal membrane oxygenation (ECMO) may be required to augment either pulmonary function (venovenous [VV]) or both heart and lung function (venoarterial [VA]). VV-ECMO is preferable due to fewer complications such as bleeding and stroke, and often hemodynamics will significantly improve with better oxygenation and correction of acidosis, negating the need for VA-ECMO support. Additionally, high VA-ECMO flows can result in insufficient flow through the newly transplanted lung, left ventricular distension from high afterload, or poor cerebral oxygenation if carotid artery perfusion occurs with poorly oxygenated transcardiac flow rather than well-oxygenated ECMO flow. VA-ECMO may be preferentially used in the subset of patients with preoperative severe pulmonary hypertension to prevent left ventricular volume overload.

CASE RESUMES

Inhaled nitric oxide is started in this patient with minimal improvement in oxygenation, so the patient is placed on VV-ECMO with right femoral vein drainage and right internal jugular vein return. With 4 L/min of ECMO flow, oxygenation and acidosis dramatically improve, and the patient hemodynamically stabilizes. Over the next few weeks, the patient requires tracheostomy for a prolonged ventilator wean, but he is able to be weaned from ECMO and inhaled vasodilators and is discharged from the ICU.

KEY POINTS TO REMEMBER

1. PGD is caused by ischemia–reperfusion injury within 72 hours of lung transplantation, leading to pulmonary edema, reduced lung compliance, and hypoxemia.
2. PGD is a diagnosis of exclusion; diagnoses such as volume overload, TRALI, infection, antibody-mediated rejection, and vascular anastomotic complications should first be ruled out.
3. PGD occurs following 30% of lung transplantations and leads to significantly higher morbidity and mortality.
4. Patients with PGD should be managed with supportive therapy such as lung-protective ventilation, targeted to the donor's ideal body weight to prevent volutrauma.
5. Inhaled pulmonary vasodilators such as inhaled nitric oxide can improve oxygenation by optimizing ventilation–perfusion matching and improve right ventricular function by reducing right ventricular afterload.

6. VV-ECMO is preferable to VA-ECMO in the management of severe cases of PGD; however, VA-ECMO may be useful in cases of severe preoperative pulmonary hypertension.

Suggested Reading
1. Snell GI, Yusen RD, Weill D, et al. Report of the ISHLT working group on primary lung graft dysfunction, part i: definition and grading—a 2016 consensus group statement of the International Society for Heart and Lung Transplantation. *J Heart Lung Transplant.* 2017;36(10):1097–1103.
2. Diamond JM, Arcasoy S, Kennedy CC, et al. Report of the International Society for Heart and Lung Transplantation working group on primary lung graft dysfunction, part ii: epidemiology, risk factors, and outcomes—a 2016 consensus group statement of the International Society for Heart and Lung Transplantation. *J Heart Lung Transplant.* 2017;36(10):1104–1113.
3. Gelman AE, Fisher AJ, Huang HJ, et al. Report of the ISHLT working group on primary lung graft dysfunction part III: mechanisms: a 2016 consensus group statement of the International Society for Heart and Lung Transplantation. *J Heart Lung Transplant.* 2017;36(10):1114–1120.
4. Diamond JM, Lee JC, Kawut SM, et al.; Lung Transplant Outcomes Group. Clinical risk factors for primary graft dysfunction after lung transplantation. *Am J Respir Crit Care Med.* 2013;187(5):527–534.
5. Van Raemdonck D, Hartwig MG, Hertz MI, et al. Report of the ISHLT working group on primary lung graft dysfunction part IV: prevention and treatment: a 2016 consensus group statement of the International Society for Heart and Lung Transplantation. *J Heart Lung Transplant.* 2017;36(10):1121–1136.

28 Intra-aortic Balloon Pump

Christopher Choi and Amirali Masoumi

A 55-year-old man with no prior medical follow-up presents to the emergency department with crushing chest pain. Workup reveals elevated troponin level and ST elevations in anterolateral electrocardiogram (ECG) leads. Emergent cardiac catheterization reveals significant left main coronary artery occlusion. Cardiothoracic surgery is consulted for emergency bypass surgery, and the patient is transferred to the intensive care unit for further care. Upon arrival, his blood pressure is 90/40s on norepinephrine 10 μg/min with ongoing chest pain.

What do you do now?

DISCUSSION

Intra-aortic balloon pump (IABP) is the single most widely used mechanical circulatory assist device available today, with over 70 000 insertions annually in the United States alone. The balloon pump system consists of 2 parts. First, there is a flexible 7.5–8.5 French catheter with one lumen that allows distal aspiration, flushing, and arterial pressure monitoring. A second lumen permits delivery of a gas to a closed polyethylene balloon. Both helium and carbon dioxide have been used; however, helium theoretically has quicker gas delivery and retrieval due to its lower density. Second, there is a mobile console, which processes the ECG and arterial waveform and triggers timing of inflation and deflation.

Hemodynamic Changes

In the setting of myocardial ischemia and cardiogenic shock, the main goal for medical and device therapies is to improve myocardial perfusion and reduce ischemic territory. The hemodynamic benefits of an IABP include (1) increased diastolic pressure (~30%) and subsequently coronary blood flow to improve myocardial perfusion; (2) reduction of heart rate (~20%) and decrease in cardiac demand; (3) decrease in afterload, especially when left ventricular function is impaired; and (4) increase in cardiac output (0.5–1.0 L/min), especially in patients with mechanical complications of acute myocardial infarction or ischemia such as mitral regurgitation or ventricular septal defect.

Principle of Counterpulsation

Counterpulsation refers to balloon inflation in diastole and deflation in early systole: this results in increased coronary blood flow, left ventricular afterload reduction, and increased end-organ perfusion. Balloon inflation occurs in the middle of the ECG T wave at the onset of diastole, and balloon deflation occurs with the R wave at the beginning of systole. When using arterial tracing, balloon inflation occurs at the dicrotic notch, and deflation occurs just before the upstroke of the waveform. Improper triggering can be counterproductive and cause the waveforms shown in Figure 28.1. In daily practice, the IABP-to-R wave trigger ratio is set to 1:1 for maximal

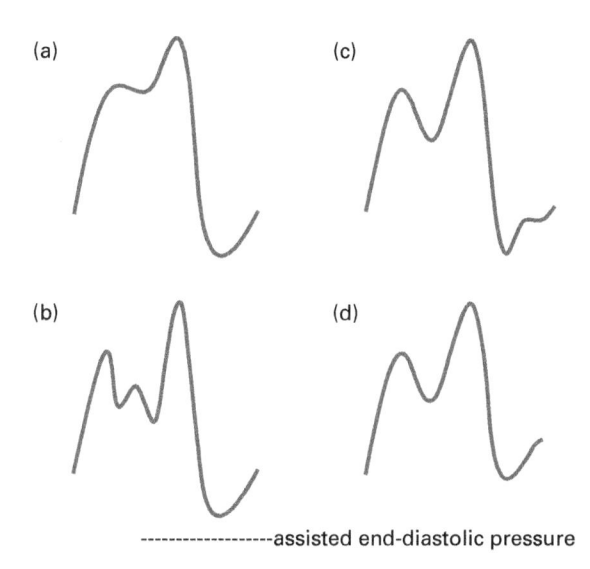

FIGURE 28.1 Arterial waveforms associated with inappropriate IABP triggering (one cardiac cycle shown for simplicity). (A) IABP inflates prior to aortic valve closure. This is reflected by the absence of the dicrotic notch. (B) IABP inflates too late. (C) IABP deflates prior to start of ventricular contraction. (D) IABP deflates too late, reflected by absence of assisted end-diastolic pressure.

Modified from Krishna M, Zacharowski K. Principles of intra-aortic balloon pump counterpulsation. *Continuing Education in Anaesthesia Critical Care & Pain.* 2009;9(1):24–28.

benefit. Ratios of 1:2 or 1:3 can be used in a protocolized fashion when weaning from the balloon pump.

On a more granular level, counterpulsation works by increasing the endocardial viability ratio, which is the ratio of oxygen supply to oxygen demand; a value of 1.0 or greater is normal. An IABP improves the oxygen supply by increasing the diastolic time pressure index, which is the time spent in diastole at a certain pressure (through augmentation). This reflects the time where the coronary arteries and the subendocardium are perfused. An IABP, in turn, lowers oxygen demand by decreasing the tension time index, which is the area under the left ventricular systolic pressure curve. Due to balloon deflation in early systole, which decreases afterload, a lower left ventricular systolic pressure is required for aortic valve opening. In other words, the length of isovolumetric contraction is less, which is the greatest period of oxygen consumption. Of note, some of the force of balloon inflation is also stored in the aortic wall, which is then converted into kinetic energy with wall recoil (Windkessel effect); this leads to improved systemic perfusion. The magnitude of all these effects depends on balloon volume, heart rate (shorter diastolic time results in less augmentation per unit time), and aortic compliance.

Patient Selection

The use of prophylactic IABP in high-risk patients undergoing coronary artery bypass is effective in the management of refractory angina and improvement of coronary perfusion flow. Therefore, inserting an IABP in this patient is reasonable, if there are no significant contraindications. Absolute contraindications for IABP placement are aortic dissection, clinically significant aortic aneurysm, severe peripheral artery disease (including bilateral femoral–popliteal grafts), significant aortic regurgitation, uncontrolled bleeding, and/or sepsis.

The role of IABP insertion in patients with myocardial infarction complicated by cardiogenic shock remains controversial. The Intraaortic Balloon Pump in Cardiogenic Shock II trial showed no difference in 30-day mortality in this population with use of IABP. Subsequently, the American College of Cardiology/American Heart Association downgraded its recommendation for IABP in these patients with cardiogenic shock post–myocardial infarction to class IIa. Importantly, <5% of the study population underwent revascularization with bypass surgery; also, the use of a left ventricular assist device was not controlled.

Other uses of balloon counterpulsation (with limited evidence) include refractory ventricular arrhythmias, inability to wean from cardiopulmonary bypass, bridge to intervention in severe/critical aortic stenosis, and refractory pulmonary edema from decompensated heart failure.

Placement

The closer the balloon is to the aortic valve, the greater the diastolic pressure elevation. However, due to the anatomy of the aortic arch, the optimal balloon position is 1–2 cm distal to the takeoff of the left subclavian artery.

The ideal balloon for any given patient would cover the length from his or her left subclavian artery to the takeoff of the celiac artery. The diameter of the balloon, when fully expanded, should not exceed 80%–90% of the diameter of the descending aorta. Currently, balloon size ranges from 25 cc to 50 cc, with 40 cc being the most prevalent.

Percutaneous placement of an IABP in the femoral artery by a modified Seldinger technique has become routine practice. Sheathless insertion and use of smaller-size catheters can decrease vascular complications. When faced with challenging anatomy, surgical cutdown may be employed. Other sites of cannulation include the subclavian or axillary artery. If placed in the cardiac catheterization lab, fluoroscopy can be used to verify proper placement. Alternatively, a chest radiograph can be used to verify the position post-procedure because the level of the carina approximates the left subclavian artery; transesophageal echocardiography can also guide IABP placement. Decreased urine output should alert the provider of balloon juxtarenal malpositioning.

Anticoagulation
Full anticoagulation with an IABP reduces the risk of thrombus formation and thromboembolic events. However, limited evidence shows that systemic heparinization increases the risk of bleeding without decreasing limb ischemic events. Advancement in balloon pump materials and smaller catheter size may explain these findings. It is reasonable to implement a selective, rather than a universal, strategy for heparinization during balloon counterpulsation therapy.

Complications
The incidence of complications associated with IABPs varies widely in the literature but can range up to 50%, with an average of 20%–30% of cases. Vascular complications include limb ischemia (most common), bleeding, dissection, and hematoma/pseudoaneurysm formation. If complications remain undiagnosed without appropriate intervention, irreversible injury and/or limb amputation may follow. During placement, there is a risk for thromboembolic events and direct vessel injury. Women have a smaller femoral artery and a higher rate of these complications with balloon counterpulsation therapy. The presence of peripheral vascular disease,

diabetes mellitus, or smoking history is also associated with higher rates of vascular complications. Duration of therapy is also linked to complications.

Mesenteric ischemia is rare and can be fatal if it is not recognized. Serial increases in lactate levels should prompt the clinician to confirm correct IABP placement. The presence of blood in the balloon tubing suggests the possibility of balloon rupture and gas embolism, an extremely uncommon but catastrophic event. Thrombocytopenia is seen in ~50% of patients, but this finding is generally mild and not associated with major bleeding or mortality.

CASE RESUMES

While awaiting surgical intervention, the patient becomes acutely tachycardiac with several beats of ventricular ectopy. He has not made urine since arrival to the unit. An in situ pulmonary artery catheter reveals a cardiac index of 1.2 L/min/m^2. An IABP is urgently placed with resolution of ventricular ectopy. His cardiac index by thermodilution improves to 1.9 L/min/m^2 followed by 30 cc of urine output. His blood pressure is support with vasopressor agents but his mentation and urine output remain stable prior to going to the operating room for coronary bypass surgery.

> **KEY POINTS TO REMEMBER**
> 1. Counterpulsation increases coronary blood flow, reduces left ventricular afterload, and increases end-organ perfusion.
> 2. Other uses of balloon counterpulsation include refractory ventricular arrhythmias, inability to wean from cardiopulmonary bypass, bridge to intervention in severe/critical aortic stenosis, and refractory pulmonary edema from decompensated heart failure.
> 3. Contraindications for IABP placement are aortic dissection, clinically significant aortic aneurysm, severe peripheral artery disease (including bilateral femoral–popliteal grafts), significant aortic regurgitation, uncontrolled bleeding, and/or sepsis.

4. Optimal positioning for IABP is 1–2 cm distal to the takeoff of the left subclavian artery.
5. Thrombocytopenia is seen in ~50% of patients.
6. Vascular complications include limb ischemia (most common), bleeding, dissection, and hematoma/pseudoaneurysm formation.
7. The presence of blood in the balloon tubing suggests the possibility of balloon rupture and gas embolism, an extremely uncommon but catastrophic event.

Suggested Reading
1. Krishna M, Zacharowski K. Principles of intra-aortic balloon pump counterpulsation. *Continuing Education in Anaesthesia Critical Care & Pain*. 2009;9(1):24–28.
2. Parissis H, Graham B, Lampridis S, et al. IABP: history–evolution–pathophysiology–indications: what we need to know. *J Cardiothorac Surg*. 2016;11:122.
3. Pucher PH, Cummings IG, Shipolini AR, et al. Is heparin needed for patients with an intra-aortic balloon pump? *Interact Cardiovasc Thorac Surg*. 2012;15(1):136–139.
4. Thiele H, Zeymer U, Neumann F, et al. Intraaortic balloon support for myocardial infarction with cardiogenic shock. *N Engl J Med*. 2012;367:1287–1296.
5. Zangrillo A, Pappalardo F, Dossi R, et al. Preoperative intra-aortic balloon pump to reduce mortality in coronary artery bypass graft: a meta-analysis or randomized controlled trials. *Crit Care*. 2015;19:10.

29 Cardiac Tamponade

Christopher Read and Emer Curran

A 69-year-old man becomes progressively more hypotensive and tachycardic 12 hours following an uncomplicated single-vessel coronary artery bypass graft and aortic valve repair. The patient is intubated, ventilated, and sedated. He develops a new sinus tachycardia of 120 beats per minute. Intra-arterial blood pressure is 75/45 mm Hg despite the administration of crystalloid boluses and an increasing dose of norepinephrine to 15 mcg/min from 2 mcg/min 2 hours ago. His central venous pressure (CVP) is increased to 25 mm Hg from 5 mm Hg in the immediate postoperative period. Hemoglobin, platelet count, international normalized ratio, activated clotting time, and core body temperature are within normal limits.

The total drain output is 100 mL and has now stopped. His blood gas shows a pH of 7.19 and a blood lactate concentration of 5.5 mmol/L. He is cool and clammy to the touch. You perform a bedside transthoracic echocardiogram, which shows a large amount of pericardial fluid around the heart.

What do you do now?

DISCUSSION

Cardiac tamponade is defined as the compression of cardiac chambers due to increased pericardial or mediastinal pressure from blood/fluid. Mediastinal bleeding following cardiac surgery can result from leaking grafts or capillary ooze from a long bypass time or coagulopathy and can present acutely or insidiously for up to 10 days. Cardiac valvular surgery and coronary bypass grafting carry a higher risk of surgical tamponade. This accumulation of blood limits the normal functioning of the heart as ventricular filling and pump function are impaired. A fall in cardiac output (CO) can ensue, leading to systemic hypoperfusion and life-threatening organ dysfunction.

During cardiac tamponade following cardiac surgery, blood accumulates in the pericardial/mediastinal space quickly, leaving little time for compensatory pericardial stretch and causes a rapid increase in pressure, as seen in Figure 29.1A. As pericardial stretch quickly reaches its limit, the pericardial pressure will initially exceed the lower right-sided chamber filling pressures, compressing the right atrium and ventricle. This results in a reduction in venous return, a rise in CVP, and a reduction in stroke volume (SV). When pericardial volume increases further due to accumulation of blood, the pressure exceeds the higher left chamber filling pressure, and there is a marked reduction in CO, leading to a state of obstructive shock and, if untreated, cardiac arrest. Therefore, vigilant assessment of postoperative mediastinal bleeding, prompt recognition of clinical and ultrasonographic features of tamponade, and early management thereof are imperative before a cardiac arrest scenario potentially ensues.

Clinical Features, Assessing Mediastinal Bleeding, and Monitors

Tamponade following cardiac surgery usually presents acutely and often without warning. Sympathetic nervous system activation resulting in tachycardia and an increase in sympathetic tone is an important physiological compensatory mechanism to maintain a mean arterial pressure in this low output state, which in turn activates the renin–angiotensin system, causing an increase in fluid retention, further compounding the problem. However, common signs of tamponade such as tachycardia, hypotension, and dyspnea are poor at discriminating between different types of shock. Historically, Beck's triad, consisting of hypotension, elevated jugular venous pressure, and muffled heart sounds, is pathognomonic of cardiac tamponade but is not always present.

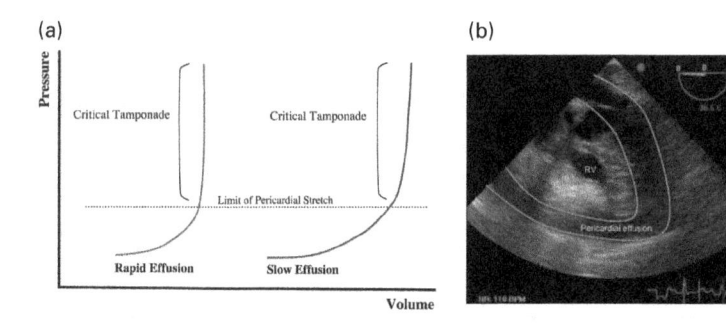

FIGURE 29.1 (A) Volume–pressure relationship in cardiac tamponade physiology.

Source: Pérez-Casares A, Cesar S, Brunet Garcia L, Sanchez-de-Toledo J. Echocardiographic evaluation of pericardial effusion and cardiac tamponade. *Front Pediatr.* 2017;5:79.

(B) TEE image showing right ventricular collapse secondary to a pericardial effusion.

Source: Odor PM, Bailey A. Anaesthesia tutorial of the week #283 cardiac tamponade. World Federation of Societies of Anaesthesiologists, 2013. https://www.wfsahq.org/components/com_virtual_library/media/1b3d4f771bc9361a73764d03a184cf76-283-Cardiac-Tamponade-RFS.pdf. Accessed July 27, 2020.

There should a high degree of suspicion for tamponade when there is hemodynamic compromise with respiratory variation (pulsus paradoxus) and elevated filling pressures, especially when found in conjunction with mediastinal bleeding that has abruptly stopped or has become excessive or the bleeding from chest drains has become minimal caused by clotted tubes.

Characteristically, the CVP waveform is raised, and all components are elevated. The a and v waves are tall, the x descent is steep, and the y descent is usually absent because early diastolic blood flow is reduced to the right side of the heart because of the compressive effect of the tamponade.

Pulsus paradoxus is defined as an "inspiratory systolic fall in arterial pressure of 10mmHg or more" in a spontaneously breathing patient, which is exaggerated in tamponade. The main mechanism of pulsus paradoxus is related to ventricular interdependence. The inspiratory increase in right ventricular filling, due to a decrease in intrathoracic pressure, results in a bulging of the interventricular septum into the left ventricle (LV) and a reduction of SV and hence CO. In tamponade, the LV chamber size can be markedly reduced, by a compressive effect, resulting in an exaggerated reduction in CO during inspiration. "Reverse" pulsus paradoxus demonstrates a fall in arterial pressure during expiration in a mechanically ventilated patient as it is in this phase in the respiratory cycle when intrathoracic pressure decreases.

Electrocardiographic features can include a compensatory tachycardia, electrical alternans, a decreased voltage, and dysrhythmias.

Radiographic evidence of tamponade which includes a widened mediastinum or enlarged cardiac silhouette may only be present in 20% of patients.

Echocardiography

If cardiac tamponade is suspected in a postoperative cardiac surgical patient, echocardiography should be performed if the clinical setting allows. A transesophageal echocardiogram (TEE) is more accurate in detecting a clot behind the heart than a transthoracic echocardiogram because of better acoustic windows. Important items to assess are the following:

1. Quantity and quality of pericardial fluid (Figure 29.1B)
2. Collapsibility of cardiac chambers (Figure 29.2A)
3. Diastolic ventricular size variability with respiratory cycle
4. Septal "bounce"

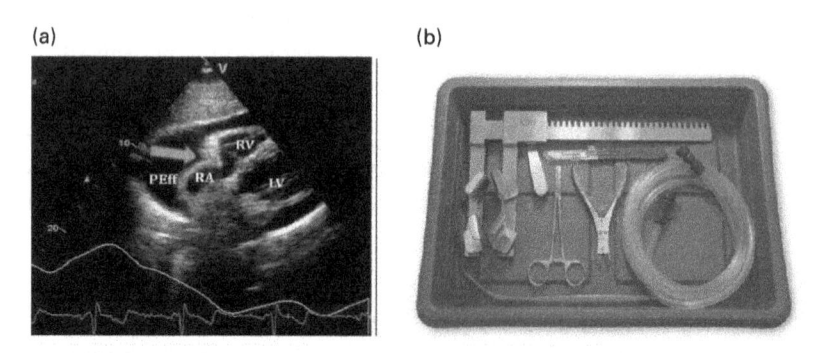

FIGURE 29.2 (A) Subcostal view of a patient with significant pericardial effusion and evidence of right atrium collapse. LV, left ventricle; Peff, pericardial effusion; RA, right atrium; RV, right ventricle.

Source: Pérez-Casares A, Cesar S, Brunet Garcia L, Sanchez-de-Toledo J. Echocardiographic evaluation of pericardial effusion and cardiac tamponade. *Front Pediatr.* 2017;5:79.

(B) Resternotomy kit.

Molnlycke Health Care.

5. Collapsibility/distensibility of the inferior vena cava with respiratory variation

Of note, the volume of pericardial effusion does not always correlate with the severity of clinical symptoms. Of all echocardiographic assessment items mentioned, the absence of cardiac chamber collapse has a higher negative predictive value to rule out cardiac tamponade. Therefore, patient management goals should always be made following a clinical assessment. There is little role for echocardiography in the cardiac arrest/peri-arrest scenario after cardiac surgery as it will cause a delay in arrest management

Management

Suspected/confirmed cardiac tamponade after cardiac surgery is an indication for urgent mediastinal exploration/resternotomy in the operating room if time allows. Emergency resternotomy in the intensive care unit is indicated in the setting of a pending arrest. Immediate involvement of cardiothoracic and anesthesiology teams is mandatory. Managing CO in tamponade causing hemodynamic compromise before mediastinal exploration can be challenging as the mainstay of therapy is relief of mediastinal pressure with resternotomy. The hemodynamic goals in maintaining an adequate CO pre-exploration include the following:

1. Inotropic therapy and augmented chronotropy (caution with inotropic therapy at time of surgical relief of tamponade)
2. Decrease in right atrial pressure
   a. avoiding excessive fluid administration, which can increase preload and worsen ventricular interdependence and CO
   b. avoiding high intrathoracic pressures by reducing positive end-expiratory pressure

Emergency Resternotomy

Emergent resternotomy is the key component of successful resuscitation following a cardiac arrest secondary to cardiac tamponade. It is a well-recognized step in standard resuscitation protocols. It allows for 3 vital steps—temporary relief of tamponade; internal cardiac massage or defibrillation, which are more effective than external massage or defibrillation; and finally, temporary stemming of the source of bleeding by direct compression until definitive surgical control is achieved. It is essential for all personnel who participate in resuscitations in cardiac critical care to be aware of the necessity of immediate resternotomy and well versed in this life-saving procedure. A small emergency resternotomy kit should be available in every cardiac intensive care unit and should include a disposable scalpel attached to the outside of the set, a wire cutter, a heavy needle holder, a single-piece sternal retractor, a sucker, and a drape, as seen in Figure 29.2B.

CASE RESUMES

On TEE you discover a large amount of pericardial fluid with compression of all cardiac chambers. In conjunction with an absent mediastinal drain output, reverse pulsus paradoxus seen on arterial line tracing, and a raised CVP waveform of 25 mm Hg, you confirm a diagnosis of cardiac tamponade. You contact the cardiothoracic team, who assess the patient and decide to take the patient for emergency resternotomy in theater and mediastinal re-exploration. A large clot is evacuated, the patient's hemodynamic status improves, and cardiovascular support is slowly weaned.

> **KEY POINTS TO REMEMBER**
> 1. Have a high degree of suspicion for tamponade when there is hemodynamic compromise with respiratory variation (pulsus paradoxus) and elevated central venous filling pressures.
> 2. Have a high degree of suspicion for tamponade if mediastinal bleeding has abruptly stopped or has become excessive or the bleeding from chest drains has been minimal caused by clotted tubes.
> 3. Prompt echocardiographic confirmation of tamponade should be performed when the diagnosis is suspected and if time allows.

4. Suspected/confirmed cardiac tamponade after cardiac surgery is an indication for urgent mediastinal exploration.
5. Emergency resternotomy in critical care is indicated in the setting of a pending arrest.
6. All healthcare providers involved with resuscitation after cardiac surgery should be aware of and well versed in the technique and preparation of the resternotomy procedure.

Suggested Reading
1. Society of Thoracic Surgeons Task Force on Resuscitation After Cardiac Surgery. The Society of Thoracic Surgeons expert consensus for the resuscitation of patients who arrest after cardiac surgery. *Ann Thorac Surg* 2017;103:1005–1020.
2. Carmona P, Mateo E, Casanovas I, et al. Management of cardiac tamponade after cardiac surgery. *J Cardiothorac Vasc Anesth.* 2012;26(2):302–311.
3. Odor P, Bailey A. Cardiac tamponade anaesthesia tutorial of the week 283. St. George's Hospital, London, UK, 2013. https://www.wfsahq.org/components/com_virtual_library/media/1b3d4f771bc9361a73764d03a184cf76-283-Cardiac-Tamponade-RFS.pdf. Accessed July 27, 2020.
4. Bojar RM. *Manual of Perioperative Care in Adult Cardiac Surgery*, 5th ed. Chichester, UK: Wiley-Blackwell; 2011.
5. Pérez-Casares A, Cesar S, Brunet-Garcia L, Sanchez-de-Toledo J. Echocardiographic evaluation of pericardial effusion and cardiac tamponade. *Front Pediatr.* 2017;5:79. doi:10.3389/fped.2017.00079.

30 Endocarditis

Ruth Boylan and Ian Conrick-Martin

It is 3 a.m., and you are called to see a 66-year-old man in the emergency department. He presents with a 2-day history of shortness of breath, fever, lack of appetite, and general malaise. His partner informs you that he underwent a mechanical mitral valve replacement 14 days previously. Significant past medical history includes immunoglobulin A nephropathy and a renal transplant 1 year previously. Despite his renal transplant, he remains on hemodialysis due to poor graft function.

On initial examination, you note an elderly man in respiratory distress, cyanosed, and cool peripherally. He is hypotensive, tachycardic, and desaturating. A bedside transthoracic echocardiogram (TTE) reveals an aberrant paraprosthetic flow, a vegetation at the site of the mitral valve prosthesis, and severely reduced left ventricular function. Blood cultures are taken and empirical antimicrobial therapy is started. You transfer the patient to the intensive care unit (ICU), initiate norepinephrine and dobutamine infusions, intubate, and order a transesophageal echocardiography (TEE).

What do you do now?

DISCUSSION

Cardiogenic Shock

Cardiogenic shock has a very high in-hospital mortality rate, ranging from 45% to 100%. Although myocardial ischemia is the most common cause of cardiogenic shock, other etiologies must always be considered. In this scenario, given the recent surgical history, acute valve dysfunction is the most probable cause of cardiogenic shock.

Acute valve dysfunction can have many causes including chordae rupture, lack of appropriate sealing of a prosthetic valve and the cardiac tissue, prosthetic valve thrombus, or valvular abscess. For this patient, one should have a high index of suspicion for paravalvular leak (PVL) with infective endocarditis (IE), resulting in a prosthetic valve abscess and acute valve dysfunction.

PVL

PVL is a relatively rare complication relating to the surgical replacement of mitral and aortic valves. The majority of PVLs are hemodynamically nonsignificant; however, large leaks lead to heart failure and increase the risk of IE. The majority of PVLs are round, oval, or crescent-shaped. Their tracks can be parallel, perpendicular, or serpiginous. PVLs are more commonly associated with mechanical valves, followed by bioprosthetic valves. PVLs (including small nonsignificant jets) occur in approximately 20% of valve replacements. PVL occurs more frequently with mitral than aortic prosthetic valves.

PVL is most commonly related to disruption of sewing ring sutures precipitated by IE and accompanied by an abscess formation. Signs and symptoms of significant PVL are heart failure, hemolytic anemia, and IE.

The most important diagnostic modality in a case of PVL is echocardiography. TTE often cannot differentiate the PVL from prosthetic regurgitation, and for this reason TEE is crucial. TEE often requires multiple projections because of the presence of thrombi, pericardial fluid, artifacts, and acoustic shadows caused by the structure of the prosthetic valves.

TEE evaluation of PVL includes the following:

- Shape and orientation of the jet
- Number of jets

- Maximum velocity
- Presence of distal flow reversal
- Pulmonary pressures

Findings on TEE suggestive of significant PVL on a prosthetic mechanical mitral valve are as follows:

- Diastolic increase of maximum velocity >1.9 m/s and mean gradient >5 mm Hg
- Velocity-time integral (VTI) across the valve prosthesis to VTI in left ventricular outflow tract ratio >2.5
- Maximum velocity of tricuspid regurgitation >3 m/s

IE

IE is caused by microbial infection of the endocardial surface or of prosthetic material in the heart. More than 80% of cases are caused by *Staphylococcus aureus* or by species of *Streptococcus* or *Enterococcus*. The total incidence of IE remains relatively constant (3–10 cases per 100,000), but there are proportionately more cases associated with prosthetic valves and secondary to hospital-acquired infections.

Risk factors for IE include the following:

- Presence of prosthetic cardiac valves
- Native cardiac valve disease
- Invasive procedure within last 60 days
- Presence of a pacemaker/defibrillator
- Presence of vascular access devices (e.g., permacath, portacath)
- Congenital cardiac disease
- Past history of IE
- Current intravenous drug use

The presence of a mechanical mitral valve alone places this patient in a high-risk group for IE. His clinical signs and symptoms are very suggestive for IE: 90% of patients with IE present with fever, often associated with systemic symptoms such as chills, night sweats, arthralgia, poor appetite, weight loss, general malaise, chest pain, and dyspnea. Heart murmurs are present in up to 85% of patients with IE, while 25% of patients have embolic complications upon presentation. IE may present as a rapidly progressive acute infection or as a subacute/chronic disease with nonspecific symptoms and low-grade fever. In-hospital mortality of patients with IE varies from 15% to 30%.

Diagnosis

The diagnosis of IE usually relies on the association between an infective syndrome and endocardial involvement. Traditionally, the modified Duke criteria were recommended for the diagnosis of IE. These criteria were based on clinical, echocardiographic, and biological findings (Box 30.1). They have a sensitivity of approximately 80% overall but are less accurate in the case of prosthetic valve endocarditis and pacemaker/defibrillator lead IE, for which additional imaging modalities improve sensitivity.

The American Heart Association and the European Society of Cardiology (ESC) published modified diagnostic criteria in 2015 for IE (Box 30.2 and

---

BOX 30.1   Definition of IE According to Modified Duke Criteria

Definite IE

Pathological criteria
- Microorganisms demonstrated by culture or on histological examination of a vegetation, a vegetation that has embolized, or an intracardiac abscess specimen; or
- Pathological lesions; vegetation or intracardiac abscess confirmed by histological examination showing active endocarditis

Clinical criteria
- 2 major criteria; or
- 1 major criterion and 3 minor criteria; or
- 5 minor criteria

Possible IE
- 1 major criterion and 1 minor criterion; or
- 3 minor criteria

Rejected IE
- Firm alternative diagnosis; or
- Resolution of symptoms suggesting IE with antibiotic therapy for ≥4 days; or
- No pathological evidence of IE at surgery or autopsy, with antibiotic therapy for ≥4 days; or
- Does not meet criteria for possible IE, as above

BOX 30.2 **Definitions of Terms Used in the Modified Criteria for Diagnosis of IE**

Major Criteria

1. Blood cultures positive for IE
   a. Typical microorganisms consistent with IE from 2 separate blood cultures
      - Viridans streptococci, Streptococcus gallolyticus (Streptococcus bovis), HACEK group, Staphylococcus aureus; or
      - Community-acquired enterococci, in the absence of a primary focus; or
   b. Microorganisms consistent with IE from persistently positive blood cultures
      - ≥2 positive blood cultures of blood samples drawn >12 h apart; or
      - All of 3 or a majority of ≥4 separate cultures of blood (with first and last samples drawn ≥1 h apart); or
   c. Single positive blood culture for *Coxiella burnetii* or phase I immunoglobulin G antibody titer >1:800
2. Imaging positive for IE
   a. Echocardiogram positive for IE
      - Vegetation
      - Abscess, pseudoaneurysm, intracardiac fistula
      - Valvular perforation or aneurysm
      - New partial dehiscence of prosthetic valve
   b. Abnormal activity around the site of prosthetic valve implantation detected by 18F-FDG PET/CT* (only if the prosthesis was implanted for >3 months) or radiolabeled leukocytes SPECT/CT*
   c. Definite paravalvular lesions by cardiac CT*

Minor Criteria

1. Predisposition such as predisposing heart condition or intravenous drug use
2. Fever defined as temperature >38°C
3. Vascular phenomena (including those detected by imaging only)
   - Major arterial emboli
   - Septic pulmonary infarcts
   - Infectious (mycotic) aneurysms
   - Intracranial hemorrhage
   - Conjunctival hemorrhages
   - Janeway lesions

> 4. Immunological phenomena
>   - Glomerulonephritis
>   - Osler's nodes
>   - Roth's spots
>   - Rheumatoid factor
> 5. Microbiological evidence: positive blood culture but does not meet a major criterion as noted above or serological evidence of active infection with organism consistent with IE
>
> * European Society of Cardiology guidelines only.
> CT = computed tomography; FDG = fluorodeoxyglucose; HACEK = *Haemophilus parainfluenzae, H. aphrophilus, H. paraphrophilus, H. influenzae, Actinobacillus actinomycetemcomitans, Cardiobacterium hominis, Eikenella corrodens, Kingella kingae,* and *K. denitrificans*; PET = positron emission tomography; SPECT = single photon emission computerized tomography.

Figure 30.1). These criteria are based on clinical, echocardiographic, biological, and radiological (magnetic resonance imaging [MRI], computed tomography [CT], positron emission tomography [PET]/CT; ESC only) findings.

Echocardiography

Echocardiography, in the form of TTE or TEE, is the technique of choice for the diagnosis of IE and plays a crucial role in the management and monitoring of these patients. TTE is the first-line imaging modality in the case of suspected IE. TEE is recommended in all patients with a clinical suspicion of IE and a negative or non-diagnostic TTE. TEE is also recommended in patients with a clinical suspicion of IE, when a prosthetic heart valve or intracardiac device is present. Figure 30.2 shows a mitral valve vegetation on TEE examination. Repeat TTE and/or TEE within 5–7 days is recommended in the case of initially negative examination when clinical suspicion of IE remains high. Echocardiography should also be considered in cases of *S. aureus* bacteremia. Intraoperative echocardiography is recommended in all cases of IE requiring surgery. TTE is recommended at completion of antimicrobial therapy for evaluation of cardiac and valve function and morphology.

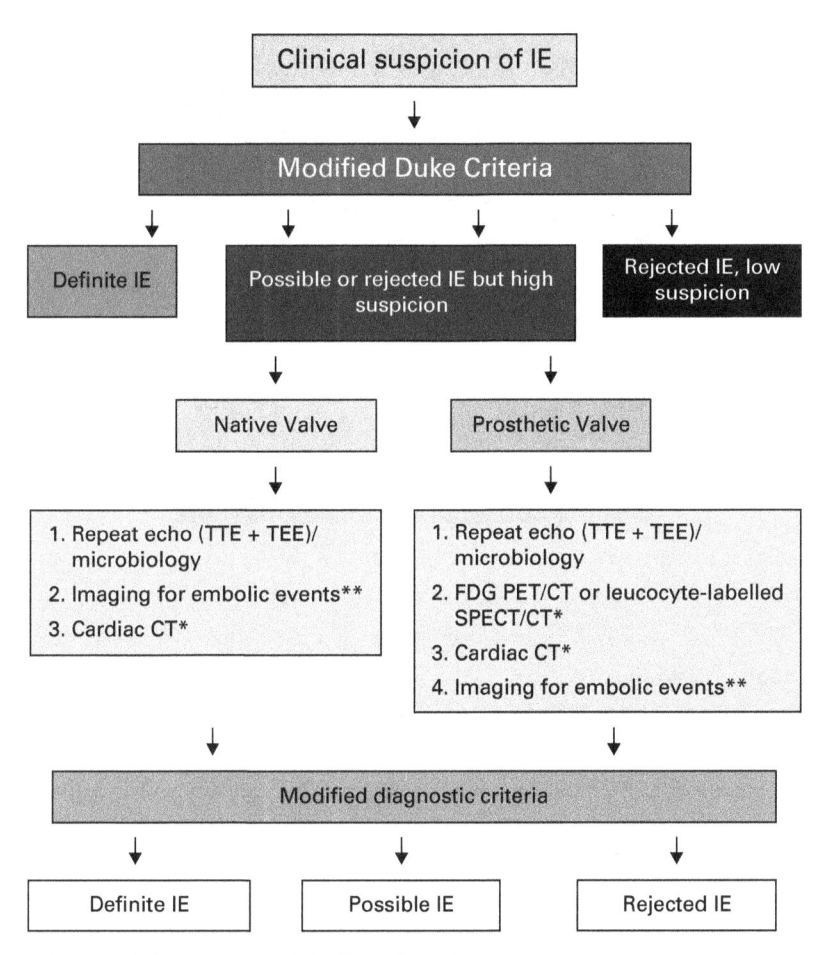

```
                    Clinical suspicion of IE
                              ↓
                    Modified Duke Criteria
        ↓                  ↓                   ↓                ↓
   Definite IE    Possible or rejected IE but high      Rejected IE, low
                              suspicion                    suspicion
                    ↓                   ↓
              Native Valve        Prosthetic Valve
                    ↓                   ↓
```

Native Valve	Prosthetic Valve
1. Repeat echo (TTE + TEE)/ microbiology 2. Imaging for embolic events** 3. Cardiac CT*	1. Repeat echo (TTE + TEE)/ microbiology 2. FDG PET/CT or leucocyte-labelled SPECT/CT* 3. Cardiac CT* 4. Imaging for embolic events**

```
                    Modified diagnostic criteria
             ↓                  ↓                   ↓
        Definite IE        Possible IE         Rejected IE
```

CT = computed tomography; FDG = fluorodeoxyglucose,

PET = positron emission tomography, SPECT = single photon emission computerized tomography,

TEE = transesophageal echocardiography, TTE = transthoracic echocardiography.

* European Society of Cardiology Guidelines 2015 only.

** May include cerebral MRI, whole body CT, and/or PET/CT.

FIGURE 30.1 Algorithm for diagnosis of IE. FDG, fluorodeoxyglucose; SPECT, single-photon emission CT.

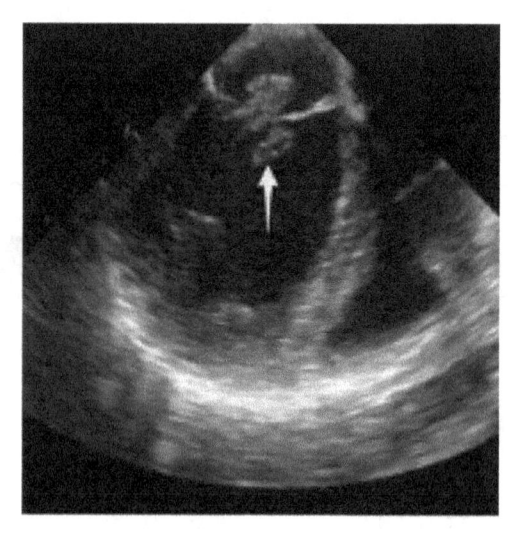

FIGURE 30.2 Mitral valve IE vegetation.
Case courtesy of Professor Frank Gaillard, Radiopedia.org, rID: 29363.

Prognostication

The rapid identification of patients at highest risk of death is an important part of the management of IE because it offers the opportunity to change the course of the disease with urgent surgery that can improve prognosis. Box 30.3 describes predictors of poor outcomes in patients with IE.

Treatment

Treatment of IE relies on the following:

1. Antimicrobial therapy to eradicate causative microbes
2. Surgical intervention to remove infected material and drain abscesses

Patients with complicated IE should be managed at an early stage in a reference center with immediate cardiothoracic surgical facilities and the presence of a multidisciplinary endocarditis team.

Antimicrobial Therapy

Antimicrobial therapy of IE should be started promptly. Three sets of blood cultures should be drawn at 30-minute intervals before initiation of empiric

> **BOX 30.3 Predictors of Poor Outcomes in Patients with Infective Endocarditis**
>
> Patient characteristics
> - Older age
> - Prosthetic valve IE
> - Diabetes mellitus
> - Co-morbidity (e.g., immunosuppressed, renal/pulmonary disease, frailty)
>
> Clinical complications of IE
> - Heart failure
> - Renal failure
> - Larger than moderate area of ischemic stroke
> - Brain hemorrhage
> - Septic shock
>
> Microorganism
> - *Staphylococcus aureus* (MSSA)
> - Fungi
> - Non-HACEK gram-negative bacilli
>
> Echocardiographic findings
> - Periannular complications
> - Severe left-sided valve regurgitation
> - Low left ventricular ejection fraction
> - Pulmonary hypertension
> - Large vegetations
> - Severe prosthetic valve dysfunction
> - Premature mitral valve closure and other signs of elevated diastolic pressures.
>
> MSSA, methicillin-sensitive *S. aureus*.

antimicrobials. The initial choice of empirical treatment depends on the following (see Table 30.1):

- The patient's previous antibiotic therapy
- Presence of native valve endocarditis (NVE) or prosthetic valve endocarditis (PVE)
- Community versus nosocomial infection
- Knowledge of local epidemiology and antibiotic resistance patterns

The choice of antimicrobial thereafter should always be based on the susceptibility of the latest recovered bacterial isolate. Bactericidal regimens are

TABLE 30.1 Proposed Antibiotic Regimens for Initial Empirical Treatment of IE in Acute Severely Ill Patients

Type of IE	Antimicrobial Dosage and Route
Community-acquired native valve or late prosthetic valve (>12 months post-surgery) endocarditis	Ampicillin 12 g/d i.v. in 4–6 doses with flucloxacillin or oxacillin 12 g/d i.v. in 4–6 doses with gentamicin 3 mg/kg/day i.v. or i.m. in 1 dose For penicillin allergy give: vancomycin 30–60 mg/kg/d i.v. in 2–3 doses with gentamicin 3 mg/kg/d in 1 dose
Early PVE (>12 months post-surgery) and non-nosocomial healthcare-associated endocarditis	Vancomycin 30 mg/kg/d i.v. in 2 doses with gentamicin 3 mg/kg/d i.v. or i.m. in 1 dose with rifampicin 900–1200 mg i.v. or orally in 2–3 doses

i.m., intramuscularly; i.v., intravenously.

more effective than bacteriostatic therapy. Aminoglycoside antimicrobials (e.g., gentamicin) synergize with cell-wall inhibitors (e.g., vancomycin) for bactericidal activity and are useful for shortening the duration of therapy. Bacterial antibiotic tolerance poses a significant hindrance to microbial eradication. Slow-growing and dormant microbes present in vegetations and biofilms display tolerance to many antimicrobials and thus justify the need for prolonged therapy (6 weeks) to fully sterilize infected heart valves. Bactericidal drug combinations are preferred to monotherapy against tolerant organisms.

Antimicrobial therapy should last at least 2 weeks for NVE and at least 6 weeks for PVE. The duration of therapy is based on the first day of negative blood culture in the case of initial positive blood culture. In NVE requiring valve replacement by a prosthesis during antimicrobial therapy, the postoperative antibiotic regimen should be that recommended for NVE and not PVE.

Aminoglycosides (e.g., gentamicin) are no longer recommended in staphylococcal NVE because they can increase renal toxicity and their clinical benefits have not been demonstrated. Rifampicin should only be used in foreign body infections such as PVE after 3–5 days of effective antibiotic therapy, once the bacteremia has been cleared.

Antimicrobial Prophylaxis

Antimicrobial prophylaxis aims to prevent the attachment of bacteria onto the endocardium after transient bacteremia following invasive procedures. In 2002, restrictions of indications for antimicrobial prophylaxis were initiated because of changes in pathophysiological concepts and multiple risk–benefit analyses.

It is currently recommended that antibiotic prophylaxis should only be considered when a high-risk dental procedure is performed on a patient with a high risk of IE.

This includes patients with the following:

- Prosthetic valves
- A previous episode of IE
- Cyanotic congenital heart disease
- Congenital heart disease repaired with prosthetic material

Surgical Intervention

Indications for surgery include the following:

- Heart failure
- Uncontrolled infection secondary to IE
- For the prevention of embolism

The objectives of surgery are the removal of infected tissues and the reconstruction of cardiac morphology, including repair/replacement of the affected valve(s). Valve repair is preferred whenever possible, particularly when IE affects the tricuspid or mitral valves without significant valve leaflet destruction. Intraoperative assessment of the valve after debridement is crucial in order to evaluate whether the remaining valve tissue is of sufficient quality to achieve a durable repair. In aortic valve IE, valve replacement with a biological or mechanical prosthesis is the technique of choice.

Complications of IE

- Heart failure
- Uncontrolled infection
- Systemic embolism
- Neurological complications

- Infectious (mycotic) aneurysms
- Splenic complications (e.g., splenomegaly)
- Myocarditis and pericarditis
- Acute renal failure
- Musculocutaneous manifestations (e.g., rash)

IE in the ICU

Admission to the ICU is often part of the patient pathway following cardiac surgery for IE. Patients with IE may also be admitted to the ICU with sepsis, heart failure, severe valvular pathology, or organ failure related to complications of IE. Morbidity is high among this cohort of patients, with most patients requiring mechanical ventilation and inotropic support and many developing renal failure. Mortality rates in critically ill patients with IE are reported to be between 29% and 84%.

Staphylococcus species followed by streptococci are the most common causative organisms among critical care patients. Fungal IE (e.g., *Candida* species) is an increasing problem in the ICU.

The clinical presentation of IE in the ICU setting may be atypical, and classic features may be masked by critical care interventions and concomitant pathology. Echocardiography can be particularly challenging in the ICU setting. There should be a low threshold for TEE in critically ill patients with *S. aureus* catheter-related bloodstream infection because of its high propensity to cause IE. Patients with sepsis should be managed according to latest international guidelines. Emergency surgery and patients with Sequential Organ Failure Assessment scores >15 on the day of surgery have the poorest outcomes.

CASE RESUMES

The TEE confirmed a large PVL at the site of the replacement mitral valve with a perivalvar abscess of the mitral valve annulus extending from the anteromedial to the posteromedial aspect of the mitral valve prosthesis. This patient underwent an excision of the mitral valve vegetation and replacement of the mechanical mitral valve. He received a 6-week course of vancomycin and rifampicin for a methicillin-sensitive *S. aureus*–positive infective endocarditis and vasopressor support for 2 weeks post-surgery and was discharged from the ICU 3 weeks postoperatively.

> **KEY POINTS TO REMEMBER**
> 1. There is a high in-hospital mortality associated with IE, especially among critically ill patients.
> 2. Rapid identification of patients at highest risk of death offers the opportunity to change the course of the disease with urgent surgery and improve prognosis.
> 3. Patients with complicated IE should be managed at an early stage in a reference center with immediate cardiothoracic surgical facilities and the presence of a multidisciplinary endocarditis team.
> 4. Echocardiography plays a key role in the diagnosis and management of IE. TTE is recommended as the first-line imaging modality in suspected IE. TEE is recommended in patients with clinical suspicion of IE when a prosthetic valve or an intracardiac device is present.
> 5. Functional imaging modalities such as multi-slice CT, MRI, and fluorodeoxyglucose PET/CT can improve the sensitivity of the modified Duke criteria when TTE/TEE findings are negative or doubtful.
> 6. *Staphylococcus* species followed by streptococci are the most common causative organisms among critical care patients, but there should be a high index of suspicion for fungal IE in the ICU setting, especially when there is failure to respond to empirical antibacterial therapy.
> 7. Empiric antimicrobial therapy should be commenced promptly if IE is suspected. The choice of antimicrobial thereafter should always be based on the susceptibility of the latest recovered bacterial isolate.
> 8. Antibiotic prophylaxis should only be considered when a high-risk dental procedure is performed on a patient with a high risk of IE.

Suggested Reading
1. Connaughton M, Rivett JG. Infective endocarditis. *BMJ*. 2010;341:6596.
2. Baddour L, Wilson WR, Bayer AS, et al. Infective endocarditis in adults: diagnosis, antimicrobial therapy, and management of complications. A scientific statement for healthcare professionals from the American Heart Association. *Circulation* 2015;132:1435–1486.
3. Habib G, Lancellotti P, Antunes MJ, et al. 2015 ESC guidelines for the management of infective endocarditis. *Eur Heart J*. 2015;36:3075–3128.
4. Li JS, Sexton DJ, Mick N, et al. Proposed modifications to the Duke criteria for the diagnosis of infective endocarditis. *Clin Infect Dis*. 2000;30:633–638.
5. Smolka G, Wojakowski W. Paravalvular leak—important complication after implantation of prosthetic valve. *ESC Council for Cardiology Practice E-Journal*. 2010;9(8).
6. Foster T, Tatco V. Infective endocarditis. Radiopaedia. https://radiopaedia.org/articles/infective-endocarditis?lang=us. Accessed July 27, 2020.

31 Postoperative Pneumothorax

Aoife Doolan and Gerard Curley

A 75-year-old male patient weighing 120 kg is admitted to the intensive care unit following 4-vessel coronary artery bypass surgery. He has a history of Global Initiative for Chronic Obstructive Lung Disease stage 3 chronic obstructive pulmonary disease with bilateral bullous disease and chronic kidney disease stage III. One mediastinal and one left pleural drain were placed intraoperatively.

Aortic cross-clamp time was long at 140 minutes. The patient is anuric for the next 12 hours, requiring continuous renal replacement therapy initiation.

Four hours later, the nurse calls to inform you that the patient's airway pressures have increased from 27 to 40 cm H_2O and that tidal volumes on assist-control ventilation have decreased from 400 mL to 250 mL. The patient now requires norepinephrine, heart rate is 130 beats per minute, and arterial oxygen saturation is 75%. Bedside lung ultrasound (US) on the right lung demonstrates the absence of lung sliding and the presence of a "lung point."

What do you do now?

DISCUSSION

Diagnosis

The patient has a right-sided tension pneumothorax, which is a life-threatening condition. It is caused by expanding intrapleural air, leading to mediastinal shift and hemodynamic compromise. Pneumothoraces may be classified into 4 groups: primary (no underlying lung disease), secondary (underlying lung disease), traumatic (penetrating and non-penetrating trauma to the chest), or iatrogenic. The incidence of pneumothoraces after cardiac surgery is 1.4%–3%. The pleural space is sometimes opened during internal mammary artery dissection. A pleural drain is inserted in the hemithorax at the end of surgery to remove air, blood, and/or fluid. The pleural space is also opened during off-pump coronary surgery to facilitate dissection. There is debate as to whether a pleurectomy is necessary during internal mammary dissection, and a literature review in 2014 suggested that maintaining the pleural integrity decreased pulmonary complications (atelectasis, pleural effusion), bleeding, pain, and hospital length of stay.

In this case, the most likely cause of pneumothorax is iatrogenic, secondary to the placement of a vascular catheter. Consideration should also be given to barotrauma from mechanical ventilation, a ruptured bulla, or accidental loss of integrity of the pleura intraoperatively during sternotomy, dissection, or closure. Other causes after cardiac surgery include kinking, blocking, disconnection, dislodgement or malposition of pleural drains, and post-pull pneumothorax.

Diagnosis is based on clinical history and examination with or without lung US (Table 31.1 and Figure 31.1). Lung US has been shown to have a better sensitivity than chest X-ray (CXR) in the diagnosis of pneumothoraces, but both are inferior to CT. Sensitivity of lung US is between 48.8% and 95% and is, clearly, operator-dependent.

Plain chest radiography is still commonly used to diagnose pneumothoraces, and if this was not a tension pneumothorax, it would be reasonable to wait for CXR. Pneumothoraces may be underappreciated on CXR. A 50% reduction in lung volume may only be visible as a 2 cm pneumothorax on CXR.

CT of the thorax has the highest sensitivity and is used as the reference standard. The 2014 American College of Radiology appropriateness

TABLE 31.1 **Lung US Signs of Pneumothorax**

Absence of lung sliding (Figure 31.1A)	The "seashore sign" (Figure 31.1B) on M mode is replaced with a "barcode sign" (horizontal lines)
Absence of B lines (Figure 31.1C)	Vertical lines that arise from the pleural line spread to the edge of the screen and move with respiration
Presence of A lines (Figure 31.1D)	Horizontal artifacts that are erased by B lines in normal lung
Presence of a lung point (Figure 31.1E)	The point where the pneumothorax ends and the pleura re-appose
Absence of the lung pulse (Figure 31.1E)	The synchronous movement of the pleura with the cardiac pulsation; vertical T lines on M mode in time with the heartbeat

criteria for blunt chest trauma recommend CT as standard for trauma with a high-energy mechanism, distracting injury, altered level of consciousness, abnormal CXR, or suspected thoracic injury. Pneumothorax size can be calculated using the light index and CT volumetrics. However, clinical features are far more important than size.

Treatment of Tension Pneumothorax

Tension pneumothorax is a clinical diagnosis and does not require CXR confirmation prior to needle decompression. However, where lung US is readily available, it may be a useful adjunct for diagnosis.

This pneumothorax requires needle decompression and placement of an underwater seal chest drain. Needle decompression can be performed in the second intercostal space midclavicular line or in the fifth intercostal space mid-axillary line. Remove the flash chamber before beginning. Insert the needle just over the third rib at a 90-degree angle. Listen for a hiss of air. The patient's hemodynamic status should improve. Remove the needle, and secure the catheter in place with tape. Then prepare for chest drain insertion.

Be mindful that needle decompression may fail. Chest wall thickness and the length of the catheter can affect success. If it is decided to insert a

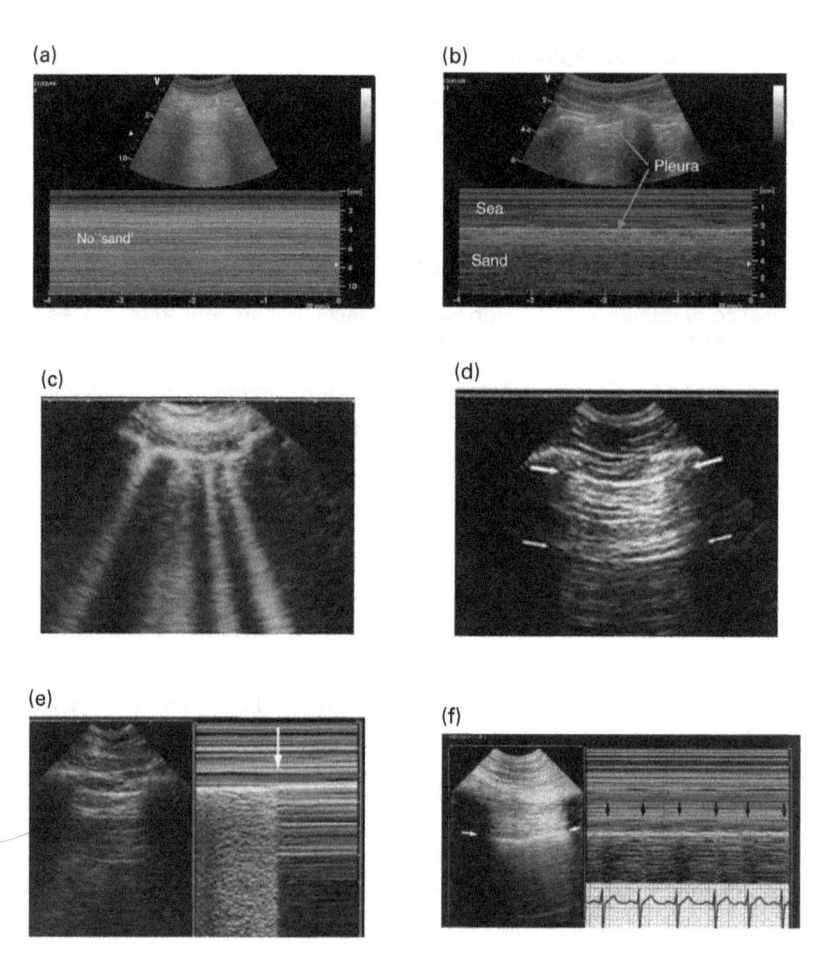

FIGURE 31.1 (A) Absent lung sliding. (B) Lung sliding. (C) B lines. (D) A lines. (E) Lung point. (F) Lung pulse.

Sources: (A, B) Miller A. Practical approach to lung ultrasound. *BJA Educ.* 2015;16(2):39–45. (C–E) Lichtenstein DA, Meziere G, Lascols N, et al. Ultrasound diagnosis of occult pneumothorax. *Crit Care Med.* 2005;33(6):1231–1238. (F) Lichtenstein DA, Meziere G, Lascols N, et al. The "lung pulse": an early ultrasound sign of complete atelectasis. *Intensive Care Med.* 2003;29(12):2187–2192.

14g cannula to decompress the pleura, it may not reach the pleural cavity. This patient is obese, and 14g cannulas are generally less than 4.5 cm in length. In a meta-analysis in 2015, a minimum catheter length of 6.44 cm was needed for a success rate at the 95th percentile. In a retrospective review in 2016, success was higher using an 8 cm catheter rather than a 5 cm catheter (69.3% vs. 20.7%). There are 14g needles specially designed for tension pneumothoraces, and they are 8.26 cm long.

Treatment of Stable Pneumothorax

If this patient was hemodynamically stable, a chest drain could be inserted after appropriate imaging. Patients undergoing positive pressure ventilation nearly always require a chest drain as positive pressure exacerbates the leak. However, if it is a small pneumothorax, causing no compromise, the clinician may decide to observe without chest drain insertion.

Chest Drain Insertion

Choosing the appropriate chest drain diameter is important. Choose a wide-bore drain (e.g., 32Fr) in this patient as he is undergoing mechanical ventilation and may have blood in his pleural space, particularly if the integrity of the pleural space was breeched during surgery.

Insert the drain into the fifth intercostal space, mid-axillary line. Placement should be directed anteriorly in the supine position in order to drain air. Make sure to advance it far enough so that the sentinel eye is within the pleural cavity. This is the most peripheral hole on a chest drain and is visible on a CXR.

Attach the chest drain to a wet or dry suction closed drainage device (Figure 31.2); the atrium oasis underwater seal drain has 3 chambers, the collection chamber, the water-seal chamber, and the wet suction control. Sterile fluid is inserted into the water seal chamber to the 2 cm mark. Check for air bubbling and oscillation. Oscillation will not occur if the chest drain is blocked, kinked, or misplaced or if the lung is fully inflated. Oscillation is easier to view when suction is turned off. In dry suction underwater drains, the graduated markings in the water seal chamber quantify the air leak. If suction is required, attach the wall suction—the chest drain dry suction regulator is preset to –20 cm H_2O but can be altered by the clinician to up to –40 cm H_2O.

Only consider suction in persistent air leaks. The theory behind suction is that air may be removed quicker via suction than by departure through the breach in integrity of the pleura. Suction should be targeted

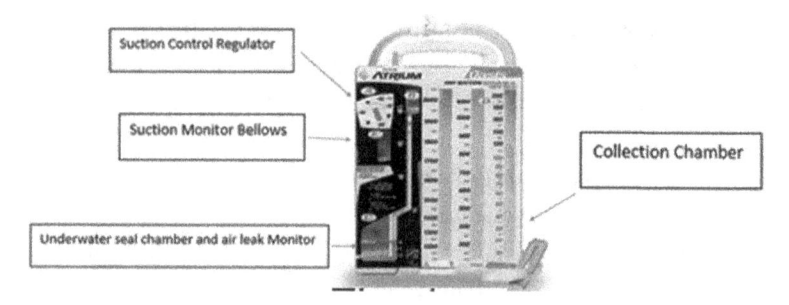

FIGURE 31.2 Atrium oasis dry suction water seal drain.

to a pressure of −10 to −20 cm H_2O. High-pressure, high-volume suction can cause worsening air leak, hypoxemia, or air stealing (a process whereby a large portion of each inspiratory breath flows out the chest drain).

Remove the drain once there is no air leak off suction and the lung is fully expanded on CXR. There is varied opinion as to whether chest drains should be kept in place in those undergoing positive pressure mechanical ventilation. In a randomized controlled trial of 92 trauma patients with chest drains, removal of the drains during positive pressure ventilation did not impact complication rates.

Troubleshooting Chest Drains

There will be no oscillation visible if there is a blockage in the chest drain. Suction can be applied to help remove the clots. The cardiothoracic surgeon may strip (compress the chest drain with the thumb and use a pulling motion down the tube away from the entry point) or milk (squeeze or twist the tube to increase the suction pressure momentarily) the chest drain. However, this can cause large negative pressure, pain, and hemodynamic instability. Fibrinolytic agents have been used to unblock small pleural catheters but not large-bore drains.

Malpositioning of the drain is more likely if there are pleural adhesions. The best way to determine the correct position of a drain is by CT imaging. It is necessary to remove intraparenchymal drains to help avoid air leaks. There is no consensus on whether to remove fissural drains.

If a drain becomes disconnected, clean it and reconnect it. Do not clamp the drain.

CASE RESUMES

Six days later the patient still has bubbling in the water chamber. He is still mechanically ventilated for a postoperative pneumonia. He is hemodynamically stable and has no signs of sepsis. There is a persistent small pneumothorax visible on CT, but there is no empyema.

Air Leaks

An air leak that persists >5–7 days is called a *persistent air leak* (PAL). The patient is clinically quite well. This PAL is likely to be caused by an alveolar–pleural fistula. In an alveolar–pleural fistula, the alveoli and the pleura are communicating. The leak is distal to the level of the subsegmental bronchi. In bronchopleural fistulas it is proximal to the subsegmental bronchi. Alveolar–pleural fistulas are caused by secondary spontaneous pneumothoraces, trauma, mechanical ventilation, and lung infections and occur after thoracic surgery.

It is less likely to be a bronchopleural fistula as he has not had surgery to his tracheobronchial tree and there is no shock or hypoxia. A bronchopleural fistula is a communication between the main stem, lobar, or segmental bronchus and the pleural space. It most commonly occurs due to stump dehiscence after thoracic surgery but can occur occasionally with malignancy, chest trauma, infection, chemotherapy, radiation, and ablation. Patients can present very unwell, with a tension pneumothorax, hypoxia, empyema, or septic shock.

Consider investigating this patient with a CT thorax, sequential balloon occlusion, and bronchoscopy in order to diagnose and locate the position of the air leak. A channel may be seen on CT between the lung/bronchus and the pleura. A balloon placed endobronchially can be sequentially advanced down through both main bronchi and lobar, segmental, and subsegmental bronchi to assess where the leak is originating. A large reduction in air leak on balloon inflation indicates the site. In a bronchopleural fistula a bronchoscopy will show a mucosal defect or bubbling at that point if saline is injected. Methylene blue injected through the chest drain will enter the pleural space and will be visible in the corresponding site in the tracheobronchial tree.

Air leaks in the postoperative setting are graded from 1 to 4 (Table 31.2.) A continuous air leak occurs in true bronchopleural fistulas.

TABLE 31.2 **Grades of Air Leak**

Grade	Definition
1	Air leak only on Valsalva maneuver
2	Air leak during expiration
3	Air leak during inspiration
4	Continuous air leak

The air leak can be measured by working out the difference between the inspiratory and expiratory volumes on the ventilator. A digital chest drainage system can also quantify the air leak. If the air leak is <20 mL/min, the chest drain can be removed. An observational study of 299 postoperative thoracic surgery patients using a digital device showed that PALs were far more common (0.5% vs. 76%) in patients with a variable air leak, persistently >20 mL/min, in the first 4 days after surgery in comparison to those with no air leak. If an air leak is >1000 mL/min at the end of the operation, surgery is usually repeated immediately. These digital devices have been shown to reduce the duration of drainage, cost, and hospital length of stay.

Treatment of Alveolar–Pleural Fistulas

Refer all PALs to thoracic surgeons. Given that this patient is still mechanically ventilated, conservative measures should be attempted initially. Reoperation in thoracic patients with air leaks is rarely needed (<2%). Minimize positive pressure ventilation, and aim to extubate as soon as possible. If there is no bronchopleural fistula present, most air leaks will resolve over a few weeks. There is still debate as to whether suction is useful in patients with air leaks; however, suction should be considered if a pneumothorax is increasing in size. A meta-analysis in 2018 showed that suction reduced the occurrence of postoperative pneumothorax in thoracic patients, but there was no difference in air leak duration, occurrence of PAL, or hospital length of stay.

If the pneumothorax is not resolving, there is a lack of consensus on how to proceed. Consider an additional chest tube, a Heimlich valve (one-way flutter valve), alternative modes of ventilation (independent lung ventilation, extracorporeal membrane oxygenation), chemical pleurodesis, and endobronchial/intrabronchial valves. The visceral and parietal pleura need to oppose after chemical pleurodesis (tetracycline, doxycycline, or talc slurry), and it should be applied only if there is a small residual pneumothorax on CXR. Endobronchial and intrabronchial valves are one-way valves placed with a flexible bronchoscope into a segmental or subsegmental bronchus and allow limited flow distally but still allow the passage of mucus and air proximally. There have been a few small studies which have shown their effectiveness. Surgery should only be considered if less invasive measures are inadequate in this mechanically ventilated patient.

Treatment of Bronchopleural Fistulas

If bronchopleural fistulas (BPFs) present late (>14 days), are caused by pleuropulmonary diseases, or occur on mechanical ventilation, management is initially conservative. Insert a chest drain, minimize mechanical ventilation, and aim to extubate the patient as soon as possible. Use minimal to no suction. Consider dependent positioning of the side with the BPF to prevent spillage and independent lung ventilation. Have a low threshold for broad-spectrum antibiotic therapy as empyema is a considerable risk. Bronchoscopic therapies should be considered. Vascular occlusion coils, the Amplatzer device, and self-expanding airway stents have successfully been used to treat larger bronchopleural fistulas (>8 mm). Sclerosants and endobronchial valves are less invasive techniques that can also be used in smaller bronchopleural fistulas (<8 mm). If these options fail, consider surgery if the fistula is localized and can be occluded.

In postoperative thoracic patients, if diagnosed early (<14 days) with no signs of instability/empyema, surgery may well be the best option with revision of the stump or stump closure with omentum or muscle. Video-assisted thoracoscopy is the preferred surgical method.

CASE RESUMES

Based on auscultation and ultrasound findings, a pneumothorax was diagnosed. The team inserted an apical 14-French thoracostomy tube which resulted in a gush of air with needle placement. The tube was left in place and a chest x-ray confirmed resolution of the pneumothorax. The tube was left in place for two days. After removal, repeat chest x-ray was obtained to ensure no further pneumothorax prior to discharge home.

> **KEY POINTS TO REMEMBER**
> 1. Lung US is a useful adjunct for diagnosing a pneumothorax.
> 2. Specially manufactured 14g catheters that are 8.25 cm in length may affect success rates for needle decompression.
> 3. Avoid suction in PALs, and only consider if initial strategies are failing.
> 4. Mechanically ventilated patients with PALs should be treated conservatively, initially with chest drains. Minimize positive pressure ventilation, and expedite extubation.

Suggested Reading
1. Miller A. Practical approach to lung ultrasound. *BJA Educ*. 2015;16(2):39–45.
2. Lichtenstein DA, Meziere G, Lascols N, et al. Ultrasound diagnosis of occult pneumothorax. *Crit Care Med*. 2005;33(6):1231–1238.
3. Lichtenstein DA, Lascols N, Prin S, Meziere G. The "lung pulse": an early ultrasound sign of complete atelectasis. *Intensive Care Med*. 2003;29(12):2187–2192.
4. MacDuff A, Arnold A, Harvey J. Management of spontaneous pneumothorax: British Thoracic Society pleural disease guideline 2010. *Thorax*. 2010;65(suppl 2):ii18–ii31.
5. Gilbert TB, McGrath BJ, Soberman M. Chest tubes: indications, placement, management, and complications. *J Intensive Care Med*. 1993;8(2):73–86.
6. Sarkar P, Chandak T, Shah R, Talwar A. Diagnosis and management bronchopleural fistula. *Indian J Chest Dis Allied Sci*. 2010;52(2):97–104.
7. Liberman M, Cassivi SD. Bronchial stump dehiscence: update on prevention and management. *Semin Thorac Cardiovasc Surg*. 2007;19(4):366–373.

32 Postoperative Cerebrovascular Injury

Naomi Quigley and Ruth-Aoibheann O'Leary

You are asked to see a 79-year-old woman who underwent elective metallic mitral valve replacement earlier the same day. Her background history is notable for hypertension, renal impairment, long-standing atrial fibrillation, and a transient ischemic attack 6 months prior to this presentation. Surgery was prolonged—cannulation of the aorta was challenging due to significant calcification of the vessel, and there was a period of hemodynamic instability coming off cardiopulmonary bypass. She has now stabilized, but the nurses are concerned that she is not waking appropriately off sedation. On examination she is obtunded despite receiving minimal sedation over the last 4 hours. Her pupils are reactive, and there are no obvious lateralizing signs.

What do you do now?

DISCUSSION

This presentation is concerning but, unfortunately, not uncommon in the postoperative period. A broad differential diagnosis should be considered in this clinical scenario, including metabolic encephalopathies, seizures, cerebrovascular accidents (CVAs), and delirium. Cardiothoracic patients in the early postoperative period often have vague presentations, and the recent use of sedation may limit clinical assessment. This patient has risk factors that make perioperative stroke more likely, and a high index of clinical suspicion is needed to ensure timely diagnosis and management.

Perioperative stroke is defined as an ischemic or hemorrhagic infarction that occurs either during surgery or in the first 30 postoperative days. They are relatively uncommon, with an incidence of 0.1%–1.9% in surgery overall. However, this increases to up to 10% in cardiothoracic and vascular surgeries. The American Society of Thoracic Surgeons quote the incidence of a perioperative neurological event as 3.3% after cardiothoracic surgery. Although perioperative strokes are relatively uncommon, they are significant, resulting in an increase in mortality and morbidity.

Risk factors for perioperative stroke can be categorized as patient- and procedure-related. In terms of procedure-related factors, mitral valve replacement has the highest risk of single valve replacement, while dual valve replacement and emergency surgery have the highest risk overall of perioperative CVA, illustrated in Table 32.1. Patient-related risk factors may be modifiable or non-modifiable, as seen in Table 32.2. Age, female gender, and previous

TABLE 32.1 **Procedure-Related Risk Factors for Perioperative Stroke**

Procedure	Incidence of Perioperative stroke (%)
Non-cardiac non-vascular surgery	0.1–1.9
Coronary artery bypass graft	1.4–1.7
Aortic valve replacement	1.5–4.8
Mitral valve	2.1–8.8
Combined valvular surgery	2.05–9.7
Coronary artery bypass graft and valve	3.3–7.4

TABLE 32.2 **Patient-Related Risk Factors for Perioperative Stroke**

Preoperative		Intraoperative Risk Factors	Postoperative Risk Factors
Modifiable	Non-Modifiable		
Carotid stenosis, especially symptomatic	Age	Type of surgery	Prolonged immobilization
Insufficient bridging	Female	Duration of surgery	Arrhythmias
Smoker	Prevention of stroke/transient ischemic attack	Redo surgery	Hyperglycemia
High body mass index		Emergency surgery	Hypotension
Hypercholesterolemia		Duration of cross-clamp and bypass	Low cardiac output state
Hypertension		Manipulation of aorta including cannulation	Uncontrolled hypertension
Peripheral vascular disease		Aortic arch disease	
Known cardiovascular disease		Dehydration	
Diabetes mellitus			
Chronic kidney disease			

history of stroke and transient ischemic attack increase perioperative risk, thus putting your patient in a higher risk group. Atrial fibrillation and carotid artery stenosis increase risk and should be optimized prior to cardiac surgery. Preoperative carotid endarterectomy should be considered particularly in patients with symptomatic disease or tight stenosis.

Perioperative strokes have a bimodal distribution, with approximately one-third occurring within the first 24 hours. Exact timing may be difficult to determine in the immediate postoperative period due to the period of anesthesia, and this can make decision-making around therapeutic options challenging. The underlying mechanism is usually embolic, related to either disruption of aortic atheromas during cross-clamping or, less frequently, air emboli during revascularization. CVA secondary to hypoperfusion is less common.

In this case, given the patient and procedural risk factors, you have a high index of suspicion for perioperative stroke. Proceed immediately with a non-contrast computed tomography (CT) brain and subsequent CT angiogram. Timely CT is key to diagnosis as CT can overrule intraparenchymal hemorrhage and demonstrate large-vessel occlusion. Magnetic resonance imaging (MRI) is also available and safe if the valve is MRI-compatible, as is the case with most recently implanted valves. Local practices vary, and it is usually recommended that patients in the acute postoperative setting wait 6 weeks to allow the valve to endothelialize. However, in the emergency setting MRI is safe to use, although a 1.5 Tesla MRI machine is preferable to a 3.0 Tesla machine.

CASE RESUMES

CT angiogram confirms an ischemic stroke with left middle cerebral artery occlusion. You urgently call the cardiothoracic surgeons, stroke physicians, and interventional radiologists to discuss management strategies.

Treatment of ischemic stroke in the perioperative period is challenging due to difficulties with accurately assessing the time of onset and concerns regarding anticoagulation and postoperative hemorrhage. Your patient is potentially within the window for interventions such as thrombolysis and thrombectomy. However, thrombolysis is contraindicated in this immediate postoperative period due to the high risk of life-threatening hemorrhage. The evidence suggests that it is absolutely contraindicated for the first 2 weeks and relatively contraindicated for 3 months. There is evidence for thrombectomy in the first 12 hours following symptom onset in anterior circulation strokes, with improved functional outcomes for thrombectomy compared to medical management but similar incidences of hemorrhagic transformation and mortality. If the patient has suffered a posterior circulation stroke, thrombectomy reduces both morbidity and mortality compared to medical management, when given within a 6-hour window.

Outside the thrombectomy window, treatments are very limited. Aspirin is safe and effective for prevention of recurrence of stroke, although there is increased risk of hemorrhagic transformation if used in conjunction with thrombolysis. Treatment with intravenous heparin has been previously recommended; but there is no evidence of revascularization, and there is an increased incidence of complications such as hemorrhagic transformation and heparin-induced thrombocytopenia. As a result, early anticoagulation is not recommended in the first 2 weeks after stroke. Beta-blockers are recommended perioperatively; however, they have not been shown to reduce the incidence of stroke. Permissive hypertension post-stroke has been recommended by the American Heart Association, with targets of less than 180/105 mm Hg.

This patient has a metallic mitral valve, which is an independent risk factor for stroke in the initial 90–180 days postoperatively as the valve becomes endothelialized. Anticoagulation reduces this risk, so there is a general consensus in the literature to target an international normalized ratio of 3.0 for up to 6 months postoperatively, with a subsequent target of 2.5. Warfarin is the anticoagulant of choice, and novel oral anticoagulants are not recommended for this patient cohort. Management of this patient's anticoagulation is complex as her risk of embolic infarct from her recent metallic valve implantation must be balanced against her risk of hemorrhagic transformation. If the infarct is >35% of the cerebral hemisphere or if there is uncontrolled hypertension, oral anticoagulation should be withheld for at least 5 days, and the patient should be bridged with intravenous heparin. CT should confirm the absence of hemorrhagic transformation prior to restarting anticoagulation.

The patient improves following the diagnosis of ischemic stroke, although she was deemed unsuitable for mechanical thrombectomy. She has marked right arm weakness but is otherwise alert and weaning from mechanical ventilation. Repeat imaging on postoperative day 3 reveals hemorrhagic transformation of her ischemic infarct, which is not associated with clinical deterioration. The surgical team is keen to start anticoagulation due to the risk of prosthetic valve thrombosis, but you are concerned about expansion of her intraparenchymal hematoma.

It is reported that 5% of patients with perioperative ischemic strokes have early hemorrhagic transformation, with another 10% becoming hemorrhagic within a few more days. Not all of these are clinically significant, and often they go undetected. Risk factors for symptomatic hemorrhagic transformation include large infarcts, anticoagulation, previous hemorrhagic infarct, increasing age, and infective endocarditis. Anticoagulation in this setting is potentially life-threatening, and evidence is limited. These decisions should be multidisciplinary, but it appears that expansion of the hemorrhage is unlikely to happen after 2 weeks; thus, cautious reintroduction of anticoagulation may be considered 14 days after symptom onset. However, close monitoring is needed, and the decision to start anticoagulation should be made on a case-by-case basis after review of appropriate imaging.

> **KEY POINTS TO REMEMBER**
>
> 1. Perioperative stroke may present atypically and requires a high index of suspicion.
> 2. Thrombectomy may be considered in the first 12 hours, especially in posterior circulation strokes.
> 3. Anticoagulation in this setting requires multidisciplinary input due to the risk of hemorrhagic transformation but is likely safe 14 days post-stroke.

Suggested Reading
1. Ko SB. Perioperative stroke: pathophysiology and management. *Korean J Anesthesiol*. 2018;71(1):3–11.
2. Libman RB, Wirkowski E, Neystat M, et al. Stroke associated with cardiac surgery. Determinants, timing, and stroke subtypes. *Arch Neurol*. 1997;54:83–87.
3. Lonchyna Vassyl A. *Difficult Decisions in Cardiothoracic Critical Care Surgery*. Chicago, IL: Springer; 2019.
4. Selim M. Perioperative stroke. *N Engl J Med*. 2007;356:706–713.
5. Kuramatsu JB, Sembill JA, Gerner ST, et al. Management of therapeutic anticoagulation in patients with intracerebral haemorrhage and mechanical heart valves. *Eur Heart J*. 2018;39:1709–1723.

33 Coagulopathy in Cardiac Surgery: Etiology and Treatment Options

Dana Teodorescu and Caroline Larkin

A 54-year-old man, without any previous known medical history, with a weight of 87 kg, presents with an ST elevation myocardial infarction. Loading doses of aspirin (300 mg) and clopidogrel (600 mg) are administered. He has numerous coronary artery lesions that are not amenable to percutaneous cardiac intervention (PCI) and undergoes an emergency 5-vessel coronary artery bypass graft (CABG) procedure. Cardiopulmonary bypass (CPB) time was 150 minutes, and he was transfused with 2 units of packed red blood cells (PRBCs), 2 units of fresh frozen plasma (FFP), and 1 pack of platelets. Following his return to the cardiothoracic intensive care unit (ICU), there is a consistent high output from his 3 chest drains with 500 mL blood loss in the first hour. His temperature is 35.4°C, and he has a metabolic acidosis with a pH of 7.25, lactate of 4 mmol/L, hemoglobin (Hb) concentration of 90.2 g/L, and platelet count of 80×10^9/L.

What do you do now?

DISCUSSION

Bleeding after sternotomy and cardiac surgery is expected up to a rate of 2 mL/kg/h for the first few hours (up to a maximum of 600 mL for the first 3 hours); however, this patient has had a significant output of 500 mL in the first postoperative hour. It is crucial that the surgical team are made aware of any issues with bleeding as the key distinction to be made at this point is determining whether the patient has had a surgical or a non-surgical bleed.

The aims of the treating ICU physician are initiating resuscitation, empirical treatment of coagulopathy, and excluding a surgical cause of ongoing blood loss as this may require urgent return to the operating room. It is important to review the handover between surgical, anesthesiology, and ICU teams to understand factors which may point toward the presence of a coagulopathy rather than a surgical bleed. Relevant information in the preoperative history includes the use of anticoagulant or antiplatelet medications and any preexisting bleeding diathesis, either congenital or acquired. Intraoperative factors include the use of CPB (i.e., "on-pump" or "off-pump" CABG), duration of CPB, use of deep hypothermic circulatory arrest (cooling to 18°C), dosage and timing of heparin, dosage and timing of protamine, use of antifibrinolytics, transfusion of blood products, surgical issues with bleeding or technical difficulties with the procedure, and any point-of-care (POC) testing results if available.

Resuscitation should start immediately with optimization of oxygenation and perfusion using fluids, blood products, inotropes, or vasopressors. Hemodynamic goal-directed therapy aiming to reduce transfusions in cardiac surgery has no proven benefit and is not recommended. Resuscitation should be initially guided by level of Hb and hematocrit, acidemia, and lactate levels, which are easily obtained with POC testing. The clinical picture is more important than an absolute Hb threshold for transfusion. One unit of PRBCs has a typical volume of 250–300 mL and is expected to increase the Hb level by approximately 1 g/dL in the euvolemic patient. Although not extensively studied, even a moderate degree of acidosis (pH <7.35), hyperlactatemia (lactate >4 mmol/L), and hypothermia are associated with increased postoperative bleeding, so maintaining normothermia and a normal pH is important.

Empirical treatment of coagulopathy involves checking, and reversing if necessary, residual or rebound heparin, transfusion of platelets if there is a clinical suspicion of platelet dysfunction, correcting fibrinogen deficits (cryoprecipitate or fibrinogen), and transfusing FFP or prothrombin complex concentrate (PCC) if dilutional coagulopathy or inadequate levels of coagulation factors are likely. Antifibrinolytics (tranexamic acid or aprotinin) should also be considered.

Persistent microvascular bleeding, in the absence of a surgical cause, suggests a coagulopathy. CPB causes a bleeding diathesis by altering the normal coagulation process. Activation of platelets occurs in the extracorporeal circuit, causing granular depletion and loss of function. The tissue factor (extrinsic) coagulation pathway is activated, leading to persistent thrombin generation despite heparin administration. The contact activation (intrinsic) coagulation pathway is activated by contact with the bypass filter fibers and leads to kinin, factor XI, and fibrinolytic system activation. In addition to this widespread activation and consumption of clotting factors, hyperfibrinolysis and hypothermia occur during CPB. Hypothermia, employed in cardiac surgery for end-organ preservation, is known to cause a coagulopathy by inhibiting platelet function and interfering with the enzymatic processes that occur in coagulation. Protamine, the heparin antagonist, has side effects of platelet inhibition and stimulation of clot breakdown. Intraoperatively, a <1:1 dosing reversal ratio with heparin should be used. Both inadequate and excessive antagonism of heparin can lead to an anticoagulant effect.

The key principles of coagulopathy management in this case are evaluation and maintenance of normal physiological conditions for hemostasis, reversal of heparin effect, maintenance of adequate levels of coagulation factors and adequate numbers of functional platelets, treatment of hyperfibrinolysis, and rescue therapy with activated factor VII or XIII if necessary.

It has been shown that algorithm-based transfusion protocols are superior to individual clinical decisions for the management of post–cardiac surgery bleeding and coagulopathy. Management includes laboratory testing with complete blood count, fibrinogen level, thrombin time, activated partial thromboplastin time (aPTT), and prothrombin time (PT) with hemostatic therapy guided by these results (Table 33.1).

TABLE 33.1 Laboratory Tests for Assessment of Coagulopathy

Test	Performed by	Utility	Prolonged by
aPTT	Adding activator of the intrinsic pathway to measure the speed of the contact pathway	Monitoring unfractionated heparin anticoagulation; sensitive to decreased levels of coagulation factors of the intrinsic and common pathways	Heparin; decreased levels of factors XI, X, IX, VII, V, and II fibrinogen; presence of inhibitors, antiphospholipid antibodies, direct thrombin inhibitors
PT/international normalized ratio	Adding thromboplastin to activate extrinsic pathway	Monitoring anticoagulation with vitamin K antagonists (warfarin); sensitive to decreased levels of factors of the extrinsic and common pathways	Vitamin K antagonists; decreased levels of factor VII (congenital or acquired liver disease), II, V, and X and fibrinogen
Thrombin time	Adding thrombin to citrated plasma to promote fibrinogen conversion to fibrin	Treatment with direct thrombin inhibitors	Factors that interfere with fibrinogen or thrombin: low levels of fibrinogen, dysfibrinogenemia, disseminated intravascular coagulation, heparin use, uremia
Activated clotting time	Adding kaolin/celite/glass beads to a non-citrated whole-blood sample to activate intrinsic pathway	Anticoagulation with high amount of unfractionated heparin (cardiac surgery, extracorporeal life support)	Heparin, hemofiltration, low levels of fibrinogen, thrombocytopenia, glycoprotein IIB/IIIa antagonists

Maintaining optimal conditions for hemostasis means keeping the patient's temperature above 36°C, an ionized calcium level >1.0 mmol/L, and normal pH. If activated clotting time is longer than 130 seconds, then an additional dose of protamine (30 IU/kg) should be administered.

POC testing of whole-blood samples has a rapid turnover and a broad diagnostic spectrum. Viscoelastic testing of clot formation is performed using thromboelastography and rotational thromboelastometry. Viscoelastic testing can suggest levels of coagulation factor activity, platelet function, and fibrinogen and plasminogen activity. The use of viscoelastic testing is now widespread in cardiac surgery centers, and they have reduced overall blood product transfusion rates. POC platelet function analyzers are also available but as yet have not been as widely studied in this area. Examples of classic thromboelastometry traces are depicted in Figure 33.1.

The formation of a platelet–fibrin clot after fibrinogen conversion to fibrin is the end product of the coagulation cascade. If the fibrinogen level is <1.5–2 g/L, it must be supplemented by using either cryoprecipitate or fibrinogen concentrate at a dose of 25–50 mg/kg (see Table 33.2 for blood products and transfusion thresholds).

If coagulopathy persists (as indicated by an international normalized ratio >1.4 or aPTT >50 seconds), then FFP, containing coagulation factors and immunoglobulins, at a dose of 15–30 mL/kg, can be transfused in persistent postoperative bleeding. Pooled plasma is widely used, and it is inactivated for viruses having a lower risk, to induce transfusion-related acute lung injury.

Although less studied, PCC may be a suitable alternative, especially when fluid loading is not desired. It can be reconstituted rapidly, without causing hemodilution, and is not associated with transfusion-associated circulatory overload or transfusion-related acute lung injury. It appears to be more effective than FFP at reducing transfusions.

At a minimum, the platelet count should be kept >50 × 10^9/L. In this case the patient has received a loading dose of the irreversible P2Y12 platelet inhibitor clopidogrel preoperatively. Additionally, he has had a prolonged CPB time, which means that his platelet function is likely to be severely impaired. In this context, transfusion to a platelet count >80 × 109/L is appropriate. Desmopressin (DDAVP) in a dose of 0.3 mcg/kg can significantly increase von Willebrand factor level and factor VIII and promote platelet

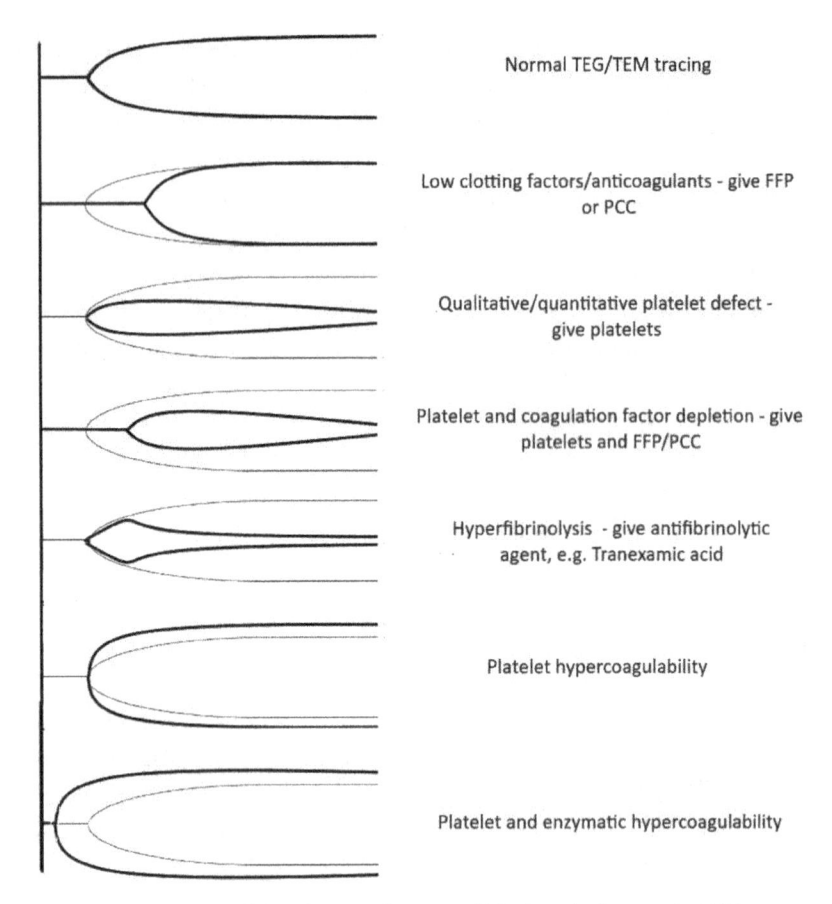

FIGURE 33.1 Examples of viscoelastic testing curves. TEG, thromboelastography; TEM, thromboelastometry.

aggregation. It is used in some institutions for the management of post–cardiac surgery coagulopathy, although evidence for its efficacy is limited.

Although hyperfibrinolysis is not detected with standard laboratory testing, the antifibrinolytics tranexamic acid (25 mg/kg), aprotinin, and ε-aminocaproic acid can be given empirically if clinical suspicion is high. Tranexamic acid is widely used but may not be as effective as aprotinin. There are safety concerns over the use of aprotinin, and it is not available in all countries.

TABLE 33.2 **Blood Products**

Blood Product	Composition	Dose Required in 70 kg Individual	Volume in Standard Unit	Suggested Transfusion Threshold Post-Cardiac Surgery if Ongoing Bleeding
PRBCs	Leukocyte-depleted red blood cells suspended in a saline–adenine–glucose–mannitol solution	1 unit will increase Hb level by 10 g/L	250–350 mL	90–100 g/L
Platelets	Pooled platelets come from 4 donors and are suspended in plasma; apheresis platelets come from 1 donor	1 pool or 1 apheresis unit is equivalent to 1 "dose" and will increase platelet count by 20–40 × 10^9/L	250–350 mL	Platelet count <50 × 10^9 L or history of anti-platelet agents
FFP	Many forms; most common is plasma separated from individual donor whole-blood donation; contains all coagulation factors but reduced levels of factors V and VIII	10–15 mL/kg will achieve a minimum of 30% of plasma clotting factor concentration; 4 units of FFP commonly administered in this scenario	250–300 mL per unit	Prolonged coagulation times suggested by aPTT/PT or thromboelastography

Continued

TABLE 33.2 Continued

Blood Product	Composition	Dose Required in 70 kg Individual	Volume in Standard Unit	Suggested Transfusion Threshold Post-Cardiac Surgery if Ongoing Bleeding
Fibrinogen	Fibrinogen concentrate is derived from pooled plasma from multiple donors	4 g will increase fibrinogen level by 1 g/L	1 g reconstituted in 50 mL sterile water	Fibrinogen <1.5 g/L
Cryoprecipitate	One unit prepared from 1 donor unit of plasma; standard unit contains 80 U of factor VIII, 200–300 mg of fibrinogen, factor XIII, von Willebrand factor, and fibronectin	2 × 5 unit "pools"; 10 units will raise the fibrinogen level by 0.7–1 g/L	50–200 mL	Primary use is for fibrinogen replacement; fibrinogen <1.5 g/L
PCC	3 or 4 vitamin K coagulation factors: II, VII, IX, and X; proteins C, S and Z; heparin; and antithrombin	20–30 IU/kg	Generally 20 mL sterile water per 500 IU	Prolonged coagulation times suggested by aPTT/PT or thromboelastography; can be used if concerned patient is fluid-overloaded

When bleeding persists despite transfusion of blood products to the previously mentioned levels, administering recombinant factor VIIa or factor XIII can be considered as an off-label use. Administration of recombinant factor VIIa at a dose of 90 mcg/kg may be considered in cases of life-threatening non-surgical coagulopathy when other measures have failed to stop bleeding. Recombinant factor VIIa has been associated with a decreased mortality rate in life-threatening hemorrhage; however, this is at the cost of an increased risk of thromboembolic events. Factor XIII increases clot stability by cross-linking fibrin monomers, and 1250–2500 units is usually the recommended dose; however, there is no significant evidence for its efficacy in this case.

CASE RESUMES

Following the transfusion of platelets, the patient's bleeding remained brisk. The decision to correct other parameters were attempted. The patient was passively warmed and fluids give for the lactic acidosis. These measures decreased chest tube output. Further laboratory assessment revealed a hemoglobin of 7.1 mg/dL and an additional packed red blood cell unit was administered. The patient remained stable and was discharged from the intensive care unit on postoperative day 1.

> **KEY POINTS TO REMEMBER**
>
> 1. Coagulopathy is often multifactorial and require evaluation with several examination and testing modalities.
> 2. A surgical cause of bleeding must be considered and excluded.
> 3. Ideally, both standard laboratory testing and a POC system should be used together.
> 4. Normal physiological conditions must be restored to treat coagulopathy: normothermia, normal pH, normal calcium level.

Suggested Reading
1. Task Force on Patient Blood Management for Adult Cardiac Surgery of the European Association for Cardio-Thoracic Surgery (EACTS), European Association of Cardiothoracic Anaesthesiology (EACTA); Boer C, Meesters MI,

Milojevic M, et al. 2017 EACTS/EACTA guidelines on patient blood management for adult cardiac surgery. *J Cardiothorac Vasc Anesth*. 2018;32(1):88–120.
2. Aneman A, Brechot N, Brodie D, et al. Advances in critical care management of patients undergoing cardiac surgery. *Intensive Care Med*. 2018;44:799–810.
3. Gerstein NS, Brierley JK, Windsor J, et al. Antifibrinolytic agents in cardiac and noncardiac surgery: a comprehensive overview and update. *J Cardiothorac Vasc Anaesth*. 2017;31(6):2183–2205.
4. Kozek-Langenecker SA, Ahmed AB, Afshari A, et al. Management of severe perioperative bleeding: guidelines from the European Society of Anaesthesiology: first update 2016. *Eur J Anaesthesiol*. 2017;34(6):332–395.

34 Postoperative Diastolic Heart Failure

Éimhín Dunne and Niall Fanning

A 60-year old male presented for urgent coronary artery bypass grafting following a myocardial infarction, with complex coronary artery disease not amenable to percutaneous coronary intervention. He has a history of poorly controlled hypertension, type 2 diabetes mellitus, and high body mass index. He underwent 3-vessel coronary artery bypass grafting. The intraoperative course was uneventful, and he was extubated shortly thereafter.

Later that evening, you are called due to respiratory distress, is tachypneic at 40 breaths per minute, and requires 60% oxygen via Venturi mask to maintain oxygen saturation at 90%. He has developed fast atrial fibrillation at 160 beats per minute. Blood pressure is 140/110 mm Hg. He is not receiving any vasoactive drug infusions. Urine output has been 25 and 30 mL/h for the last 2 hours.

What do you do now?

DISCUSSION

This is a scenario of near cardiorespiratory collapse in the acute postoperative period. It is a potentially life-threatening situation and requires urgent investigation and treatment, carried out in parallel, to avoid a downward spiral to cardiorespiratory arrest. A logical approach needs to be taken when managing acute deterioration in the post–cardiac surgery patient. Life-threatening complications need to be considered and addressed immediately (Table 34.1). Surgical complications such as cardiac tamponade are generally progressive and warrant immediate reoperation. Once life-threatening complications have been excluded or identified and addressed, a systematic approach to the remaining differential diagnoses can be undertaken.

TABLE 34.1 **Differential Diagnoses to Consider in Acute Deterioration Post–Cardiac Surgery**

Surgical	Graft failure (spasm/occlusion)
	Valve failure
	Tamponade
	Systolic anterior motion of the mitral valve
	Myocardial rupture (preceding ischemic event)
	Pneumothorax
	Hemothorax
	Endotracheal tube malposition
Medical	Inadequate preload
	—Volume deficit
	—Bleeding
	—Systemic inflammatory response syndrome (postoperative, post-bypass, sepsis)
	Pump failure (preexisting, new ischemia)
	Excessive afterload
	—Hypertension
	—Hypothermia
Electrical	Dysrhythmias

Investigations

An electrocardiogram (ECG) can help reveal precipitants (e.g., ischemia, arrhythmias). Morphological and electrical abnormalities consistent with diastolic dysfunction may be evident on the ECG; these include left ventricular (LV) hypertrophy and P wave abnormalities (mitral valve disease, elevated filling pressures).

Immediate echocardiography is mandatory in acute heart failure patients with either hemodynamic instability or suspected life-threatening structural or functional cardiac abnormality. Echocardiography in this patient is of paramount importance and will facilitate the commencement of appropriate targeted therapy. Focused echocardiographic assessment in this patient is necessary to exclude tamponade, estimate ventricular function, and assess valvular integrity.

A focused echo is carried out and reveals concentric LV hypertrophy (Figure 34.1). Left atrial (LA) size cannot be reliably assessed due to the presence of atrial fibrillation, but there is an impression of LA dilation. Left heart function is maintained, and the estimated ejection fraction is >50%. Advanced echocardiographic assessment will help establish the severity of diastolic dysfunction through estimates of pulmonary artery systolic pressure and LV filling pressures.

Chest X-ray (CXR) can be a useful test in the diagnosis of acute heart failure. Venous congestion, pleural effusions, and frank pulmonary edema can all help to confirm a diagnosis. However, a normal CXR does not exclude a diagnosis of heart failure. Position of hardware (chest drains, pacing wires, endotracheal tube if present) should be noted. A pneumothorax is unlikely in this patient at this time but should not be forgotten as a potential cause of deterioration in a postoperative patient. The CXR can also help to exclude some competing diagnoses, such as hemothorax or lung consolidation.

Lung ultrasound can help to provide a more immediate answer for those clinically skilled in identifying the diffuse B lines of pulmonary edema and the characteristic ultrasonographic features of pneumothoraces. This can be carried out at the bedside at the time of echocardiography and avoids the potential delay in obtaining a portable CXR.

Full blood testing to exclude anemia and a raised white cell count may point toward an alternative cause of deterioration. Renal function and

(a) Thick left ventricular wall   (b) Left ventricular cavity during systole (a) and diastole (b)

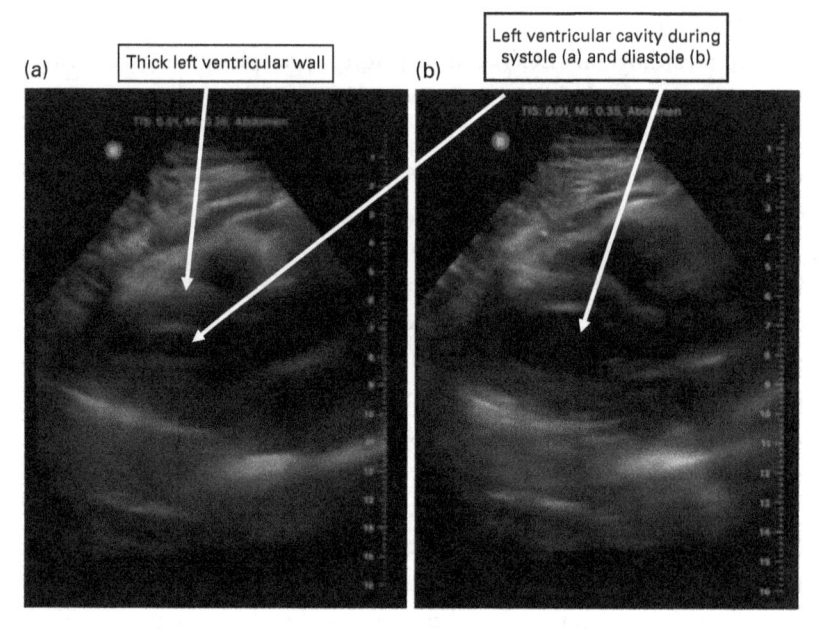

FIGURE 34.1 Transthoracic echocardiography imaging demonstrating diastolic heart failure. The patient has a thickened, concentric hypertrophic left ventricle. During systole (a), the left ventricle has normal ability to eject blood and may even nearly obliterate the cavity when hypovolemia exists. During diastole (b), the left ventricle is too stiff to properly relax impairing the ability of the ventricle to fill with blood.

electrolytes should be examined to investigate any change from baseline and may require electrolyte replacement in the treatment and/or prevention of arrhythmias. Cardiac enzymes and brain natriuretic peptide can be difficult to interpret in the post–cardiac surgery patient, but an observation of trends may be useful. Liver function tests can help to identify liver congestion, which can predict a poorer prognosis if present.

The development of atrial fibrillation following coronary artery bypass grafting is common, with reported incidence rates varying between 16% and 45%. This is a transient phenomenon for the majority of patients, with 90% reported to be in sinus rhythm at 6 weeks postoperatively. However, it should be noted that the development of atrial fibrillation post–coronary artery bypass grafting is associated with a higher risk of stroke during long-term follow-up and is linked to a higher 30-day mortality when compared to those patients who do not develop atrial tachyarrhythmias.

Diastolic Heart Failure

Diastolic heart failure is also called Heart Failure with preserved Ejection Fraction, or HFpEF, since systolic function is preserved. Diastole is the component of the cardiac cycle when ventricular filling occurs. The degree to which the LV will fill with blood is dependent on the rate of ventricular relaxation and the compliance of the LV. The ability of the LV to accommodate a volume of blood is dependent on the intrinsic stiffness and viscoelastic properties of the myocardium coupled with the restraint of the pericardium. Figure 34.2 illustrates the decrease in size of the left ventricular pressure-volume loop with decreased compliance as seen in diastolic heart failure.

The onset of ventricular relaxation brings about a rapid decline in intracavitary LV pressure. As the pressure continues to drop, it eventually falls below LA pressure, causing the mitral valve to open and allowing passive filling of the LV. In the normal LV, the pressure will gradually rise, slowing the rate of blood flow from the LA until the pressure between the 2 chambers equalizes and diastasis occurs. Atrial contraction then occurs, leading to a rise in LA pressure. This allows for the addition of a further

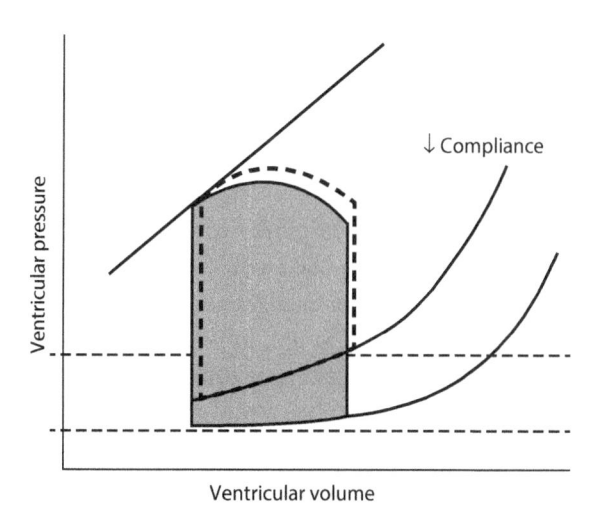

FIGURE 34.2 The left ventricular pressure-volume loop seen in diastolic heart failure with loos of ventricular compliance (dotted line). The pressure inside the cavity is increased while the volume is decreased.

20%–30% into the LV volume. In the compliant LV, this additional volume will lead to a minimal pressure rise, just above LA pressure, forcing the mitral valve to close.

The maintenance of low LV filling pressures throughout the period of diastole is of pivotal importance to optimal cardiorespiratory function. The complex interplay of the dynamic and overlapping processes of diastole minimizes oxygen demand of the left heart and ensures that pulmonary capillary hydrostatic pressures are maintained at a low level, allowing for a high degree of lung distensibility. These processes have the capacity to compensate for the increased diastolic pressure exerted on the LV at times of hemodynamic stress such as during exercise, in hypertension, and in atrial fibrillation.

The fundamental problem in diastolic dysfunction is the increased resistance to LV filling. The stiff LV cannot accommodate the same volume unless there is a compensatory increase in intracavity pressure.

Diastolic dysfunction can be identified at both microscopic and macroscopic levels. Often, not evident clinically until the later stages of the process, it can be assessed and severity graded non-invasively by echocardiography. Where the diagnosis remains uncertain, more invasive testing, including cardiac catheterization, can prove useful.

At the microscopic level, there is an increase in myofibrillary density and an increase in myocyte diameter without a concomitant increase in myocyte length. Cardiomyocyte degeneration and apoptosis leads to varying degrees of interstitial fibrosis, ultimately leading to cardiomyocyte stiffness. These changes are more common with advancing age but, when seen in the under 65-year age group, tend to be associated with non-cardiovascular comorbidities such as obesity, metabolic syndrome, and renal impairment.

Macroscopically, these cellular changes result in a concentric hypertrophy with an increase in relative wall thickness in the presence of normal or near normal LV volumes. There is impaired myocardial relaxation and abnormal distensibility of the LV. This intrinsic stiffness means that higher filling pressures are required to accommodate the same volume. When the mitral valve opens, these higher pressures are transmitted from the LV to the LA and, with time, back into the pulmonary vasculature. This can result in LA dilation and pulmonary hypertension. These changes become more pronounced at times of hemodynamic stress and can precipitate decompensated heart failure as the compensatory mechanisms are exhausted. Loss of atrial contraction in atrial fibrillation can be hugely detrimental to these patients as it dramatically reduces LV filling and limits stroke volume.

Diastolic dysfunction often remains asymptomatic until late in the disease process. When it presents clinically, it can be associated with an abnormal ejection fraction or, more commonly, with preserved ejection fraction. The diagnosis of diastolic dysfunction requires 3 conditions: the presence of signs and/or symptoms, normal LV systolic function (ejection fraction >50%), and increased diastolic filling pressures. It is often accompanied by LV remodeling, commonly in the form of concentric hypertrophy.

Treatment

Fluid therapy: A thick LV surrounding a small cavity requires an adequate preload volume to help generate these higher pressures. Even in the setting of pulmonary edema, judicious fluid therapy is sometimes required to optimize preload.

Diuretics: Titrated intravenous loop diuretics may be beneficial in those with signs/symptoms of fluid overload. Doses as low as 20–40 mg of furosemide can be sufficient, especially in the diuretic-naive patients. Depending on the clinical response, bolus dose therapy or continuous infusion can be utilized. Ultrafiltration may be necessary in those who remain congested and failed a trial of diuretic therapy.

Vasoactive medicines: Consider vasodilator therapy for symptomatic relief in those with systolic blood pressure >90 mm Hg. Vasodilators are thought to decrease venous tone to optimize preload and decrease arterial tone to reduce afterload. However, the evidence to support the use of vasodilator therapy in acute diastolic heart failure is limited. On the contrary, these patients often require vasopressor therapy to increase the afterload of the LV. Inotropic agents may further impair cardiac relaxation and should probably be avoided in the management of diastolic dysfunction.

Control of ventricular rate in atrial fibrillation: Restoration of sinus rhythm is recommended for those who are hemodynamically compromised or symptomatic. For asymptomatic patients, rate control and rhythm control strategies seem to be comparable and choice of agent should take into account patient factors, side effects of the agent, and physician preference. The optimal ventricular rate in atrial fibrillation is uncertain. It is likely less than 110 beats per minute. Aggressive rate control may be deleterious.

Amiodarone: Amiodarone is widely used and generally considered safe. It has concerning pulmonary complications, particularly if used for prolonged duration; however, it is well tolerated in the acute setting. Most commonly it is used as a bolus dose followed by an infusion. The mechanism of action is debated, but most likely amiodarone in the acute setting functions as a low-dose beta-blocker. Digoxin may be considered, usually in a 0.25–0.5 mg intravenous bolus dose. As digoxin has a narrow therapeutic index, a smaller dose such as 0.0625–0.125 mg may be adequate in those with moderate to severe renal impairment. There are concerns around the negative inotropic effect of beta-blockers, but used cautiously they may have a role.

CASE RESUMES

The patient was evaluated with auscultation and bedside echocardiography performed. The right ventricle demonstrated fluid and pressure overload. Intravenous diuretic was administered with improvement in urine output. His oxygen requirements decreased over the next few hours of diuresis. Serial bedside echocardiographic assessments were made to ensure LV filling was adequate with repeat dosing of intravenous diuretic. He was able to ambulate the following morning and released from the intensive care unit.

KEY POINTS TO REMEMBER

1. Acute diastolic heart failure presents a difficult management scenario in the early post–cardiac surgery period.
2. Initial diagnosis is assisted by knowledge of the patient's medical history and intraoperative course.
3. Diagnosis is made using both clinical and echocardiographic parameters.

4. Treatment of the precipitating cause, such as atrial fibrillation, is vitally important along with the exclusion of other potentially serious complications.
5. Individualized treatment aiming to optimize heart rate and rhythm, systemic vascular resistance, and fluid status will facilitate ventricular relaxation, minimizing the effects of diastolic dysfunction.

Suggested Reading
1. Ricard JD, Roux D. Invasive ventilation and acute heart failure syndrome. In: Mebazaa A, Gheorghiade M, Zannad FM, Parrillo JE, eds. *Acute Heart Failure*. London, UK: Springer; 2008:486–493.
2. Ponikowski P, Voors AA, Anker SD, et al.; ESC Scientific Document Group. 2016 ESC guidelines for the diagnosis and treatment of acute and chronic heart failure: the Task Force for the Diagnosis and Treatment of Acute and Chronic Heart Failure of the European Society of Cardiology (ESC). Developed with the special contribution of the Heart Failure Association (HFA) of the ESC. *Eur Heart J*. 2016;37(27):2129–2200.
3. Nohria A, Tsang SW, Fang JC, et al. Clinical assessment identifies hemodynamic profiles that predict outcomes in patients admitted with heart failure. *J Am Coll Cardiol*. 2003;41:1797–1804.
4. Nishimura RA, Borlaug BA. Diastology for the clinician. *J Cardiol*. 2019;73(6):445–452.
5. Borlaug BA, Jaber WA, Ommen SR, Lam CS, Redfield MM, Nishimura RA. Diastolic relaxation and compliance reserve during dynamic exercise in heart failure with preserved ejection fraction. *Heart*. 2011;97(12):964–969.

35 Postoperative Vasodilatory Shock

Fiona Roberts and Alan Gaffney

A 65-year-old man is admitted following elective aortic valve replacement surgery for severe aortic stenosis. He has a history of ischemic heart disease with an ejection fraction of 40%–45%, tobacco abuse (30 pack/year history), and moderate chronic obstructive pulmonary disease.

He remains intubated until postoperative day 2 due to low arterial oxygen saturations, poor respiratory mechanics, and the requirement for frequent suctioning. On postoperative day 3 he develops a fever, his white blood cell count increases to 18.6×10^9/L, and he has a productive cough. A chest radiograph demonstrates a new opacification in the left lung. Heart rate is 125 beats per minute, norepinephrine is required to maintain an adequate perfusing blood pressure, serum lactate increases to 3.6 mmol/L, and urine output is <0.5 mL/min. He is more obtunded compared to the previous day.

What do you do now?

DISCUSSION

There are some clinical features that are common to all types of shock and help with initial diagnosis. Hypotension requiring vasopressor support, oliguria, abnormal mentation, and deranged acid–base balance (classically a raised anion gap metabolic acidosis) are the main features of shock and end-organ dysfunction.

Next, the underlying condition must be considered. Are there signs of sepsis, such as in our patient (e.g., pyrexias, raised inflammatory markers, and a productive cough with associated chest X-ray changes)? Or is there a rash or bronchospasm that may indicate an anaphylactic reaction, for example?

On clinical examination, vasodilatory shock can often be distinguished from other types of shock by the presence of warm-to-touch peripheries. Both cardiogenic and hypovolemic shock will likely, but not always, present with cold and possibly mottled peripheries.

The hallmark of vasodilatory shock is hypotension with normal or increased cardiac output. The hyperdynamic circulatory state of vasodilatory shock results in a tachycardia and an increased pulse pressure. Of course, it is important to be aware that up to 30% of patients with septic shock can develop myocardial depression and thus a reduced cardiac output.

Radiological and biochemical investigations can assist with determining the diagnosis of shock. Metabolic acidosis with a negative base excess and elevated serum lactate is ubiquitous in a shocked state. Lactate can be an important indicator of end-organ perfusion and tissue hypoxia. A high lactate foretells a particularly grave prognosis in the presence of shock.

Raised white blood cell and C-reactive protein counts can support the diagnosis of septic shock, whereas raised tryptase or an eosinophilia could point to an anaphylactic cause. Blood cultures and samples from sputum, urine, and drain fluid can help isolate a causative organism. Similarly, a chest X-ray or computed tomography scan can help locate a septic source or rule out other pathology such as tension pneumothorax.

If history, clinical examination, and basic clinical investigations do not shine any light on the cause of shock, then further hemodynamic investigation with an echocardiogram or sometimes invasive hemodynamic monitoring may be necessary. A transthoracic echocardiogram (TTE) can be helpful in further distinguishing a vasodilatory shock from a cardiogenic or hypovolemic shock. It can also help guide treatment. It is usually readily available and non-invasive and thus a valuable adjunct. It can visualize right and left cardiac chamber size and contractility, inferior vena cava diameter, and collapsibility (in the assessment of hypovolemia) and rule out the presence of pericardial fluid. If TTE is unsatisfactory due to technical issues (body habitus, chest drains, dressings) a transesophageal echocardiogram may be indicated.

Invasive devices such as pulmonary artery catheters (PACs) can estimate cardiac output and measure mixed venous oxygen saturations as well as other parameters. It can be useful in distinguishing between different types of shock as well as guiding resuscitation and treatment response. Although a PAC was once the gold standard for septic shock, its use has declined greatly worldwide over recent years. This is largely due to a lack of mortality benefit displayed by several well-designed trials over since 2010. PAC use is controversial, but the general consensus would be that it may aid management of septic shock patients with myocardial dysfunction or right ventricular failure.

Pathophysiology

Shock is characterized by a significant reduction in systemic tissue perfusion resulting in an imbalance between oxygen consumption and oxygen delivery. This leads to cellular dysfunction and derangement of vital biochemical processes.

Vasodilatory shock—also known as *vasoplegic shock*—is relatively common following cardiac surgery and can be challenging to manage. Despite being a well-recognized complication, clinical features and spectrum of severity are poorly described.

The causes of vasodilatory shock are diverse. They include sepsis, surgical insult, anaphylaxis, and others including trauma, burns, and pancreatitis. Sepsis is by far the most common cause of vasodilatory shock. It accounts for more than 200 000 cases per year in the United States. It is also frequently encountered in the postoperative cardiac surgery patient. It is also important to remember that vasodilatory shock may be the final common pathway for shock of all types.

Vasodilation is the end result of inappropriately increased vasodilatory mechanisms coupled with failure of vasoconstrictor mechanisms.

The pathophysiology of vasodilatory shock is complex and multifactorial. Although still not fully understood, it is widely accepted that it includes activation of several intrinsic vasodilatory pathways and a vascular hyporesponsiveness to vasopressors. Septic shock is the most studied cause of vasodilatory shock; however, similar mechanisms are thought to play a pivotal role in all causes of vasodilatory shock. Gram-negative bacterial endotoxin was discovered to cause vascular collapse in 1899. Our understanding of the pathophysiology of septic shock has evolved slowly since then.

Systemic vascular resistance is determined by changes in arteriolar diameter, controlled by the contractile activity of the vascular smooth muscle cells (VSMCs) in the tunica media. The contractile state of the VSMCs, or vascular "tone," is regulated through intracellular calcium (Ca^{2+}) concentration. It is dependent on the rate of Ca^{2+} influx versus expulsion, which in turn is regulated by intrinsic and extrinsic mechanisms. Intrinsic mechanisms include induction of nitric oxide (NO) synthases and release of prostacyclin and endothelin as well as vasoactive metabolites (hydrogen peroxide) and autacoids (serotonin, prostaglandins, and thromboxane A2). Extrinsic regulation is mostly maintained via sympathetic neural control and vasoactive hormones, including adrenaline, angiotensin II, and vasopressin.

NO was originally described as an endothelium-derived relaxing factor of vascular smooth muscle. Since then, NO has been widely recognized as a vasodilator during sepsis. NO also plays a very important role in blood pressure and organ blood flow regulation, mainly by reducing intracellular calcium as it diffuses freely from the endothelium into the neighboring VSMCs, thus causing relaxation of vascular smooth muscle and vasodilation. Furthermore, the role of NO in vascular hyporesponsiveness during vasodilatory shock seems to be of great importance. One possible mechanism is the direct activation by NO of potassium channels that are sensitive to cytosolic calcium. NO overproduction during sepsis may also be the cause of direct myocardial depression.

Prostacyclin—also known as *prostaglandin I_2*—is produced by the endothelium constitutively and induces cyclic adenosine monophosphate/protein kinase A–mediated vasodilation.

Extrinsic regulation plays an important role in vasodilatory shock. Plasma catecholamine concentrations are elevated, and the renin–angiotensin system is activated in vasodilatory shock of all causes; however, it appears to be catecholamine resistance that is the problem. Both animal and human studies appear to support the idea that expression of alpha-1 adrenoreceptors falls as sepsis progresses. This, in turn, leads to peripheral noradrenaline resistance.

Vasopressin, an endogenous hormone, increases intracellular calcium levels via interaction with specific V1 receptors. This in turn drives contraction. In sepsis, after 24-hours, vasopressin levels fall below normal. This may be a mechanism for the development of vasoplegia. Furthermore, V2 receptors on endothelial cells may provoke loss via the increased synthesis of NO.

The vasodilation provoked by these intrinsic and extrinsic mechanisms leads to hypotension, venous pooling, and therefore reduced oxygen delivery to the mitochondria. Initially, the tissues can compensate for reduced flow by increasing the oxygen extraction ratio. The reduced blood flow also causes activation of the sympathetic nervous system, which in turn increases the heart rate and initially provides a degree of vasoconstriction, shunting blood away from the splanchnic circulation. Oxygen consumption soon surpasses oxygen delivery, and increased lactate production and end-organ dysfunction being to occur. Increasing glucose liberation from the liver can overwhelm the struggling mitochondria, thus causing further lactate production.

Management

Shock is a clinical emergency, and prompt recognition and initiation of treatment is crucial. The time between shock onset and shock resolution is a key factor that defines the extent of organ dysfunction and the likelihood of death as prolonged shock causes inflammation and irreversible tissue injury.

In vasodilatory shock, identification of the underlying cause is of paramount importance. Management strategies are aimed not only at resuscitation, which maintains organ perfusion, but also at the underlying driving cause. For example, if the cause of vasodilatory shock happened to be anaphylaxis, then the treatment of choice would be intramuscular epinephrine. However, in the more common scenario of septic shock, source control and early initiation of appropriate antimicrobials are crucial. For our patient, antimicrobial therapies targeting the most likely causes of hospital-acquired pneumonia in our particular hospital should be commenced. Other sources of sepsis in a post–cardiac surgery patient (not necessarily our patient) should always be considered, including line sepsis from indwelling catheters and urinary tract infection.

The mortality rate of septic shock has been steadily decreasing. This is mainly attributed to increased awareness and recognition of sepsis and therefore more timely intervention. Although early goal-directed therapy was shown to be beneficial in the Rivers trial of 2001, more recent randomized controlled trials have not shown a mortality benefit when compared to standard care.

Treatment response goals are not well described. It is generally accepted to aim for a mean arterial pressure >65 mm Hg; however, that does not account for patient variability such as preexisting uncontrolled hypertension.

Treatment begins with the administration of fluids in an attempt to restore intravascular volume and cardiac preload. Crystalloids are first line for fluid management in shock; however, there is no definitive evidence as to which crystalloid is superior The most common crystalloid used worldwide is 0.9% normal saline, which has a supraphysiological chloride content. Other crystalloids, such as Ringer's lactate, resemble human plasma more closely.

Colloids such as albumin, dextrans, gelatin, and hydroxy-ethyl starch are commonly used in critically unwell patients. ALBIOS (Albumin Italian Outcomes Study) compared albumin with crystalloids versus crystalloids alone in septic shock and found no difference in 28-day mortality. The CRISTAL (Colloids versus Crystalloids for the Resuscitation of the Critically Ill) trial compared crystalloids with colloids in 2857 adults in shock and found no difference in 28-day mortality. Albumin appears to be a very reasonable alternative to crystalloid; however, it has disadvantages in terms of cost, its delivery via glass bottles, and the small potential risk of viral infections. Hydroxy-ethyl starches have been shown consistently to increase the risk of renal failure and even all-cause mortality in sepsis.

When a fluid resuscitation (e.g., up to 30 mL/kg) is not sufficient to maintain an adequate mean arterial pressure of >65 mm Hg, vasopressor therapy is indicated to maintain organ perfusion. Examples of vasopressors include norepinephrine, epinephrine, vasopressin, dopamine, phenylephrine, and angiotensin. All differ in their receptor target as well as their half-life and effects. Norepinephrine is considered the first-line agent in septic shock. It is also first line in other forms of shock. A Cochrane review in 2011 of 23 randomized controlled trials assessed 6 different vasopressors (alone or in combination with dobutamine or dopexamine) and showed no evidence of superiority. However, there were increased arrhythmias in the dopamine group.

Vasopressin is considered second line and is recommended in patients on norepinephrine doses >0.15–0.5 mcg/kg/min. It has been shown to be safe and to reduce norepinephrine requirements but not to infer a mortality benefit. The rationale for vasopressin use in septic shock is a relative deficiency of endogenous vasopressin.

Phenylephrine should be used with caution in septic shock. It has purely alpha-1 adrenergic activity and can cause splanchnic vasoconstriction. It is a weaker vasopressor than norepinephrine and has even been shown to increase mortality.

Epinephrine has both chronotropic and inotropic effects. Hence, it improves contractility and provides vasoconstriction. Despite this, its clinical benefits are limited by its side effects, including tachycardia and hyperlactatemia.

Additional therapies can act as adjuncts to vasopressors; however, their efficacy has not been proven. As discussed, excess production of NO may be a driving factor in vasodilatory shock. Therefore, methylene blue, which prevents NO overproduction, may have a role in vasodilatory shock. The use of methylene blue has been proposed not only for septic shock but also for vasodilatory shock post–cardiac surgery and in the anaphylactic patient.

Other adjunctive treatments include corticosteroids. Corticosteroids are commonly used in the treatment of septic shock without much evidence to support them. Steroids have an undesirable side effect profile, including immunosuppression and insulin resistance; thus, use should be considered on a patient-to-patient basis. Consensus guidelines suggest low-dose glucocorticoid therapy only in patients with vasopressor-dependent septic shock and removal once vasopressor requirements cease.

CASE RESUMES

The patient had sputum, urine and blood cultures drawn. While awaiting results, empiric antibiotics were started for gram positive and negative bacteremic coverage. Within 24 hours, pressor requirements decreased. The sputum culture speciated a pansensitive gram negative bacteria associated with community acquired pneumonia. Antibiotics were tapered to single agent and the patient continued to improve.

> **KEY POINTS TO REMEMBER**
>
> 1. Shock is the physiologic state characterized by significant reduction of systemic tissue perfusion, resulting in poor tissue delivery and therefore cellular dysfunction and derangement of cellular processes.
> 2. Shock post–cardiac surgery carries a high morbidity and mortality.
> 3. Sepsis is by far the most common cause of vasodilatory shock worldwide.
> 4. The hallmark of vasodilatory shock is hypotension with normal or increased cardiac output; however, it is important to remember that 30% of patients will develop myocardial depression and thus reduced cardiac output.
> 5. Shock is a clinical emergency, and prompt recognition and treatment initiation is crucial.
> 6. The time between shock onset and shock resolution is a key factor that defines the extent of organ dysfunction and the likelihood of death.
> 7. Early fluid resuscitation and appropriate antimicrobial therapy are the most crucial treatment interventions in septic shock.
> 8. Noradrenaline is the first-line vasopressor of choice in septic shock.

Suggested Reading
1. Levy MM, Evans LE, Rhodes A. The Surviving Sepsis campaign bundle: 2018 update. *Intensive Care Med.* 2018;44:925–928.
2. Lambden S, Creagh-Brown BC, Hunt J, Summers C, Forni LG. Definitions and pathophysiology of vasoplegic shock. *Crit Care.* 2018;22:174.
3. Hauffe T, Krüger B, Bettex D. Shock management for cardio-surgical ICU patients—the golden hours. *Card Fail Rev.* 2015;1(2):75–82.

4. Gyawali B, Ramakrishna K, Dhamoon AS. Sepsis: The evolution in definition, pathophysiology, and management. *SAGE Open Med*. 2019;7:2050312119835043.
5. Rivers E, Nguyen B, Havstad S, et al.; Early Goal-Directed Therapy Collaborative Group. Early goal-directed therapy in the treatment of severe sepsis and septic shock. *N Engl J Med*. 2001;345(19):1368–1377.

36 Postoperative Cardiogenic Shock

Maurice Hogan

A 62-year-old woman is admitted to the intensive care unit (ICU) for management immediately following coronary artery bypass grafting (CABG). She had presented approximately 2 weeks previously with symptoms of dyspnea and increased leg swelling. Her preoperative left ventricular ejection fraction was 40%. She also has diabetes, hypertension, chronic kidney disease stage II, and dyslipidemia.

On arrival to the ICU she has a heart rate of 80 bpm, sinus rhythm, and blood pressure (BP) of 110/50 mm Hg. Her serum lactate is 2.5 mmol/L, cardiac index is 2.8 L/min/m^2, and mixed venous oxygen saturation is 62%. Approximately 2 hours later the BP is 75/40 mm Hg. Despite a fluid bolus and the addition of a norepinephrine infusion, the patient remains anuric. The arterial blood gas analysis shows a lactate of 6 mmol/L, and the cardiac index has dropped to 1.5 L/min/m^2. The patient is cool peripherally.

What do you do now?

DISCUSSION

Diagnosis

The patient is hypotensive, profoundly so, and that the situation is refractory to initial management steps. Hemodynamic lability early in the postoperative period is not unusual; however, this is more sinister. In addition to hypotension, there is evidence of low cardiac output and hypoperfusion with rising lactate and anuria. Clinically the patient is cool to touch, which is a sign of peripheral vasoconstriction. The patient is in shock in the early postoperative period and the differential diagnosis is diverse (Table 36.1).

The key management steps are to resuscitate and stabilize the patient, inform the cardiac surgical team, continue assessment to determine any specific cause, and prepare for emergency chest opening or mechanical support if the situation does not improve or deteriorates. The immediate priority

TABLE 36.1 **Classification, Etiology, and Investigations of Shock**

Shock Classification	Possible Etiology Post–Cardiac Surgery	Investigations
Cardiogenic	Myocardial ischemia, LCOS, arrhythmia, valvular dysfunction	Clinical examination: hemodynamic assessment, electrocardiogram, echocardiography, arterial blood gas
Hypovolemic	Bleeding, fluid shift	Clinical examination: chest drain output assessment, chest X-ray, echocardiogram, arterial blood gas, complete blood count, coagulation profile
Obstructive	Pericardial tamponade, tension pneumothorax, pulmonary embolism	Clinical examination: echocardiogram, chest X-ray, computerized tomography angiogram
Distributive	Postoperative systemic inflammatory response syndrome, septic shock, anaphylaxis	Clinical examination: hemodynamic assessment, microbiological cultures, serum tryptase concentration

is to support the hemodynamics with pharmacological and possibly mechanical support while simultaneously assessing for and treating the specific cause. The patient has demonstrated a significant and sudden deterioration since the surgery was completed, and it is possible that the scenario may further evolve, even to full cardiac arrest. In that case, management would proceed per the Society of Thoracic Surgeons consensus for resuscitation of patients who arrest after cardiac surgery.

In this case there is no actual evidence of bleeding or acute blood loss, there has been minimal chest drain output, and a repeat chest X-ray performed does not show any evidence of fluid collection or pneumothorax. The patient is already intubated and sedated, and resuscitation can appropriately focus on the hemodynamic situation. An electrocardiogram is immediately performed, which shows evidence of new ischemia with ST elevation in lead I and the augmented vector left lead. A transesophageal echocardiography (TEE) probe is inserted and excludes a pericardial effusion; however, new akinesis of the lateral wall, with left ventricular ejection fraction approximately 20%, and new moderate mitral regurgitation are diagnosed. Echocardiography is essential in the assessment here. It is appropriate to perform transthoracic echocardiography initially, but if the images attained are not satisfactory, then TEE is mandatory.

The patient is in cardiogenic shock and has deteriorated very quickly and significantly since surgery was completed. The underlying cause seems almost certainly to be acute graft failure. The surgical team are informed of the emergency and instruct that the patient is to return to the operating room (OR). Hemodynamic stabilization is ongoing with preparation for emergency return to the OR. Cardiogenic shock is essentially a clinical diagnosis based on the presence of persistent hypotension (systolic BP <90 mm Hg) and signs of impaired organ perfusion:

- altered mental state
- cold, clammy skin and extremities
- oliguria, urine output <30 mL/h
- serum lactate >2 mmol/L

While some of the other possible causes of shock can be excluded, it remains possible that the etiology could be multifactorial. Some degree of postoperative systemic inflammatory response or vasoplegia is likely.

The pulmonary artery catheter is helpful in this regard and in terms of monitoring response to treatment. This patient is also at potential risk for developing low cardiac output syndrome (LCOS) after cardiac surgery; however, a number of features of the case are atypical for LCOS. Firstly, she has deteriorated very early postoperatively and quite suddenly and profoundly, which suggests a new, specific mechanism for the deterioration. LCOS should always be considered as a diagnosis of exclusion. Never attribute postoperative shock or hemodynamic instability to LCOS without excluding the other potential causes listed in Table 36.1. LCOS by definition requires some period of pharmacological or mechanical support. The underlying etiology is usually not defined; however, it most likely predominantly relates to ischemia–reperfusion myocardial injury, and dysfunction may vary from lasting only a few hours in the case of stunning to being potentially persistent in the case of myocardial infarction (MI). Conditions such as valvular dysfunction (native or prosthetic), pulmonary hypertension, or systemic comorbidities also contribute to LCOS. The deterioration in left ventricular ejection fraction in this case can be attributed to the presumed graft failure. New mitral regurgitation is also not uncommon in this situation; the mitral valve apparatus becomes dysfunctional due to the regional myocardial wall abnormality, and leaflets fail to coapt correctly during systole, thus leading to acute ischemic mitral regurgitation. Undoubtedly, the regurgitation is contributing to the hemodynamic instability, essentially as a maladaptive response; however, the primary treatment strategy should still be to restore coronary perfusion and then re-examine the mitral valve function.

Support: Fluids and Pharmacology

Despite over 2 million open cardiac surgery procedures being performed annually worldwide, there are no definitive guidelines on fluid resuscitation or pharmacologic support of hypotensive or shocked patients postoperatively, and individual and institutional practices can vary considerably. Some fluid boluses are indicated for almost every patient post–cardiac surgery—within the first hours at least. There has been no conclusive demonstration of benefit for administration of colloid over crystalloid post–cardiac surgery; in fact, most colloids have been shown to be harmful in comparison. Even packed red blood cells, that is, fluid with the absolute colloidal effect and additional presumed benefit of increased oxygen carrying capacity, are not associated with benefit unless given to correct concurrent severe anemia. The optimal response to both vasopressors and inotropes, however, is only achieved after optimization of intravascular volume status, something again which can be challenging to ascertain in this scenario. Real-time TEE guidance may be the best guide to fluid resuscitation in this case and more helpful than any isolated hemodynamic parameter. Secondary right ventricular failure in response to overzealous fluid administration is a risk in this scenario and would likely precipitate full cardiac arrest. Right ventricular dilatation or vena caval enlargement may become evident on echo in response to fluid administration.

Currently available clinical evidence supports the use of norepinephrine as a first-line treatment for the hypotensive patient in cardiogenic shock; when compared directly, it is shown to be favorable to dopamine, epinephrine, phenylephrine, and vasopressin. Cardiogenic shock is associated with inflammatory response and vasodilation, and associated hypotension may respond very well to norepinephrine. There may still be theoretical opposition to the concept of increasing afterload in a patient with cardiogenic shock; however, the actual consequences of hypotension are worse, hence the clinical benefit in responsive patients. Norepinephrine also has some positive effect on cardiac output, with the least, and possibly a negligible, effect on coronary perfusion, again given that restoration of systemic pressure also restores coronary perfusion. In cases where BP does not respond to norepinephrine and the patient is euvolemic, a second agent should be added. Vasopressin may be most appropriate. Shock refractory to norepinephrine or combination vasopressors is serious and may indicate that mechanical support is required.

This patient has cardiogenic shock, and use of an inotropic agent in addition to a vasopressor is also indicated. Available inotropes generally fall into 3 categories: β agonists (e.g., dobutamine, epinephrine, dopamine), phosphodiesterase III inhibitors (e.g., milrinone, enoximone), and calcium sensitizers (e.g., levosimendan). Dobutamine is the most suitable agent in this setting as it has rapid onset, has cardiac effects which are directly titratable along its dose range, and can increase cardiac output by increasing both stroke volume and heart rate. Epinephrine may achieve the same end points; however, its cardiac effects are not directly titratable along the dose range (i.e., as the dose is increased, the vasopressor effect dominates). In addition, it is associated with lactic acidosis, making assessment of response difficult to interpret. The downside of β agonists generally in this setting is that they increase myocardial oxygen demand, something which may ultimately worsen the effect of the ischemic insult. However, the alternative of persistent shock is potentially imminently fatal. Milrinone is not favored as in therapeutic doses it will worsen hypotension and has a delayed onset unless a bolus dose is administered, compared with dobutamine. Direct titration is challenging in the acute situation; in addition, milrinone clearance is greatly prolonged in renal failure, further complicating its management. Milrinone is also associated with a higher risk of ventricular arrhythmia compared to dobutamine, although one advantage of phosphodiesterase III inhibitors and levosimendan is that they may be somewhat more efficacious in a beta-blocked patient. Levosimendan, like milrinone, is limited in this setting as it also will worsen hypotension and have a delayed response, making titration difficult. For all vasopressors and inotropes, the principle of use is the same: use the lowest dose required, for the least duration possible.

Support: Mechanical

The marginal benefit of inotropes in this scenario is relatively low. They have no intrinsic therapeutic value; their only use is to aim to achieve hemodynamic stability and prevent multiorgan failure. Stabilization of hemodynamics enough to facilitate treatment of the underlying cause is the primary goal. Support of cardiac output and BP to maintain organ function until cardiac function is restored after treatment is the secondary goal. At either stage, pharmacological support alone may be inadequate, and use of mechanical support must be considered. The complications of inotropes and vasopressors are dose-dependent: the higher the doses required, generally the less favorable the outcome is likely to be. When the patient continues to demonstrate signs of shock despite increasing doses of medication, the situation is considered refractory to pharmacological support. As much as the dose at any given point can indicate this, the trend over hours or even minutes may be more telling. Patients may recover quickly from cardiogenic shock once the underlying cause is treated. In contrast, they may deteriorate quickly despite increasing doses of vasopressors and inotropes unless the cause can be reversed.

There are 3 forms of mechanical support which may be practically considered here: the intra-aortic balloon pump (IABP), the percutaneous pump (Impella), or full mechanical support with venoarterial extracorporeal membrane oxygenation (VA-ECMO). Similar to pharmacological support, outcomes with mechanical support are best if the underlying cause of shock is reversible and treated successfully. Traditionally, the IABP has been liberally utilized for such patients in cardiogenic shock post–acute coronary syndrome or CABG surgery, with the rationale being that it both increases coronary perfusion and improves cardiac output by decreasing systemic afterload. It can be inserted quickly, carries a low risk of vascular complications, and is relatively cheap; however, no difference in mortality was found between patients who had IABP after early revascularization for MI complicated by cardiogenic shock in a randomized controlled trial.

Use of Impella in patients with isolated left ventricular failure and cardiogenic shock represents a very attractive hypothesis; however, there is little robust clinical evidence currently to support its use. In addition, it is associated with significant risk of vascular injury and hemolysis and higher rates of transfusion, without any mortality benefit, specifically when compared with IABP. VA-ECMO represents the maximal supportive therapy which can be offered. Mortality associated with VA-ECMO for post-cardiotomy shock ranges 60%–80%; however, from retrospective analyses at least, it does seem possible to salvage some patients who would otherwise die without such support. Case selection and good clinical decision-making are thus extremely important. This patient would be an appropriate candidate for VA-ECMO given her age, potential reversibility of the cause of shock, and short duration of the shock state, minimizing the risk of extra-cardiac organ failure. The decision to proceed and initiate VA-ECMO depends essentially on her response to pharmacologic support. The best prognosis for her relies on prompt, successful revascularization. Indeed, this may even be best facilitated by initiation of VA-ECMO or even cardiopulmonary bypass prior to intervention. Failure to maintain systemic BP, increasing signs or markers of malperfusion (increasing lactate), and echocardiographic findings are all important indicators that ECMO may be necessary. In cases where there is sustained severe hemodynamic compromise, it may be appropriate to initiate emergency VA-ECMO even without knowing what the cause of shock is, as the most effective systemic support available.

Treatment

Cardiogenic shock post-MI is an emergency, and the only effective treatment is early revascularization. The mortality for patients with cardiogenic shock post-MI is up to 80% and drops to approximately 40% with successful early revascularization of the culprit lesion. A good outcome for this patient depends on prompt restoration of coronary flow to the culprit vessel. Whether this is achieved by surgical revision or percutaneous stenting does not seem to matter. In this case, there is a question as to how best to define the nature of the ischemia and how to deal with it. The surgical team could reopen the chest in the ICU. This is the quickest access to inspect the grafts; however, unless a graft is simply kinked, definitive treatment options are limited. If stable enough, the patient may be taken either to the coronary angiogram suite or back to the OR, where all surgical options including return to cardiopulmonary bypass are available. In this case, the patient was returned to a hybrid OR, and the surgical team reopened the chest primarily, with the interventional cardiology team preparing simultaneously for coronary angiogram and possible percutaneous intervention. The vein graft to the obtuse marginal branch had no flow and was thrombosed. Such an event so early postoperatively is considered a technical complication of surgery. The surgical team made one attempt to revise the graft on a beating heart; however, a subsequent coronary angiogram still showed no flow. At this stage the decision was made to stent the native left circumflex vessel, and 2 drug eluting stents were successfully deployed, with thrombolysis in MI grade 2 flow; this was considered satisfactory.

CASE RESUMES

By this stage the patient had required a moderate dose of norepinephrine to maintain a normal perfusion pressure, and dobutamine 10 mcg/kg/min had been added and titrated up to increase cardiac output. After stent deployment, the heart rate was 96 bpm and BP was 92/52 mm Hg. Lactate remained elevated at 8 mmol/L, and the patient remained anuric. Cardiac index was measured at 2.0 L/min/m^2. At this point, the surgeon suggested inserting an IABP, which was enthusiastically endorsed by the cardiologist. The IABP was set at 1:1 support on full augmentation. The patient was then returned to the ICU with this combined pharmacologic and mechanical support and made a satisfactory recovery. She did develop acute renal failure, which resolved without need for dialysis. The IABP was removed on day 1, and vasopressor and inotrope support was discontinued on day 2, with BP maintained in the normal range and cardiac index 2.5 L/min/m^2. Echocardiography at that stage showed mild hypokinesia of the lateral wall, with an ejection fraction of 35% and only mild mitral regurgitation.

KEY POINTS TO REMEMBER

1. Cardiogenic shock is a clinical diagnosis.
2. Always work to identify the specific cause(s) of postoperative shock, while managing hemodynamics; LCOS is a diagnosis of exclusion.
3. The only effective treatment for cardiogenic shock post-MI is revascularization.
4. Categorically state that the patient is in cardiogenic shock as soon as the diagnosis is made, and inform the surgical team immediately.

Suggested Reading

1. van Diepen S, Katz JN, Albert NM, et al. Contemporary management of cardiogenic shock: a scientific statement from the American Heart Association. *Circulation*. 2017;136(16):e232–e268.
2. Lomivorotov VV, Efremov SM, Kirov MY, Fominskiy EV, Karaskov AM. Low-cardiac-output syndrome after cardiac surgery. *J Cardiothorac Vasc Anesth*. 2017;31(1):291–308.
3. Thiele H, Zeymer U, Neumann F-J, et al. Intraaortic balloon support for myocardial infarction with cardiogenic shock. *N Engl J Med*. 2012;367(14):1287–1296.
4. Hajjar LA, Teboul JL. Mechanical circulatory support devices for cardiogenic shock: state of the art. *Crit Care*. 2019 Mar 9;23(1):76.
5. Hochman JS, Sleeper LA, Webb JG, et al. Early revascularization in acute myocardial infarction complicated by cardiogenic shock. SHOCK Investigators. Should we emergently revascularize occluded coronaries for cardiogenic shock. *N Engl J Med*. 1999;341(9):625–634.

6. Society of Thoracic Surgeons Task Force on Resuscitation After Cardiac Surgery. The Society of Thoracic Surgeons Expert Consensus for the Resuscitation of Patients Who Arrest After Cardiac Surgery. *Ann Thorac Surg.* 2017;103(3):1005–1020.

37 Cardiac Surgery–Associated Acute Kidney Injury

Coilin Smyth and Sinead Galvin

A 76-year-old man presented with worsening exertional dyspnea over the preceding year. A transthoracic echocardiogram demonstrated severe aortic stenosis with an estimated mean transvalvular gradient of 46 mm Hg and a valve area of 0.6 cm^2. Coronary angiography showed high-grade proximal circumflex and left anterior descending lesions. The right coronary artery had a 30%–40% distal lesion. He was scheduled for a tissue aortic valve replacement (AVR) and 2-vessel coronary artery bypass grafting. His background medical history was significant for hypertension, chronic kidney disease (CKD), hypercholesterolemia, and obesity (body mass index 38). His baseline creatinine was 140 μmol/L (1.58 mg/dL). His estimated glomerular filtration rate (eGFR) using the CKD Epidemiology Collaboration equation was 42 mL/min/1.73 m^2. Preoperative medications included aspirin 75 mg daily, atorvastatin 40 mg nocte, ramipril 10 mg daily, and bisoprolol 5 mg daily. His CKD was due to long-standing hypertensive disease. His recent ambulatory blood pressure (BP) study confirmed an average daytime mean arterial pressure of 70 mm Hg.

What do you do now?

DISCUSSION

What do we tell this patient about his risk of kidney injury at his preoperative visit?

The patient attended the preoperative assessment clinic 10 days prior to his scheduled surgery.

This patient's risk factor profile for cardiac surgery–associated acute kidney injury (CS-AKI) includes preexisting stage 3 CKD, obesity, hypertension, and impaired left ventricular function. This is now considered in the context of surgical risk factors. Table 37.1 demonstrates a comprehensive list of perioperative risk factors for CS-AKI. These risk factors can be categorized by modifiable, non-modifiable, surgical, and non-surgical. The preoperative assessment clinic provides a key opportunity to highlight these risks with the patient. It allows time for discussion with the patient regarding the significance of these risk factors and to consent accordingly. It also allows modifiable risks to be addressed.

Preexisting CKD is this patient's most significant non-modifiable risk factor. It implies both suboptimal function and a lack of renal reserve. Studies indicate that 10%–20% of patients with elevated preoperative

TABLE 37.1 **Perioperative Risk Factors for AKI Post–Cardiac Surgery**

Preoperative	Intraoperative	Postoperative
Advanced age	Complex surgery	Vasopressor exposure
Chronic kidney disease	CPB duration	Inotrope exposure
Hypertension	Need to return to CPB	Diuretic exposure
Hyperlipidemia	Low hematocrit during CPB	Blood transfusion
Female gender	Aortic cross-clamp time	Anemia
Liver disease	Hypoperfusion	Hypovolemia
Peripheral vascular disease	Hypovolemia	Venous congestion
Previous stroke	Venous congestion	Cardiogenic shock
Smoking history		

baseline creatinine between 2 and 4 mg/dL will require renal replacement therapy (RRT) postoperatively, whereas, 30% of those patients with preoperative creatinine >3.4 mg/L will require RRT. AKI or acute on chronic kidney injury increases the risk of RRT postoperatively. Where possible, surgery should be carried out when any acute decline in function has recovered to baseline.

Modifiable risk factors can be addressed to reduce the risk of CS-AKI. Preoperative coronary angiography was indicated here to assess coronary arterial status prior to valve replacement. To mitigate a patient's risk of contrast-induced AKI, ramipril was held for 48 hours around the angiographic procedure, and he was adequately hydrated. A 2017 meta-analysis has shown that *N*-acetylcysteine is ineffective at preventing contrast-induced AKI.

Comorbidities such as hypertension, chronic obstructive pulmonary disease, congestive cardiac failure, and diabetes should be optimized preoperatively.

Surgical factors also impact the risk of CS-AKI. The least invasive surgery should be considered in patients who are at high risk of CS-AKI. This patient required coronary bypass grafting as well as an AVR. This ruled out a less invasive option, such as percutaneous AVR. Emergency surgery carries a greater risk of CS-AKI. Such patients are more acutely unwell and will have endured low-flow periods as well as myocardial ischemia.

CASE RESUMES

The patient had a hemodynamically stable induction of anesthesia in the pre–cardiopulmonary bypass (CPB) period. Mean arterial pressure (MAP) was targeted at 70 mm Hg throughout the procedure and in the intensive care unit (ICU). This MAP was initially achieved with fluid loading (800 mL lactated Ringer's), after which a low-dose norepinephrine infusion was commenced. There was intraoperative transesophageal echo monitoring, with detailed pre- and post-bypass studies. Two arterial conduits were fashioned, left internal mammary artery to left anterior descending and right radial to left circumflex, with good targets reported by the surgical team. The native aortic valve was replaced with a 25 mm tissue AVR. CPB time was 142 minutes, with a cross-clamp time of 120 minutes. The patient weaned easily from bypass. He received 2 units of packed red cells to maintain a hemoglobin concentration >8–9 g/dL, along with plasma, fibrinogen concentrate, and platelets.

MITIGATING THE RISK OF CS-AKI INTRAOPERATIVELY

No single intervention has been shown to mitigate the risk of CS-AKI in the perioperative period. The usual MAP target of 65 mm Hg, below which there is an association with an increased risk of stroke, was adjusted to 70 mm Hg. This was because a 24-hour ambulatory BP study demonstrated premorbid poorly controlled hypertension. A pulmonary artery catheter was placed to aid cardiac output optimization. Management of hypovolemia and preload optimization intraoperatively and on return to the ICU were with restrictive chloride solutions (lactated Ringer's solution or Plasmalyte). Chloride-rich solutions have been associated with increased risk of AKI. Blood or 5% albumin was chosen for any potential emergent rapid volume expansion, due to the association between AKI and synthetic starch-based colloids.

Low-flow states, irrespective of the etiology (ventricular dysfunction, tamponade, ongoing bleeding, dysrhythmias, pacing dysfunction, ongoing ischemia) as well vasoplegic states postoperatively impact negatively on renal perfusion. In the ICU, hemodynamic monitoring, targets, and interventions are designed to identify and then to offset the major hemodynamic fluxes that are common in the initial days after cardiac surgery. The perioperative goals for this patient are to favorably manipulate renal metabolic supply–demand balance and to ensure that there is no ongoing renal ischemia or insult. Timely rescue is an important concept for this patient given his poor renal reserve.

On postoperative day 1, the patient developed oliguria (0.2 mL/kg/h) for 6 hours and a worsening metabolic acidosis, despite meeting hemodynamic targets. By postoperative day 2 serum creatinine concentration had risen significantly to 2.7 mg/dL, with a serum potassium of 5.2 mEq/L and a positive fluid balance of 3 L in 24 hours. According to the Kidney Disease Improving Global Outcomes (KDIGO) definition of renal function, the patient had a level 1 AKI (Table 37.2).

TABLE 37.2 **Kidney Disease Improving Global Outcomes (KDIGO)**

Stage	Serum Creatinine	Urine Output
1	1.5–1.9 × baseline creatinine or >26.5 μmol/L increase	<0.5 mL/kg/h for 6–12 h
2	2.0–2.9 × baseline creatinine	<0.5 mL/kg/h for >12 h
3	3.0 × baseline	<0.3 mL/kg/h

DIAGNOSING CS-AKI

The diagnosis of AKI and the assessment of its severity are key determinants of immediate therapies and overall prognosis. There are 3 diagnostic scoring systems for AKI: RIFLE (risk, injury, failure, loss, end-stage kidney disease), KDIGO, and AKIN (Acute Kidney Injury Network). The KDIGO scoring system has a higher sensitivity than AKIN and/or RIFLE. Table 37.2 shows the KDIGO diagnostic tool.

Serum concentrations of creatinine, urea output, and urine output (UO) are the parameters most frequently used to monitor renal function. Acid–base status in the postoperative patient, while not specific, can also be an early indicator of renal dysfunction. These markers all have limitations.

Serum creatinine concentration will only exceed normal values when >50% of nephron function is already lost. Serum creatinine concentration also varies depending on muscle mass, gender, age, ethnicity, and diet. eGFR equations have attempted to correct for some of these variabilities. Table 37.3 highlights 3 of these formulae, while Table 37.4 compares the components of each equation. The Cockcroft-Gault formula tends to overestimate GFR in healthy individuals, while the Modification of Diet in Renal Disease (MDRD) underestimates it. The MDRD is more accurate at estimating GFR in patients with CKD but is less accurate with patients at the extremes of body mass index. A newer formula, that of the CKD Epidemiology Collaboration, is thought to be more accurate than the MDRD, especially for patients with near-normal renal function. In the preoperative patient, this formula would be advised to highlight patients with normal or mild renal impairment. Using serum creatinine as the primary

TABLE 37.3 **eGFR Equations**

MDRD	GFR = 186 × serum Cr-1.154 × age-0.203 × 1.212 (if patient is black) × 0.742 (if female)
Cockcroft-Gault	CrCl (mL/min) = (140 age) × weight (kg) × (0.85 if female)/(72 × Cr)
CKD Epidemiology	CrCl = A × (serum Cr/B)C × 0.993age × (1.159 if black)
	A, B, and C are based on baseline creatinine (Cr) and gender

diagnostic marker is also limited by the 48-hour to 7-day interval between initial renal insult and elevation of serum creatinine.

UO is another diagnostic marker of AKI. UO of <0.5 mL/kg/h is an indicator of declining GFR. The limitations of UO include the possibility of AKI with preserved UO and pharmacological manipulation of UO using diuretic therapy.

Serum or urinary biomarkers for early diagnosis of AKI have been and continue to be researched. Table 37.5 shows renal-specific biomarkers and their origin within the kidney. A meta-analysis in 2016 concluded that current biomarkers exhibit at best modest discrimination for cardiac surgery–associated AKI in the early postoperative period in adults. Although renal biomarkers hold potential benefit for the future, there is no biomarker currently available that has led to a clinical advantage for the post–cardiac surgery patient cohort.

RRT was commenced on postoperative day 3 due to worsening oligo-anuric renal failure with an associated metabolic acidemia (pH 7.22) and mild hyperkalemia (5.8 mEq/L).

TABLE 37.4 **eGFR Equation Comparisons**

eGFR Equation	Serum Cr	Gender	Age	Race	Weight
MDRD	Y	Y	Y	Y	N
Cockcroft-Gault	Y	Y	Y	N	Y
CKD Epidemiology	Y	Y	Y	Y	N

TABLE 37.5 **Plasma and Urinary Biomarkers of Renal Injury and Their Origin in the Kidney**

Biomarker	Origin	Biomarker	Origin
NGAL	Glomerulus, distal tubule, collecting duct	Urine BGST	Distal tubule
Cystatin C	Glomerulus, proximal tubule	Netrin-1	Proximal tubule
Interleukin-18	Proximal tubule	Hepcidin	Proximal tubule
KIM-1	Proximal tubule	Urinary calprotectin	Collecting duct
L-FABP	Proximal tubule	TIMP-2	Proximal tubule
NAG	Proximal tubule, distal tubule	IGFBP7	Proximal tubule
Urine aGST	Proximal tubule	TLR 3	Proximal tubule
β2-Microglobulin	Glomerulus		

IGFBP, insulin-like growth factor binding protein; KIM-1, kidney injury molecule 1; L-FABP, liver-type fatty acid binding protein; NAG, N-acetyl-β-D-glucosaminidase; NGAL, neutrophil gelatinase-associated lipocalin; TIMP, tissue inhibitor if metalloproteinase; TLR, toll-like receptor.

INDICATIONS FOR TIMING OF RRT

The clear indications to commence RRT include failure of intravascular volume control, electrolyte abnormalities, acid–base dysregulation, and uremia. These complications can be temporized medically prior to the initiation of RRT or renal function recovery. In post–cardiac surgery patients, a stunned myocardium is at increased risk of arrhythmia and has less reserve to adapt to fluxes in intravascular volumes. This usually necessitates earlier definitive intervention with RRT.

Evidence of pulmonary edema in the setting of CS-AKI usually requires RRT for ultrafiltration, particularly if volume status is delaying ventilatory weaning and thus liberation from the ventilator. The use of diuretics is discussed in the following section.

Potassium levels >6 mEq/L require treatment. Any intracellular shift of potassium via insulin infusions or bicarbonate therapy will provide a temporary decrease in serum [K$^+$]. RRT will be required as a definitive step in most critically ill patients. Hyperkalemia in the post–cardiac surgery patient is common secondary to blood transfusions and reperfusion metabolites.

A pH of <7.1–7.2 is a reasonable trigger for RRT for acidemia due to AKI in these patients. Postoperative cardiac surgery patients are less capable of respiratory compensation for metabolic acidosis. They are also less able to tolerate the associated volume expansion when sodium bicarbonate is administered. Finally, acidemia is associated with impaired myocardial contractility.

Less commonly, complications of uremia such as pericarditis or encephalopathy may require RRT.

DIURETIC THERAPY IN THE MANAGEMENT OF AKI

Diuretic therapy can be used to increase UO. This does not reflect an increase in renal function. The benefits include optimizing intravascular volume. There is also a hypothesis that by decreasing the activity of the adenosine triphosphate (ATP)–dependent pump (Na/K/Cl pump), the kidney may require less ATP and therefore tolerate low-flow states slightly better.

Loop diuretics are used first line. It is important to remember that furosemide's action is from the luminal side and therefore requires filtration through the glomerulus. Increased doses are required when GFR is decreased.

The negative effect of diuretics is the impact on electrolyte balance. Sodium, chloride, and potassium should all be monitored closely.

TIMING OF INITIATION OF RRT

The decision to commence RRT was based on worsening renal indices including acidemia, hyperkalemia, and oliguria. These 3 concomitant consequences of AKI, in a patient with a fragile myocardium, influenced the decision in this clinical scenario.

Studies have looked at the optimal timing for RRT by assessing early versus late strategies. An early initiation strategy can prevent and reverse the metabolic sequelae of a developing AKI. A late strategy may allow time for renal function recovery without need for this intervention, which has complications and costs associated. A meta-analysis published in 2017 looking at "early" versus "late" RRT strategies in the general ICU patient cohort concluded that there has been no mortality benefit demonstrated by the early initiation of RRT. The study also demonstrated no difference in length of stay or ventilator days. This meta-analysis advocates a "watchful waiting" approach. The post–cardiac surgery patient does not fit neatly into the general ICU cohort. A study looking specifically at post–cardiac surgery patients demonstrated a survival benefit in early RRT, though it was a much smaller study than the one previously quoted.

MODALITY AND DOSING OF RRT

A continuous mode of RRT (CRRT) is most intuitive in hemodynamically unstable patients. This is due to the decreased rate of blood flow and subsequent reduction in fluid shifts compared to intermittent dialysis. There is, however, no evidence that filtration, dialysis, or a combination of both filtration and dialysis is superior.

For CRRT techniques, the dose is the sum of all effluent fluids expressed as milliliters per kilogram per hour. Two large randomized controlled trials have compared intensive dosing (35–40 mL/kg/h) to less intensive dosing (25 mL/kg/h) in critically ill patients, concluding that there was no mortality benefit to a higher dosing of RRT. Overall daily filter time is a key determinant of effective CRRT. Filter down time, secondary to clotting or other interruptions (radiological, surgical, etc.) can have a significant impact on the overall 24-hour dosing. In post–cardiac surgical patients, there is no evidence to deviate from the evidence supporting 25 mL/kg/h as the initial dose for CRRT in CS-AKI.

ANTICOAGULATION

Regional citrate anticoagulation was used to reduce the risk of post-surgical bleeding while also maximizing filter life.

Anticoagulation options include no anticoagulation, regional citrate anticoagulation, and systemic heparin anticoagulation. The life of the filter is markedly shorter if no anticoagulation is used. Two randomized controlled trials published in 2015 showed that citrate was associated with longer filter life in critically ill patients compared to heparin. This impacts effective daily dialysis time and blood loss due to circuit clotting without recirculation. Cardiac patients are at risk of postoperative bleeding, and regional citrate anticoagulation is associated with fewer bleeding complications than systemic heparin. A meta-analysis in 2019 confirmed its safety profile as an alternative to heparin.

DIALYSIS ACCESS: WHEN AND WHICH SITE

The timing and site of insertion of a dialysis catheter are important considerations. The benefits of preoperative insertion include the controlled theater environment, the ease of patient positioning under general anesthesia, and the ability to maintain strict asepsis. This approach also avoids the crisis insertion of a dialysis catheter in a potentially unstable postoperative ICU patient. The disadvantages of this preemptive approach include insertion-related complications for an intravascular device that may not ultimately be needed.

The optimal site for the catheter is one that allows optimal flow rate with the lowest risk of infection and the lowest risk of complications during insertion. Rates of infection are highest in femoral lines and lowest in subclavian lines. The internal jugular vein carries a slightly higher infection risk than the subclavian vein. The rates of pneumothorax and arterial puncture are highest in subclavian lines compared to internal jugular or femoral lines. Subclavian lines are associated with increased risk of vessel stenosis. This is a major consideration for patients who may need longer-term central access for chronic RRT.

Regarding flow rates, a study in 2010 looking at femoral versus internal jugular sites concluded that jugular site did not significantly outperform femoral site placement. The femoral vein also offers easier access in the unstable patient and does not require the Trendelenburg position, which can cause further cardiorespiratory decompensation in acute volume overload. The KDIGO guidelines recommend using the right internal jugular vein as first choice, followed by the femoral vein. The third option would be the left internal jugular and finally the subclavian veins.

The tip of an internal jugular or subclavian central venous catheter should be at the right atrium to achieve optimal flow, while a femoral line should reach the inferior vena cava.

MANAGEMENT OF THE ESTABLISHED DIALYSIS PATIENT PRESENTING FOR CARDIAC SURGERY

Patients with end-stage renal disease (ESRD) present for cardiac surgery due to a shared risk profile. These patients are challenging to manage.

Patients with CKD stage 5 (eGFR <15, not dialysis-dependent) and ESRD (dialysis-dependent) have additional preoperative needs. Hemoglobin concentration should be kept >9 g/dL, similar to patients with coronary artery disease. A study in 2014 showed a link between preoperative hemoglobin and postoperative outcomes in patients with CKD. Decreased endogenous erythropoietin and chronic dialysis both result in decreased hemoglobin levels. Exogenous erythropoietin and supplemental iron are used to achieve this. Blood transfusions in this population may increase immunological complexity for future transplantation. Parathyroid hormone, calcium, and phosphate levels should be measured at the preoperative visit to assess the presence and/or extent of electrolyte abnormalities. These patients are likely to be more vulnerable to positioning injuries and fractures in the event of advanced renal bone disease. The subset of dialysis patients who experience significant hypotension after dialysis or chronically is a complex group to manage for major surgery. They tend to be older, frailer, and predominantly female. They tend to become profoundly vasoplegic around major surgery.

Patients with ESRD should have high-efficiency dialysis in the weeks leading up to surgery, with the last dialysis the day before surgery. Hemodialysis on the morning of major surgery is associated with perioperative vasoplegia and hypovolemia. Dry weight (target weight post-dialysis) should be noted and achieved on the last dialysis session preoperatively. In patients maintained on peritoneal dialysis (PD), extra vigilance should be paid to the efficacy of the mode. If there is concern regarding the efficiency of the established PD regimen, consideration should be given to switching to hemodialysis preoperatively. This should be decided in collaboration with the attending nephrologist.

Postoperative dialysis should be scheduled for the day after surgery. This will usually be a continuous mode to avoid the higher flow rates and hemodynamic shifts associated with intermittent hemodialysis.

Arteriovenous fistula care commences preinduction with examination of the fistula to ensure flow. Protective labeling, wrapping, and prevention of compression during surgery are imperative. Intra- and postoperatively, the risk of thrombosis increases due to the relative low-flow state associated with cardiopulmonary bypass and any impaired myocardial function.

PROGNOSIS POST-CS-AKI

CS-AKI is common and a strong predictor of mortality. In its most severe form, CS-AKI increases the odds ratio of operative mortality 3- to 8-fold, length of stay in the ICU and hospital, and costs of care. In one study of over 47 000 patients, the incidence of AKI requiring CRRT was 1%. The mortality in this cohort was 65% compared to 4.3% in patients without this complication.

Patients who are discharged from hospital after CS-AKI continue to have a significant additional morbidity and mortality compared to the general post–cardiac surgery population. ESRD and associated dialysis dependence is the most common morbidity. Even in those patients who recover renal function, there is an increased rate of major adverse cardiovascular events. This prognosis reinforces the fact that optimal renal care, from risk stratification to prevention to early diagnosis to treatment, is paramount in the cardiac surgical patient.

Knowledge and communication of these outcomes play a central role in counseling patients preoperatively, who are at significant risk of CS-AKI. It is also important in patient and family discussions during the postoperative period after a CS-AKI has occurred.

KEY POINTS TO REMEMBER

1. The preoperative visit should be used to optimize all modifiable risk factors for CS-AKI and to counsel the patient regarding their individual risk for CS-AKI.
2. In the preoperative setting, the CKD Epidemiology equation should be used to assess eGFR. It is the most sensitive for marginally impaired renal function.
3. Diuretics should be used to optimize intravascular volume status and not solely to increase UO. Loop diuretics should be used first line.
4. The timing of RRT should be on a case-by-case basis with no mortality benefit to an early strategy or a late strategy.
5. The dialysis time per 24 hours is the key determinant of effective daily dialysis. Interruptions should be minimized. An appropriate initial dosing is 25 mL/kg/h.
6. Regional anti-coagulation with citrate carries benefits of increased filter life and decreased bleeding risk.
7. The right internal jugular should be the first choice for a dialysis catheter, but there is only a small benefit over the use of femoral veins.
8. Patients previously established on RRT should have effective dialysis on the day prior to surgery and commence CRRT on postoperative day 1.
9. There is a significant increase in morbidity and mortality in patients who require RRT. This increased risk extends beyond the hospital stay and includes patients who successfully wean from RRT.

Suggested Reading
1. Yamauchi T, Miyagawa S, Yoshikawa Y, Toda K, Sawa Y; Osaka Cardiovascular Surgery Research (OSCAR) Group. Risk index for postoperative acute kidney injury after valvular surgery using cardiopulmonary bypass. *Ann Thorac Surg*. 2017;104(3):868–875. doi: 10.1016/j.athoracsur.2017.02.012.
2. Besen BAMP, Romano TG, Mendes PV, et al. Early versus late initiation of renal replacement therapy in critically ill patients: systematic review

and meta-analysis. *J Intensive Care Med.* 2019;34(9):714–722. doi:10.1177/0885066617710914.
3. Zhang W, Bai M, Yu Y, et al. Safety and efficacy of regional citrate anticoagulation for continuous renal replacement therapy in liver failure patients: a systematic review and meta-analysis. *Crit Care.* 2019;23(1):22. doi:10.1186/s13054-019-2317-9.
4. Lee S, Park S, Kang MW, et al. Postdischarge long-term cardiovascular outcomes of intensive care unit survivors who developed dialysis-requiring acute kidney injury after cardiac surgery. *J Crit Care.* 2019;50:92–98. doi:10.1016/j.jcrc.2018.11.028.
5. Hayes W. Ab-normal saline in abnormal kidney function: risks and alternatives. *Pediatr Nephrol.* 2019;34(7):1191–1199. doi:10.1007/s00467-018-4008-1.
6. Ho J, Tangri N, Komenda P, et al. Urinary, plasma, and serum biomarkers' utility for predicting acute kidney injury associated with cardiac surgery in adults: a meta-analysis. *Am J Kidney Dis.* 2015;66(6):993–1005. doi:10.1053/j.ajkd.2015.06.018.

Index

For the benefit of digital users, indexed terms that span two pages (e.g., 52–53) may, on occasion, appear on only one of those pages.

Tables, figures, and boxes are indicated by *t*, *f*, or *b* following the page number.

acetaminophen, 52–53, 53*t*, 54
acid-base equations
  anion gap, 89–90
  Henderson–Hasselbalch equation, 87–88
  Winter's formula, 88–89
acidosis
  metabolic acidosis in the ICU, 85–95
  respiratory acidosis in the ICU, 73–84
Acquired von Willebrand Disease (aVWD), 198–99, 208–9, 242
acute cellular rejection (ACR), 248–49, 250–52
acute kidney injury (AKI)
  anticoagulation, 361–62
  dialysis access site selection, 362–63
  diuretic therapy in management of, 360
  indications for timing of RRT, 359–60
  management of established dialysis patients, 363–64
  mitigating risks intraoperatively, 356
  modality and dosing of RRT, 361
  prognosis, 364
  risk factor for CS-AKI, 354*t*, 354–55
  timing of initiation of RRT, 360–61
acute respiratory distress syndrome (ARDS)
  evidence for ECMO, 223–24
  how ECMO works, 225–27, 226*f*
  management during ECMO, 227
  patient selection, 224–25, 225*f*
  weaning from ECMO, 228
advanced cardiovascular life support (ACLS)
  airway considerations, 158–59
  bradycardia and systole, 156–57
  cardiac arrest with intra-aortic balloon pump in situ, 157–58
  consensus guidelines, 155*f*
  pulseless electrical activity (PEA) arrest, 157*t*, 157
  resternotomy, 158
  ventricular fibrillation, 155–56
American Heart Association, ACLS guidelines, 154, 159
analgesia
  additional techniques, 55
  multimodal analgesia, 52–55, 53*t*
  neuraxial techniques, 50
  opioids, 52
  other regional techniques, 50–51, 51*f*, 52*b*
anion gap, 89–90
antibody-mediated rejection (AMR), 249–50
aortic stenosis
  neurological injuries, 166–67
  paravalvular leak (PVL), 165–66
  postprocedure arrhythmias, 165
  TAVR postoperative management and pitfalls, 162–64, 163*t*
  valve options for TAVR, 164
  vascular complications, 167–68
arterial blood gas (ABG)
  4 types of respiratory and metabolic derangements, 74*t*
  acid-base nomogram for human plasma, 76*f*
  in respiratory acidosis, 74–75
arteriovenous malformations (AVMs), 209
atrial fibrillation, postoperative, 129–36

Bayes model, 3
bleeding and thrombosis
　etiology and treatment of coagulopathy, 313–21
　evaluation of suspected post-op bleeding, 198
　evaluation of suspected thrombosis, 199f
　gastrointestinal bleeding, 207–14
　parameters of life-threatening physiology, 243t
　pulmonary embolism, 59–70
　troubleshooting with LVADs, 197–204
blood products, 317, 319t
bradycardia, ACLS response, 156–57
bronchopleural fistulas (BPFs), 305

cardiac surgery
　acute kidney injury associated with, 353–65
　coagulopathy etiology and treatment, 313–21
　glycemic control following, 37–46
　pulmonary artery catheterization in, 13–23
　risk assessment scores in, 1–11
cardiac surgery–associated acute kidney injury (CS- AKI). *See* acute kidney injury (AKI)
cardiac tamponade
　clinical features, 276–78
　echocardiography, 243t, 278f, 278–79
　emergency resternotomy, 278f, 279–80
　management of, 279
cardiogenic shock
　classification, etiology, and investigations of, 344t
　fluid and pharmacology support, 346–48
　mechanical support, 231–38, 348–50
　treatment of, 350–51
cerebrovascular injury
　bimodal distribution of, 309–10
　incidence of, 308
　risk factors, 308t, 308–9, 309t

chest drains
　air leaks, 303–4
　assessment in hypovolemic shock, 344t, 345
　in BPFs, 305
　inserting, 301–2
　in stable pneumothorax, 301
　in tension pneumothorax, 299
　troubleshooting, 302
CKD Epidemiology Collaboration, 357–58
Cleveland Clinic score, 3
coagulopathy, etiology and treatment in cardiac surgery. *See also* bleeding and thrombosis
　algorithm-based transfusion protocols, 315–17
　blood products and transfusion thresholds, 317, 319t
　empirical treatment, 315
　expected bleeding, 314
　fibrinolysis, 318
　key principles of management, 315
　laboratory testing, 315, 316t
　persistent microvascular bleeding, 315
　platelet count, 317–18
　prothrombin complex concentrate (PCC), 317
　recombinant factor VIIa or factor XIII, 321
　resuscitation guidelines, 314
　thromboelastometry traces, 317, 318f
Cockcroft-Gault formula, 357–58
continuous mode of RRT (CRRT), 361, 364, 365
counterpulsation, 149, 157–58, 268–70, 269f, 271–72

dialysis
　access site selection, 362–63
　anticoagulation, 361–62
　indications for timing of RRT, 359–60
　management of established patients, 363–64

mitigating risks intraoperatively, 356
modality and dosing of RRT, 361
timing of initiation of RRT, 360–61
diastolic heart failure
    diastolic dysfunction, 325
    initial approach, 324
    investigations, 325
    treatment of, 329–30

early goal-directed therapy (EGDT), for septic shock, 115–16
ECMO (extracorporeal membrane oxygenation)
    ECMO cannulation strategies, 99–100
    rhabdomyolysis due to
        causes of, 101–4, 102t
        ischemia-reperfusion injury, 100–1
        ischemic changes secondary to hyperemia, 98f, 98
        monitoring, 105
        risk factors for limb ischemia, 99b
    venoarterial (VA-ECMO)
        following lung transplantation, 263–65
        indication and contraindications, 232–33
        management of patients, 234–37
        patient selection, 233–34
        weaning from, 237
    venovenous (VV-ECMO)
        evidence for ECMO, 223–24
        following lung transplantation, 263–65
        how ECMO works, 225–27, 226f
        management during ECMO, 227
        patient selection, 224–25, 225f
        weaning from ECMO, 228
eGFR equations, 357–58, 358t
end-stage renal disease (ESRD), 363–64
European Resuscitation Council, consensus guidelines, 154, 155f
European System for the Cardiac Operative Risk Evaluation (EuroSCORE), 4–7, 5t

extracorporeal life support (ECLS). *See* VA-ECMO (venoarterial ECMO)

Fick equation, 26, 244
frailty, risk assessment scores and, 7–10, 9f

gabapentinoids, 52–53, 53t, 55–56, 57
gastrointestinal bleeding (GIB)
    multifactorial pathogenesis of, 208–9
    risk factor for LVAD-related GIB, 208
    treatment and secondary prophylaxis, 211–13
glycemic control
    diabetes versus HbA1c and outcomes, 41
    incidence of acute hyperglycemia, 38
    perioperative hyperglycemia and morbidity and mortality, 39–40, 40t
    stress hyperglycemia, 38–39
    treatment guidelines, 41–44, 42b, 44f

HbA1c, 39, 41, 42
heart failure. *See* diastolic heart failure
heart transplantation
    management of orthotopic, 241–46
    rejection and immunosuppression in orthotopic, 247–55, 250t
Henderson–Hasselbalch equation, 87–88
hyperacute rejection, 248
hyperglycemia, 38–40, 40t, 42b. *See also* glycemic control
hyperlactatemia
    causes of, 31t, 35, 91t
    increased postoperative bleeding and, 314
    pathophysiology of, 91t
    as side effect of epinephrine, 339
hypotension and LVAD function
    clinical examination, 192–93
    incidence of, 195–96
    potential causes of hypotension, 193–95
    treatment, 195

INDEX   369

hypoxemia
  due to primary graft dysfunction, 257–65, 262f
  primary graft dysfunction grading system, 262t

immunosuppression, 252–55
Impella, 217f, 217–19, 218t, 349–50
infective endocarditis (IE)
  cause of, 285
  complications, 293–94
  in the ICU, 294
  mitral valve vegetation, 290f
  prognosis, 290, 291b
  prophylaxis, 293
  risk factors, 285
  signs and symptoms, 285–86
  surgical intervention, 293
  treatment, 290–92
intra-aortic balloon pumps (IABP)
  ACLS response to cardiac arrest, 157–58
  anticoagulation, 271
  cardiac arrest with, 157–58
  complications, 271–72
  hemodynamic changes, 268
  patient selection, 270
  placement, 271
  in postoperative cardiogenic shock, 349–50
  principle of counterpulsation, 268–70, 269f
  risk of embolic phenomena with, 101
ischemia-reperfusion injury
  limb ischemia, 99
  prevention and management, 69, 175
  primary graft dysfunction and, 259, 264
  rhabdomyolysis due to ECMO, 100–1
  unilateral pulmonary edema (UPE), 173f, 174–75, 176

ketamine, 52–53, 53t, 54
Kidney Disease Improving Global Outcomes (KDIGO), 356–57, 357t, 362–63

left ventricular assist devices (LVAD)
  gastrointestinal bleeding and
    multifactorial pathogenesis of, 208–9
    risk factor for LVAD-related GIB, 208
    treatment and secondary prophylaxis, 211–13
  implantation and management
    contraindications, 181
    device management, 185–86
    early complications, 186–88
    indications for LVAD implantation, 180–82
    intraoperative management, 183–85
    perioperative evaluation, 180
    second- and third-generation LVADs, 188, 189t
  troubleshooting bleeding and thrombosis
    Acquired von Willebrand's syndrome, 198–99
    etiology, 198
    evaluation of thromboembolic events, 201–2
    flow-chart for evaluation of post-op bleeding, 198
    flow-chart for evaluation of suspected thrombosis, 199f
    pump thrombosis, 202–3
    treatment of, 199–201
  troubleshooting hypotension
    clinical examination, 192–93
    incidence of, 195–96
    potential causes of hypotension, 193–95
    treatment, 195
low cardiac output syndrome, 344t, 345–46, 351
lung transplantation, pulmonary infiltrates and hypoxemia following, 257–65, 260t, 262f, 262t
lung ultrasound, 298, 299t, 299, 306
LVAD suction events, 186

Mayo Clinic model, 3
mechanical ventilation
    hyperglycemia and, 40*t*, 40, 42*b*
    management of, 80–83
    post-thoracotomy care, 48
    in respiratory acidosis, 79–80
    SvO_2 calculations and, 27
Medtronic CoreValve, 164
Medtronic Evolut, 164
metabolic acidosis
    acid-base equations
        anion gap, 89–90
        Henderson–Hasselbalch equation, 87–88
        Winter's formula, 88–89
    assessment of, 91–92
    lactic acidosis, 90, 91*t*
    treatment of, 93
mitral valve surgery, unilateral pulmonary edema and, 171–76, 172*f*, 173*f*
Modification of Diet in Renal Disease (MDRD), 357–58

neuraxial analgesia techniques, 50
non-invasive ventilation (NIV), 79, 84
non-sustained ventricular tachycardia (NSVT), 144, 145*f*
Northern New England score, 3
NSAIDS (non-steroidal anti-inflammatory drugs), 52–54, 53*t*

opioids, 52
orthotopic heart transplantation (OHT)
    management of
        hemodynamic and echocardiographic parameters, 242–43
        initial evaluation, 244–45
        primary graft dysfunction, 245
        risks of OHT, 242
        RV failure, 243, 244*f*
    rejection and immunosuppression
        acute cellular rejection (ACR), 248–49, 250*t*
        antibody-mediated rejection (AMR), 249–50
        hyperacute rejection, 248
        immunosuppression, 252–53
        maintenance immunosuppression, 253–55
        management of acute rejection, 250–52
oxygen consumption and delivery
    in critical illness
        causes of decreased SvO_2, 29*t*
        causes of increased SvO_2, 29*t*
        hyperlactatemia, 30–32, 31*t*
        other delivery assessments, 30
        sampling locations for $ScvO_2$ and SvO_2, 33*f*
        SvO_2 calculations, 14–22
        thermodilution measurements, 28–30
        utility of $ScvO_2$, 32–34
    pulmonary infiltrates and hypoxemia following lung transplantation, 257–65, 260*t*, 262*f*, 262*t*
    VA-ECMO (venoarterial ECMO)
        following lung transplantation, 263–65
        indication and contraindications, 232–33
        management of patients, 234–37
        patient selection, 233–34
        weaning from, 237
    VV-ECMO (venovenous ECMO)
        evidence for ECMO, 223–24
        following lung transplantation, 263–65
        how ECMO works, 225–27, 226*f*
        management during ECMO, 227
        patient selection, 224–25, 225*f*
        weaning from ECMO, 228

paravalvular leak (PVL), 284–85
Parsonnet score, 3

pneumothorax
    air leaks, 303–4, 304t
    chest drain insertion, 301–2, 302f
    treatment of alveolar-pleural fistulas, 304–5
    treatment of bronchopleural fistulas, 305
    treatment of stable pneumothorax, 301
    treatment of tension pneumothorax, 299–301
    troubleshooting chest drains, 302
point of care cardiac ultrasound (POCUS), 30
postoperative atrial fibrillation (POAF)
    atrial flutter, 135
    initial management, 131–32
    prophylaxis, 130–31, 131b
    refractory cases, 134
    risk factors, 130b
    summary of POAF treatments, 133t
    treatment of hemodynamically stable, 132–33
    treatment of hemodynamically unstable, 133–34
postoperative care
    advanced cardiovascular life support (ACLS), 153–60
    analgesia, 47–57
    atrial fibrillation, 129–36
    cardiogenic shock, 343–51
    cerebrovascular injury, 307–12
    diastolic heart failure, 323–31
    differential diagnoses to consider, 324t
    pneumothorax, 297–306
    pulmonary embolism, 59–70
    right ventricular failure, 121–28
    septic shock, 111–19
    vasodilatory shock, 333–40
    ventricular fibrillation, 143–50
post-thoracotomy analgesia
    additional techniques, 55
    multimodal analgesia, 52–55, 53t
    neuraxial techniques, 50
    opioids, 52
    other regional techniques, 50–51, 51f, 52b
primary graft dysfunction (PGD)
    following heart transplantation, 245
    following lung transplantation, 258–65, 260t, 262f, 262t
Protek Duo system, 217f, 217–19, 218t
pulmonary artery catheters (PACs)
    placement of, 15–18
    pressure measurements and waveforms provided by, 14–15, 17f, 18t
    thermodilution measurements, 15, 19t
    utility of PACs, 18–21
    ventricular ectopy, 14, 15f, 16t
pulmonary edema, robotic mitral valve surgery and, 171–76, 172f, 173f
pulmonary embolism
    assessing RV function in, 61–64, 63f
    mortality risk associated with original PESI score, 65t
    mortality risk associated with sPESI score, 65t
    postoperative care, 67–69
    severity assessment in, 64, 65t
    treatment of, 64–67
Pulmonary Embolism Severity Index (PESI), 64, 65t
pulmonary infiltrates, following lung transplantation, 257–65
pulseless electrical activity (PEA) arrest, 157

QTc prolongation
    causes of, 138–39
    common QTc prolonging medications, 139t
    treatment of, 139–40

renal function, monitoring, 357. *See also* acute kidney injury (AKI)
renal replacement therapy (RRT)
    dialysis access site selection, 362–63
    indications for timing of, 359–60
    modality and dosing of, 361

prognosis post CS-AKI, 364, 365
required postoperatively, 354–55
timing of initiation, 360–61, 365
respiratory acidosis
  ABG interpretation, 74t, 74–75, 76f
  airway pressures, 81–83, 82f
  assessment of, 75–78, 77f
  hypoxia in, 78–79
  mechanical ventilation in, 79–80
  mechanical ventilation management, 80–81
resternotomy
  ACLS response, 158, 160
  emergency in cardiac tamponade, 278f, 279–80, 281
rhabdomyolysis
  causes of, 101–4, 102t
  ECMO cannulation strategies, 99–100
  ischemia-reperfusion injury, 100–1
  ischemic changes secondary to hyperemia, 98f, 98
  monitoring, 105
  risk factors for limb ischemia, 99b
  treatment of, 105–8
right ventricular assist devices (RVAD)
  RVAD options, 217f, 217–19, 218t
  RV failure, 216–17
right ventricular failure (RVF)
  assessing RV function in PE, 61–64
  clinical presentation, 124f, 124
  management of
    afterload, 126
    contractility, 125–26
    key management points, 124–25
    perfusion, 126–27
    preload, 125
    rate and rhythm, 126
  mechanisms of right ventricular failure, 122–23, 123f
  monitoring and additional measures, 127
  parameters of life-threatening physiology, 243t
  perioperative RVF risk factors, 122

risk assessment scores
  common risk assessment systems, 3–7
  frailty as a risk factor, 7–10, 9f
robotic mitral valve surgery, unilateral pulmonary edema and, 171–76, 172f, 173f

Sapien 3, 164
Sequential Organ Failure Assessment (SOFA) score, 112, 113t
shock
  cardiogenic shock
    classification, etiology, and investigations of, 344t
    endocarditis, 284
    fluid and pharmacology support, 346–48
    mechanical support, 231–38, 348–50
    treatment of, 350–51
  septic shock
    early goal-directed therapy (EGDT), 115–16
    treatment, 114–18, 118t
    urine output in, 113t
  vasodilatory shock
    management of, 337–39
    pathophysiology of, 335–37
SIRS criteria, 112
Society of Thoracic Surgeons (STS)
  consensus guidelines, 154, 155f
  glycemic control guidelines, 41–44, 42b
  risk assessment scores, 4–7, 6t
stroke
  bimodal distribution of, 309–10
  incidence of, 308
  risk factors, 308t, 308–9, 309t
  SAVR and, 166, 169
surgical aortic valve repair (SAVR)
  incidence of parivalvular leak with, 165–66
  incidence of stroke, 166, 169
  mortality with PM post-SAVR, 165
  versus TAVR, 2, 8, 162, 167
  vascular complications, 167

systemic inflammatory response syndrome (SIRS), 112
systole, ACLS response, 156–57

Tandem Heart, 217*f*, 217–19, 218*t*
thermodilution measurements, 15, 19*t*, 22, 28–30, 92
torsades de pointes (Tdp)
    causes of, 138–39
    common QTc prolonging medications, 139*t*
    treatment of, 139–40
transaortic valve replacement (TAVR)
    frailty and mortality following, 8, 11
    neurological injuries, 166–67
    paravalvular leak (PVL), 165–66
    postoperative management and pitfalls, 162–64, 163*t*
    postprocedure arrhythmias, 165
    versus SAVR, 1
    STS scoring system and, 4
    valve options, 164
    vascular complications, 167–68
transfusions, 317, 319*t*
transplantation
    management of orthotopic heart transplantation, 241–46
    pulmonary infiltrates and hypoxemia following lung transplantation, 257–65, 260*t*, 262*f*, 262*t*
    rejection and immunosuppression in orthotopic heart transplantation, 247–55
type A lactic acidosis, 30–31, 35, 90
type B lactic acidosis, 30–32, 35, 90, 91*t*

unilateral pulmonary edema (UPE)
    etiology, 174–75
    incidence of, 173
    physiologic changes during lung ischemia-reperfusion injury, 173*f*
    postoperative chest X-ray, 172*f*
    prevention and management, 175
    treatment of, 175

urine output
    decreased as sign of balloon juxtarenal malpositioning, 271
    decreased as sign of hypoperfusion, 131–32, 345
    decreased as sign of RV failure, 216
    decreased necessitating hemodialysis, 107–8
    as diagnostic marker of AKI, 358
    increasing with diuretic therapy, 105–7, 108, 360, 365
    KDIGO definition of renal function, 357*t*
    as marker for perfusion, 244
    monitoring, 357
    in postoperative septic shock, 113*t*

VA-ECMO (venoarterial ECMO)
    following lung transplantation, 263–65
    indication and contraindications, 232–33
    management of patients, 234–37
    patient selection, 233–34
    peripherally cannulated, 245
    in postoperative cardiogenic shock, 349–50
    primary graft dysfunction and, 263–64, 265
    RVAD options, 217*f*
    weaning from, 237
vasodilatory shock
    management of, 337–39
    pathophysiology of, 335–37
ventricular ectopy
    causes of, 18
    ECG strip showing, 15*f*
    hemodynamic instability resulting from, 22
    risk factors and treatments for, 16*t*, 22
ventricular fibrillation
    ACLS response, 155–56
    etiology
        adrenergic medications and inotropes, 148

antiarrhythmic medications, 148
electrolyte abnormalities, 146–47
hypothermia and acid base
abnormalities, 148
ischemia, 146
pacing wires, 148–49
pulmonary artery catheters
(PACs), 147
incidence of, 144
treatment of
cardioversion and defibrillation, 149
identification and treatment of
ischemia, 149–50
lidocaine, 150
types of arrhythmia
mimickers of ventricular arrhythmias,
145–46

non-sustained ventricular tachycardia
(NSVT), 144, 145*f*
premature ventricular complexes
(PVCs), 144*f*, 144
ventricular fibrillation, 145*f*, 145
ventricular tachyarrhythmias (VT), 145
VV-ECMO (venovenous ECMO)
evidence for ECMO, 223–24
following lung transplantation, 263–65
how ECMO works, 225–27, 226*f*
management during ECMO, 227
patient selection, 224–25, 225*f*
weaning from ECMO, 228

Winter's formula, 88–89

Yale Insulin Infusion Protocol, 43–44, 44*f*